Patient Zero and the Making of the AIDS Epidemic

Patient Zero and the Making of the AIDS Epidemic

RICHARD A. McKAY

THE UNIVERSITY OF CHICAGO PRESS   CHICAGO AND LONDON

The University of Chicago Press, Chicago 60637
The University of Chicago Press, Ltd., London
© 2017 by The University of Chicago
Published 2017
Printed in the United States of America
26 25 24 23 22 21 20 19 18 17   1 2 3 4 5

ISBN-13: 978-0-226-06381-2   (cloth)
ISBN-13: 978-0-226-06395-9   (paper)
ISBN-13: 978-0-226-06400-0   (e-book)
DOI: 10.7208/chicago/9780226064000.001.0001

Library of Congress Cataloging-in-Publication Data
Names: McKay, Richard Andrew, 1978– author.
Title: Patient zero and the making of the AIDS epidemic / Richard A. McKay.
Description: Chicago : The University of Chicago Press, 2017. | Includes bibliographical
    references and index.
Identifiers: LCCN 2017018054 | ISBN 9780226063812 (cloth : alk. paper) |
    ISBN 9780226063959 (pbk. : alk. paper) | ISBN 9780226064000 (e-book)
Subjects: LCSH: aids (Disease)—North America—History. | Epidemics—North America.
    | AIDS (Disease)—North America—Historiography. | Dugas, Gaétan, 1952–1984. |
    AIDS (Disease)—Patients.
Classification: LCC RA643.86.N7 M46 2017 | DDC 362.19697/920097—dc23
LC record available at https://lccn.loc.gov/2017018054

what's your name
what's your sign
what's your disease

i saw you standing there
pretty as you please
and couldn't help wondering
which of these
afflicts you:

sores around the mouth
or further south
swelling of the joints
or other points
lesions or lumps
blisters or bumps
or feeling generally queasy
from being too easy

seems everyone has something
and is avoiding something more
from the saints among us
to those who are hor-
monally imbalanced
and can't get enough
of that funky stuff

i'm not casting aspersions
or condemning diversions
just a prudent inspection
to compare your infection
with mine

i'm in no position
to judge your condition
or condemn you
and call you a sleaze

but before we're encased
in something debased
please tell me
what's your disease

BILL RUSSELL, "EPITAPH FOR
THE SEXUAL REVOLUTION,"
Christopher Street,
December 1982

Contents

Acknowledgments

I am greatly indebted to my funding agencies, without whose financial support this work would not have been possible. These include the J. Armand Bombardier Foundation for an Internationalist Fellowship and the Wellcome Trust for a master's studentship—both of which supported the early stages of this research. The bulk of the project was made possible with a generous award from the Wellcome Trust (080651) and support from the University of Oxford's Clarendon Fund. Travel awards from Green Templeton College, the American Association for the History of Medicine, and the Canadian Society for the History of Medicine also helped enable me to visit North America for research trips and conferences. In addition, research fellowships from the Economic and Social Research Council (PTA-026–27–2838) and the Wellcome Trust (098705) provided opportunities for further research and writing.

For their early support and enthusiasm, I owe a great debt to Gareth Davies and Sloan Mahone. Their thoughtful questions and insightful feedback have improved this book immeasurably. At times when matters appeared particularly bleak, their encouragement made all the difference. Also heartening were discussions with Allan Brandt, Dorothy Porter, George Rousseau, Judith Leavitt, Virginia Berridge, Margaret Pelling, Pietro Corsi, Jason Szabo, Jacalyn Duffin, Naomi Rogers, and John Harley Warner. For their wonderful early teaching that helped put me on this path, I will always be grateful to Betty Anne Rivers Wang and the late Jerry Falk in South Surrey, British Columbia.

I would like to recognize the generous time and effort put in by each of my interviewees, whose trust and heartfelt reminiscences have enriched my work tremendously. I hope that I have succeeded in representing their views accurately and, where our interpretations have diverged, handled this with fairness and tact. I would like to thank Bill Darrow, Jean Robert, Joseph Sonnabend, Michael Brown, and Ray Redford for allowing me to consult copies of documents in their personal collections, and the siblings of Gaétan Dugas for granting me permission to quote from their brother's correspondence. I must also thank the archivists and staff at the following archives and libraries for their time, patience, and assistance: Archives gaies de Québec; Bibliothèque et Archives nationales du Québec; the British Columbia Gay and Lesbian Archives (BCGLA); the Canadian Lesbian and Gay Archives (CLGA); Columbia University's Center for Oral History Archives; the Gay, Lesbian, Bisexual, Transgender Historical Society; the John Hay Library; Library and Archives Canada; the Lesbian, Gay, Bisexual and Transgender Community Center National History Archive; the National Library of Medicine; the New York Public Library; ONE National Gay and Lesbian Archives at the USC [University of Southern California] Libraries; the Parish of Notre-Dame-de-L'Annonciation, Ancienne-Lorette; Ronald Reagan Presidential Library; San Francisco Public Library (SFPL); Sir James Dunn Law Library; the Toronto International Film Festival Group's Film Reference Library; and the University of California–San Francisco (UCSF) Library and Center for Knowledge Management, Archives and Special Collections Division. Special mention must go to Alan Miller at CLGA; Josué Hurtado, formerly of UCSF; Ron Dutton at BCGLA; and Tim Wilson at SFPL for their exceptionally high level of assistance, as well as to the dedicated volunteer staff members at LGBT archives across North America, whose commitment to preserving and sharing records of the past are fundamentally important for historical endeavors like this one.

My time at Oxford would not have been the same without the wonderful people at the Wellcome Unit (particularly Carol Brady and Belinda Michaelides) and at Green—and later Green Templeton—College. I cannot imagine better-suited environments for carrying out several years of research and reflection—particularly when fueled by the tremendous food and interdisciplinary collegiality of Green's legendary lunches—and I will always feel fortunate to have lived and studied there. Out of this incredibly stimulating and welcoming community, a special thank-you is due to Pat Markus and her late husband Andrew for their ongoing guidance, support, and warm friendship. Mark Harrison and John Howard generously helped shape this book with their careful readings of an earlier iteration, as did two anonymous reviewers for the University of Chicago Press.

This work has accompanied me through several institutional moves: from Oxford to King's College London (KCL), and on again to the University of Cambridge's Department of History and Philosophy of Science. For my time at KCL I owe an enormous debt to Ludmilla Jordanova, for her attentive mentorship and inspirational historical practice. I am grateful as well for the friends and colleagues I met there, and for their contributions to my thinking: Katherine Foxhall, Keren Hammerschlag, Florence Grant, Rosemary Wall, Sophie Mann, Dennis Stathakopoulos, and Anne Marie Rafferty. At Cambridge, I feel lucky to have been able to share enjoyable and productive conversations about this research with Lauren Kassell, Nick Hopwood, Jesse Olszynko-Gryn, Dmitriy Myelnikov, Andrew Buskell, Helen Curry, Chitra Ramalingam, Clare Griffin, Margaret Carlyle, Sarah Bull, Stephen John, Anna Alexandrova, Lukas Engelmann, Tamara Hug, and the late John Forrester. More generally, my collegial thanks go to Claire Jones, Sally Sheard, Flurin Condrau, Anne Kveim Lie, Gayle Davis, Gerard Koskovich, Matthew Weait, Harold Jaffe, and Michael Worobey. Their questions, feedback, and encouragement have made this work much stronger; any errors that may remain are my own responsibility.

I am grateful for thought-provoking comments and questions from copanelists and audience members at a whole host of seminars and conference presentations between 2007 and 2014, including seminars and symposia at Oxford's Green College and the Wellcome Unit, and at Cambridge, Warwick, Liverpool, Exeter, KCL, UCSF, and Concordia; conference panels hosted at the meetings of the Canadian Society for the History of Medicine, the American Association for the History of Medicine, the Society for the Social History of Medicine, the European Association for the History of Medicine and Health, the Committee on Lesbian, Gay, Bisexual, and Transgender History of the American Historical Association, at the 80th Anglo-American Conference of Historians, and the wonderful group assembled for We Demand: History / Sex / Activism in Canada; as well as community presentations in Toronto and San Francisco. Traveling for research and presentations meant that I frequently needed to find a place to sleep, so warm thank-yous go to the Welshes, the Kowalczyks, the Walters, the Brodskys, Jen Coens (and roommates), Vic and Ginevra Syperek, Lila McDowell and Lynn

Crimando, Kate Mannle, Paul Gedye, Jeffrey Lancaster, and Lynne LeBlanc for offering me welcoming places to stay over the years. At the University of Chicago Press, I'm grateful to Doug Mitchell for believing in this project from the early stages and for his wonderfully encouraging and edifying e-mails; to Kyle Wagner, Tim McGovern, Yvonne Zipter, Kathleen Raven, and Ashley Pierce for their assistance in shepherding the book from submission through production and beyond; to Lori Meek Schuldt for her insightful copyediting work; to Isaac Tobin for designing a stunningly evocative cover; and to Jan Williams for her efforts in compiling the index.

My family and friends have been a source of encouragement, humor, and perspective throughout this long project—one which could have lasted twice as long if Mum had not generously and tirelessly transcribed the interviews with total discretion. I thank Mum, Dad, Blythe, Susan, Mark, Chris, Sue, Giles, Antoinette, Isabella, and Enya and Zelda for their love, patience, and support. My work and I have particularly benefited from friendship and conversations—AIDS-related and not—with many people, including Erica Charters, Henry Meier, Simon Pooley, Phil Tiemeyer, Tamson Pietsch, Jamie Salo, Anders Krarup, Mandisa Mbali, Rebecca Hodes, Lauren Brodsky, Jackie Cheng, Will Motley, Dave Bagby, Tyler and Erie Lane, Aaron and Julia Morinis Orkin, Mari Webel, Paul Steinberg, Lindsey Richardson, Sophie Walker, Anna Renou, Pete Goult, Madeline Fowler, Charles Laurie, Rebekah Braswell, Ben and Fiona Irving, Jenn DeLucry, Christine Dandy, Jocelyn Parr, Angela Danyluk, Keri Laughlin, Derek and Samantha Creech, and Josh Raymond. Kate Mannle's assistance with image research was invaluable, as were the skilled translating efforts of Leila Merouchi and A. Landry. Crucially, Theo Raymond has provided common sense, a keen reader's eye, a much-needed ability to find humor, and unfaltering love since the project's inception—I would not have been able to complete this project without him in my corner.

Thank you, all.

Abbreviations

ACT	AIDS Committee of Toronto
ACT[-]UP	AIDS Coalition to Unleash Power
AID	Acquired Immune Deficiency
AIDS	acquired immune deficiency syndrome, *also called* acquired immunodeficiency syndrome
APA	American Psychiatric Association
ARV	AIDS-related virus
ASO	AIDS Service Organization
Band	*And the Band Played On*
BAR	*Bay Area Reporter*
BCGLA	British Columbia Gay and Lesbian Archives
CAJ	Canadian Association of Journalists
CAS	Canadian AIDS Society
CBC	Canadian Broadcasting Corporation
CDC	Centers for Disease Control
CEH	Center for Environmental Health
CID	Center for Infectious Diseases
CIJ	Centre for Investigative Journalism
CLGA	Canadian Lesbian and Gay Archives
CMV	cytomegalovirus
CPS	Center for Prevention Services
EIS	Epidemic Intelligence Service
EPO	Epidemiology Program Office
GMHC	Gay Men's Health Crisis
GRID	gay related immune deficiency
HAART	highly active antiretroviral therapy
HIV	human immunodeficiency virus

HLTV-III	human T-cell lymphotropic virus type III
IV	intravenous
KCL	King's College London
KS	Kaposi's sarcoma
KS/OI	Kaposi's sarcoma and opportunistic infections
LAV	lymphadenopathy-associated virus
LCDC	Laboratory Centre for Disease Control
LGBT	lesbian, gay, bisexual, and transgender/transsexual
MMWR	*Morbidity and Mortality Weekly Report*
NAC-AIDS	National Advisory Committee on AIDS
NCAB	National Cancer Advisory Board
NCI	National Cancer Institute
NIH	National Institutes of Health
NYN	*New York Native*
NYU	New York University
OI	opportunistic infection
OPV	oral polio vaccine
ORTEP	Oak Ridge Thermal Ellipsoid Plot
PCC	Portland Community College
PCP	*Pneumocystis carinii* pneumonia
PLWH	person living with HIV/AIDS
PHS	[United States] Public Health Service
PWA	person with AIDS *or* the group People with AIDS
SARS	severe acute respiratory syndrome
SES	socioeconomic status
SFAF	San Francisco AIDS Foundation
SFPL	San Francisco Public Library
SIV	simian immunodeficiency virus
STDs	sexually transmitted diseases
STIs	sexually transmitted infections
TB	tuberculosis
UCSF	University of California–San Francisco
UN	United Nations
VD	venereal disease
VDCD	Venereal Disease Control Division

Introduction

"He Is Still Out There"

He is a living man with Kaposi's sarcoma. He is still out there. — *James Curran*, chief, AIDS Task Force, Centers for Disease Control (CDC), 1982

On a rainy day in December 1982, some of the most distinguished cancer researchers and health advocates in the United States gathered in a darkened National Institutes of Health conference room in Bethesda, Maryland, to listen to an update on the acquired immune deficiency syndrome (AIDS) epidemic. Projected slides of graphs and figures broke through the somberness to support the speakers' points as first Dr. Bruce Chabner, acting director of the National Cancer Institute (NCI), and then Dr. James Curran, head of the CDC's AIDS Task Force, addressed the National Cancer Advisory Board during the board's final meeting of the year.[1] The transcript of an audio recording captured that day offers an entry point into the contemporary state of scientific knowledge regarding the then newly recognized and recently named AIDS epidemic, following eighteen months of concerted investigation. This record also documents an early instance of the type of attention attracted by the man who would later become known as "Patient Zero."

---

1. The transcript is available online through the National Institute of Health's website devoted to AIDS history. See "Presentations at the NCAB Meeting, December 1, 1982," meeting transcript, December 1, 1982, http://history.nih.gov/NIHInOwnWords/assets/media/pdf/unpublished/unpublished_38.pdf.

The meeting's transcript serves as a useful "spine" for this introductory chapter, as it presents in microcosmic form many of the questions and concerns that would be expressed over the following decade and a half and which will be explored in this book.

As host of the meeting, Chabner spoke first, detailing developments in AIDS research that had occurred since the syndrome had first come to the attention of the NCI and presented both "the possibility of an unusual new form of cancer and also an opportunity to study a disease from the prodromal symptoms."[2] He explained how a decrease in the number of "helper T-cell[s]"—crucial actors in the immune system's efforts to control infection—had resulted in clinical displays of immune deficiency for a number of patients. This deficiency was characterized by Kaposi's sarcoma (KS), a skin cancer, and a series of opportunistic infections, most notably *Pneumocystis carinii* pneumonia (PCP).[3] The condition, Chabner went on, had first been noticed in the homosexual male population of New York, as early as 1978, though there were now cases in most major US cities, with the highest numbers in New York, Los Angeles, and San Francisco, and in several other countries.[4]

In addition to this stricken "sub-population" of the gay community, which he observed was characterized by "a very high level of sexual activity," Chabner proceeded to list the other "affected groups" under investigation. He mentioned intravenous drug users, most of whom were young African American or Hispanic heterosexuals living in New York City or the adjacent New Jersey area.[5] The scientist made a special note of the third group, Haitian immigrants, who were of interest because they had both KS and the "overwhelming infections" of PCP and irregu-

---

2. Ibid., 1.

3. Ibid., 1, 3 (page 2 missing).

4. Ibid.

5. Ibid., 4. "Affected groups" would soon be replaced, controversially, by "high risk group" in early 1983; see CDC, "Prevention of Acquired Immune Deficiency Syndrome (AIDS): Report of Inter-Agency Recommendations," *Morbidity and Mortality Weekly Report* 32, no. 8 (1983): 101–3 (hereafter *MMWR*). For a critique of how "risk groups" served a social function of marking out certain individuals as beyond the moral concern of the "general population," see Jan Zita Grover, "AIDS: Keywords," in *AIDS: Cultural Analysis, Cultural Activism*, ed. Douglas Crimp (Cambridge, MA: MIT Press, 1988), 27–28. For more on the problematic categorization of "4-H risk groups" (homosexuals, "heroin addicts," hemophiliacs, and Haitians), see Paula Treichler, "AIDS, Gender, and Biomedical Discourse: Current Contests for Meaning," in *AIDS: The Burdens of History*, ed. Elizabeth Fee and Daniel M. Fox (London: University of California Press, 1988), 194, 198.

lar tuberculosis, and yet in general they admitted no history of homosexuality or drug use.[6] Rounding out this list of affected groups was a small number of hemophiliac patients. Chabner spent the rest of his presentation discussing the clinical manifestations of the syndrome, advancing the likelihood of a "virally caused agent" similar to hepatitis B, and outlining the funds and efforts that the NCI had devoted to AIDS research.[7]

* * *

This book examines the origins, emergence, dissemination, and consequences of one "fact" that took shape during the early years of the North American AIDS epidemic, drew discussion at the 1982 NCAB meeting, and proliferated in words and images in the years that followed: that of "Patient Zero." For years, several successive editions of a top-selling medical dictionary—a type of publication frequently considered to bear the ultimate imprimatur of authority—contained an entry for *Patient Zero* which read: "an individual identified by the Centers for Disease Control and Prevention (CDC) as the person who introduced the human immunodeficiency virus in the United States. According to CDC records, Patient Zero, an airline steward, infected nearly 50 other persons before he died of acquired immunodeficiency syndrome in 1984."[8]

While this definition is inaccurate on several counts, for reasons that will become evident in the following chapters, it serves as an adequate summary of the resilient popular understanding of the "Patient Zero" story. This book seeks to answer four questions. What were the origins of this idea, including its precipitating causes and historical antecedents? How did it achieve its rapid diffusion into North American social consciousness and beyond in the course of the early years of the AIDS epidemic and with what consequences? What factors can explain the idea's continued resilience and widespread cultural significance across

6. "NCAB Meeting," 5.

7. Ibid., 9. The CDC advanced a single-agent theory in earnest in the summer of 1982, though added support would come in December of that year, shortly after the NCAB meeting, with reports of transmission through a blood transfusion case in San Francisco; see Arthur J. Ammann et al., "Acquired Immunodeficiency in an Infant: Possible Transmission by Means of Blood Products," *Lancet* 321, no. 8331 (1983): 956–58.

8. "Patient Zero," in *Mosby's Medical Dictionary*, 9th ed., ed. Marie T. O'Toole (St. Louis: Mosby Elsevier, 2013), 1346. The entry appeared for the first time in the dictionary's fifth edition (1998) and remained unchanged until the tenth edition (2017).

disciplinary and national boundaries? And finally, what can we learn about the lived experience of Gaétan Dugas, the flight attendant who was labeled as "Patient Zero," who was publicly vilified several years after his death, and whose own perspective has effectively been silenced? Understanding the construction and widespread appeal of "Patient Zero" offers insight into the complicated ways in which societies respond to the threat of deadly epidemics and, more generally, how they make sense of complex events. This book traces the development of this idea from "Patient O" to "Patient 0" and finally to "Patient Zero," through several communities of practice in public health and the media, illuminating the flows of power and struggle at play in the process. It will also challenge some of the damaging meanings the term took on, particularly in the wake of the publication of *And the Band Played On* (1987), the influential history of the American epidemic written by the journalist Randy Shilts that brought the story to a wide audience.[9] In following this path, this book embarks on a social, cultural, and medical history of the early AIDS epidemic in Canada and the United States.

In addition to the efforts of physicians, scientists, and epidemiologists—who dominated the NCAB meeting in 1982 as well as the initial investigations into the syndrome—how AIDS has been understood and experienced has been shaped by academics, writers, artists, and activists, who drew upon diverse backgrounds including cultural and art theory, political science, sociology, legal studies, and history.[10] Since it was

9. Randy Shilts, *And the Band Played On: Politics, People, and the American AIDS Epidemic* (New York: St. Martin's Press, 1987). Shilts also offers an account of the NCAB meeting in *Band*, 201, though drawing as he did on the reminiscences of Curran and Dr. Robert Gallo, he was not aware of any mention at that meeting of the man he would call "Patient Zero."

10. A few key works from each discipline help sketch the contours of this enormous coverage: in epidemiology, see James W. Curran et al., "Epidemiology of HIV Infection and AIDS in the United States," *Science* 239, no. 4840 (1988): 610–16; in cultural criticism and art theory, see Cindy Patton, *Sex and Germs: The Politics of AIDS* (Boston: South End Press, 1985); Simon Watney, *Policing Desire: Pornography, AIDS and the Media* (Minneapolis: University of Minnesota Press, 1987); Cindy Patton, *Inventing AIDS* (New York: Routledge, 1990); Susan Sontag, *Illness as Metaphor and AIDS and Its Metaphors* (New York: Picador USA, 1990); Paula Treichler, *How to Have Theory in an Epidemic: Cultural Chronicles of AIDS* (London: Duke University Press, 1999); Cindy Patton, *Globalizing AIDS* (Minneapolis: University of Minnesota Press, 2002); Douglas Crimp, *Melancholia and Moralism: Essays on AIDS and Queer Politics* (London: MIT Press, 2002); Priscilla Wald, *Contagious: Cultures, Carriers, and the Outbreak Narrative* (London: Duke Univer-

first recognized as a newly emerging and deadly epidemic more than thirty years ago, AIDS has generated a truly vast literature across the medical sciences, social sciences, humanities, and law. The AIDS epidemic, as the cultural scholar Paula Treichler has perceptively noted, was at the same time both an epidemic of transmissible disease and "an epidemic of signification"—where meanings reproduced rapidly, with vital consequences for the way in which the condition was understood, experienced, and addressed.[11]

This epidemic of transmissible disease was first recognized during a period in the late twentieth century when knowledge claims by practitioners of science and medicine had come under increasing attack from humanistic circles in many parts of the world. This trend formed part of a broader questioning of authority, objectivity, and the use of grand narratives—such as a confident belief in historical progress—and encouraged some observers to consider how humans, as social actors, went about creating scientific knowledge.[12] Critics argued that scientific and medical knowledge claims, rather than representing a transparent depiction of the natural world, were instead the product of meaning-making practices. Thus, they reasoned, these claims, and the work underpinning them, ought to be submitted to investigation and analysis much as any other cultural activity would be.[13]

---

sity Press, 2008); in political science, see Dennis Altman, *AIDS in the Mind of America: The Social, Political, and Psychological Impact of a New Epidemic* (Garden City, NY: Anchor Press, 1986); Ronald Bayer, *Private Acts, Social Consequences: AIDS and the Politics of Public Health* (New Brunswick, NJ: Rutgers University Press, 1991); in sociology, see Steven Epstein, *Impure Science: AIDS, Activism, and the Politics of Knowledge* (Berkeley: University of California Press, 1996); in legal studies, see Matthew Weait, "Taking the Blame: Criminal Law, Social Responsibility and the Sexual Transmission of HIV," *Journal of Social and Family Law* 23, no. 4 (2001): 441–57; Lawrence O. Gostin, *The AIDS Pandemic: Complacency, Injustice, and Unfilled Expectations* (London: University of North Carolina Press, 2004). A separate listing of historical studies follows.

11. Triechler's famous quote comes from a paper first published in 1988; see Triechler, *Theory in an Epidemic*, 11. Her work has had a significant influence on this book's approach.

12. Jan Golinski, *Making Natural Knowledge: Constructivism and the History of Science* (London: University of Chicago Press, 2005), 6; M. R. Bury, "Social Constructionism and the Development of Medical Sociology," *Sociology of Health and Illness* 8, no. 2 (1986): 137–69; Ludmilla Jordanova, "The Social Construction of Medical Knowledge," *Social History of Medicine* 8, no. 3 (1995): 363.

13. Golinski, *Making Natural Knowledge*, 5, 16. Critics have alleged that some practitioners of social construction went too far in their attempts to unsettle the status quo. The

Not only did this intellectual tradition influence activist responses to AIDS in the 1980s and 1990s, but it also raises important questions for this book. In our daily lives we most frequently use words, stories, and images to interpret external phenomena and express our understanding of the world, and so it is vital to see these elements as an essential, constitutive part of our reality and not simply a neutral, natural label or a depiction of how things "actually" are in the world. Who gets to name? How do they see the world? What type of word or image do these speakers choose to represent the phenomena they observe? What preexisting frameworks, narratives, and experience do they draw on? How do they tell their stories? To whom? These are questions that illuminate flows of power in society, so it is vital that we do not take names, images, and stories to be self-evident. In moral terms, such representations shape in profound ways our notions of right and wrong, safety and risk, cause and effect, as well as responsibility, blame, and culpability. Rather than viewing "knowledge" as a sum of facts identified by experts, or an accumulation of common sense, it is important to think of it as an uneasy, unstable, and time-bound truce in an ongoing and unending struggle for understanding. At stake are questions of authority, expertise, and representation, not to mention the agency and treatment of those who lack the power, ability, or interest to adequately represent themselves. These are evidently historical questions as well, as meanings change, intermix, and are recycled over time, while ebbs and flows of power affect who

---

medical historian Charles Rosenberg, for example, criticized the work of one scholar for asserting that all that mattered in the case of a cholera epidemic were cultural practices and denying the existence of "disease" itself; see Charles E. Rosenberg, "Disease and Social Order in America: Perceptions and Expectations," in Fee and Fox, *AIDS: The Burdens of History*, 13. Rosenberg was critiquing François Delaporte's *Disease and Civilization: The Cholera in Paris, 1832*, trans. Arthur Goldhammer (London: MIT Press, 1986). Rosenberg suggests, by contrast, that AIDS is a "postrelativist phenomenon," exposing the limitations of a purely biological model divorced from social interpretations, while at the same time showing the inadequacy of an extreme focus on the creation of social meanings that denies the existence of biological disease; Charles E. Rosenberg, "What Is an Epidemic? AIDS in Historical Perspective," in *Explaining Epidemics and Other Studies in the History of Medicine* (Cambridge: Cambridge University Press, 1992), 292. Taking Rosenberg's point, the approach adopted in this book is one of "moderate" social construction. It recognizes the existence of an underlying pathological process causing the disease that became known as AIDS, yet also emphasizes the vital importance of investigating the socially produced meanings surrounding it.

can speak (or stay silent) and what they can say (or not). I shall return to these questions near the end of this introduction, when I consider in greater detail my own position as a historian in the construction of this historical account.

* * *

The initial geographic focus, as Chabner mentioned, on New York, Los Angeles, and San Francisco soon expanded to include Haiti, Canada, and countries in Western Europe. By 1983, the syndrome was recognized to exist at substantial levels in several countries in sub-Saharan Africa. This ominous distribution became easier to monitor with the discovery and isolation of a causative virus—eventually named the human immunodeficiency virus (HIV)—during 1983 and 1984 and the development and distribution of a test for antibodies to the virus in 1985.[14] Reports from the Joint United Nations Programme on HIV/AIDS chart the devastating consequences of this condition from then until now. They estimate that HIV was responsible for the deaths of approximately twenty-nine million people worldwide between 1970 and 2009, and that nearly thirty-seven million people were living with the virus in 2014, the most recent year for which data were available at the time of this writing.[15]

HIV infection has traversed the world and infected people from all races and ethnicities, exposing in the process the extreme difficulties in

14. The virus—variously named lymphadenopathy-associated virus (LAV) by French scientists in 1983, human T-cell lymphotropic virus type III (HTLV-III) by Robert Gallo's team in 1984, and AIDS-related virus (ARV) by another American team led by Jay Levy in 1984—was eventually named HIV in 1986; for a review of the politics involved in such a decision, see Paula Treichler, "AIDS, Homophobia, and Biomedical Discourse: An Epidemic of Signification," in Crimp, *AIDS*, 31–70; Epstein, *Impure Science*, 45–78.

15. Joint United Nations Programme on HIV/AIDS, *Outlook 30* (Geneva: UNAIDS, 2011), 17, http://www.unaids.org/sites/default/files/media_asset/20110607_JC2069_30Out look_en_0.pdf; Joint United Nations Programme on HIV/AIDS, *AIDS by the Numbers 2015* (Geneva: UNAIDS, 2015), 4, http://www.unaids.org/sites/default/files/media_asset/AIDS_by_the_numbers_2015_en.pdf. Hereafter, the word *epidemic* is used to describe a higher than usual number of cases in areas as small as a single community and as large as a single continent, and *pandemic* to refer to the global spread of AIDS across several continents.

addressing its spread across barriers of language and culture.[16] In contrast to the diversity of social, cultural, and political reactions to the virus, within each individual body there is a relatively similar continuum from infection to early death—particularly in the absence of antiretroviral therapy.[17] When a person has become infected with HIV, the virus enters the bloodstream and the individual's cells. Many people develop flu-like symptoms during the primary, acute-infection stage, which can last for up to two weeks, before returning to feeling normal. The virus travels to the lymph nodes and replicates rapidly in the absence of antibodies, which can take the body between one and three months to produce. After a person has seroconverted—that is, after his or her body has begun to produce antibodies to combat the virus—the immune system enters into a slow, silent, and gradually losing struggle with HIV. This process, during which the body's T cells are slowly depleted, happens over a period of years, and in many cases the only external sign is an eventual swelling of the lymph nodes.

At a certain point, the T cells deplete more rapidly, allowing virus levels in the body to rise substantially. Poverty, malnutrition, and co-infections can bring on this stage sooner.[18] At earlier stages of HIV disease, often within five to seven years of infection, the compromised immune system might give rise to such moderate symptoms as rash, tiredness, night sweats, weight loss, and fungal infections. As time passes, more severe medical difficulties might emerge, including recurrent thrush and herpes, persistent diarrhea, and extreme loss of weight. Finally, severe damage to the immune system occurs, roughly ten years following infection. This development will allow the invasion of opportunistic infections—illnesses that would not normally occur in healthy

16. The massive scope of the challenge and variety in the responses can be gleaned from a review of the thousands of abstracts of the posters and presentations at each biennial International AIDS Conference. See, for example, the abstracts presented at the 21st International Conference in Durban, South Africa, in 2016: http://www.aids2016.org/Portals/0/File/AIDS2016_Abstracts_LOW.pdf?ver=2016-08-10-154247-087.

17. The description that follows holds true for most infected individuals, though about 5 percent of this population may become long-term nonprogressors, remaining healthy with no apparent loss of T cell function for many years; see Jay A. Levy, "HIV Pathogenesis: 25 Years of Progress and Persistent Challenges," *AIDS* 23, no. 2 (2009): 158.

18. Marie-Marcelle Deschamps et al., "HIV Infection in Haiti: Natural History and Disease Progression," *AIDS* 14, no. 16 (2000): 2515–21.

individuals—often in rapid succession. The most common of these conditions, which now herald the designation of late-stage HIV disease or AIDS, include PCP, *Mycobacterium avium* complex, cytomegalovirus, toxoplasmosis, and candidiasis.[19] An aggressive form of KS—a previously rare and relatively benign cancer typically affecting older men—was also one of the most common complications seen in the gay communities when the epidemic was first recognized, and it was the chief reason why the National Cancer Institute had expressed such interest in the new syndrome.[20] In the absence of effective treatment, the risk of death increases with each passing year after seroconversion, with nearly two-thirds of untreated patients in resource-rich countries dying within fifteen years of infection.[21]

The Origins of HIV/AIDS

"As I mentioned," Chabner emphasized to the meeting's attendees, "the first cases were seen in homosexual males in New York." He continued, "There are now cases in most major US cities and foreign countries. In some of these instances the patients in foreign countries have known contacts, homosexual contact, with people in New York or other American cities. There are fewer cases in number in foreign countries than in the United States." Alluding to the dramatic rise in reported cases, Chabner explained, "At this point when the slide was made we had 600

19. This description of the stages of HIV infection has been drawn from the informative online HIV/AIDS resource, *The Body*. See San Francisco AIDS Foundation, "The Stages of HIV Disease," The Body: The Complete Online HIV/AIDS Resource, August 22, 2008, http://www.thebody.com/content/whatis/art2506.html.

20. Studies would note that the proportion of gay and bisexual men with AIDS who developed Kaposi's sarcoma decreased from 79 percent in 1981 to 25 percent in 1989. In 1994, a new herpes virus was isolated which was found to be a contributing factor for developing KS; see Yuan Chang et al., "Identification of Herpesvirus-Like DNA Sequences in AIDS-Associated Kaposi's Sarcoma," *Science* 266, no. 5192 (1994): 1865–69. One likely hypothesis is that this virus was more widespread in the gay community in the late 1970s, leading to a higher proportion of KS in the first cases of AIDS in men who had sex with men.

21. Beryl A. Koblin et al., "Long-Term Survival after Infection with Human Immunodeficiency Virus Type 1 (HIV-1) among Homosexual Men in Hepatitis B Vaccine Trial Cohorts in Amsterdam, New York City, and San Francisco, 1978–1995," *American Journal of Epidemiology* 150, no. 10 (1999): 1027.

known patients that had the disease, now the number is closer to 800 patients."[22]

* * *

From the time he spoke those words to the present day, attempting to locate the origins of HIV/AIDS has been a contentious issue—and one which would be central to discussions of "Patient Zero" in the 1980s. As readers shall see in chapter 1, epidemics throughout history have repeatedly been accompanied by attempts to locate origins and to lay blame. Initially, with the vast majority of people diagnosed with AIDS located in New York City, or with ties to that city, many observers assumed that the origins of the epidemic lay there. Soon, the appearance of cases among Haitian immigrants led to speculation that the immune disorder was endemic in their home country, or, perhaps, that vacationing American homosexuals from New York had unwittingly spread an etiological agent there.[23] A joint Belgian and American research trip to Zaire in 1983 established that a similar condition, predominantly affecting heterosexual men and women, was widespread there. This realization challenged the notion that the etiological agent thought to cause AIDS had initially come into existence in the United States or that the disease was predominantly one affecting gay men.[24] Primate hosts of a more ancient deadly virus that might have been passed to humans were sought. African green monkeys were proposed as likely hosts, before eventually ceding this position to chimpanzees in central Africa.[25]

After scientists developed a blood test for HIV, attempts to locate the

22. "NCAB Meeting," 3.

23. See Renée Sabatier, *Blaming Others: Prejudice, Race and Worldwide AIDS* (London: Panos Institute, 1988); Paul Farmer, *AIDS and Accusation: Haiti and the Geography of Blame*, rev. ed. (Berkeley: University of California Press, 2006).

24. Peter Piot et al., "Acquired Immunodefiency Syndrome in a Heterosexual Population in Zaire," *Lancet* 324, no. 8394 (1984): 65–69. Piot, the Belgian physician who headed this trip and later became the head of the United Nations AIDS Programme, describes the experience in his memoir, *No Time to Lose: A Life in Pursuit of Deadly Viruses* (W. W. Norton, 2012), 121–32.

25. This appears to be true for HIV-1; HIV-2, a far less widely distributed form of the virus, is believed to have crossed into humans from the sooty mangabey monkey; Justin Stebbing and Graeme Moyle, "The Clades of HIV: Their Origins and Clinical Significance," *AIDS Reviews* 5, no. 4 (2003): 205–13.

virus in decades-old stored samples yielded contested results. In October 1987, preserved samples from a teenaged male from St. Louis who died of an AIDS-like condition in 1969 were reported to have tested positive for HIV antibodies. Samples from a British sailor who had died in 1959 after a devastating series of infections including *pneumocystis carinii* pneumonia yielded similar positive rest results.[26] Experts would later cast doubt on the validity of these two examples due to subsequent difficulties in reproducing the results with tests that searched for the actual genetic presence of the virus, as opposed to antibodies.[27] However, tests repeatedly detected the virus in another archival sample: blood drawn in 1959 from an individual in the vicinity of Léopoldville, the capital of what was then the Belgian Congo.[28]

Throughout the 1980s and 1990s, suggestions that HIV had originated in Africa were met from a number of quarters as a further example of Western fascination with the continent as a diseased and dangerous landmass. Meanwhile, during this period, most scientists came to believe that HIV had resulted from the cross-species transmission of a simian immunodeficiency virus (SIV) to a single human during the hunting and/or consumption of chimpanzee meat. Some AIDS activists and African officials mounted resistance, however, citing a lack of evidence and racist insinuations of bestiality.[29] An alternative and more marginalized explanation to this "cut hunter" theory also arose, which alleged that a laboratory based in the Belgian Congo unwittingly used SIV-infected chimpanzee tissue in the local preparations of an oral polio vaccine (OPV) in the late 1950s. Between 1957 and 1960, these oral doses were fed to several hundred thousand individuals in the Belgian Congo and in the Belgian-administered areas near Lake Victoria and

26. John Crewdson, "Case Shakes Theories of AIDS Origin," *Chicago Tribune*, October 25, 1987, 1, 20; Gerald Corbitt, Andrew S. Bailey, and George Williams, "HIV Infection in Manchester, 1959," *Lancet* 336, no. 8706 (1990): 51.

27. Edward Hooper and William D. Hamilton, "1959 Manchester Case of Syndrome Resembling AIDS," *Lancet* 348 (1996): 1363–65; Edward Hooper, *The River: A Journey Back to the Source of HIV and AIDS* (London: Allen Lane, 1999), 133–37, 741, 1006n5.

28. A. Nahmias et al., "Evidence for Human Infection with an HTLV-III/LAV-like Virus in Central Africa, 1959," *Lancet* 1 (1987): 1279–80. Following decolonization, Léopoldville was renamed Kinshasa and the former colony took on the name Zaire, before changing its name again in 1997 to the Democratic Republic of the Congo.

29. Treichler, *Theory in an Epidemic*, 121–22.

Lake Tanganyika, regions which would later see early and extensive HIV epidemics.[30]

Mainstream scientists have rejected the OPV theory, particularly following reports describing a scientific debate in 2000 at the Royal Society in London, which declared that there was no firm evidence to support it.[31] The theory's most prominent supporter, Edward Hooper, continues to vigorously defend the theory and respond to its critics from his personal website.[32] Some scientists, including several associated with the OPV research, have answered forcefully with counterclaims and legal threats. They asserted that the OPV theory was dangerous and that it directly contributed to fears worldwide about the dangers of vaccination campaigns and jeopardized the global eradication of polio.[33] Other researchers have pushed past Hooper's increasingly lonely objections. Some have used computer models of HIV mutation rates to estimate the date of the crossover event, that of an immunodeficiency virus passing from a chim-

30. A lengthy account of this theory of accidental iatrogenic introduction, as well as many other origin theories, is Edward Hooper's *The River*. A more succinct and up-to-date version of his main points in support of the OPV theory can be found in his article "The Origins of the AIDS Pandemic: A Quick Guide to the Principal Theories and the Alleged Refutations," *AIDS Origins* (blog), April 25, 2012, http://www.aidsorigins.com/origins-aids-pandemic.

31. Brian Martin offers an intriguing analysis of the ways in which the scientific community has worked to discredit Hooper and the OPV theory: "The Politics of a Scientific Meeting: The Origin-of-AIDS Debate at the Royal Society," *Politics and the Life Sciences* 20, no. 2 (2001): 119–30.

32. In her book *The AIDS Conspiracy: Science Fights Back* (New York: Columbia University Press, 2012), 29–31, Nicoli Nattrass suggests that Hooper's actions—which include personal attacks and often verbose and angry writing on his personal website—resemble those of a conspiracy theorist. Some fairness to Hooper, though, might allow the acknowledgment that someone like him—who has undertaken extensive research, who has seen some of his interviewees subsequently retract their recorded testimony, and whose opponents have misrepresented and then ignored his points—might have genuine concerns that he was witnessing something resembling a cover-up.

33. For example, Hilary Koprowski, "Hypotheses and Facts," *Philosophical Transactions of the Royal Society of London B: Biological Sciences* 356, no. 1410 (2001): 832; Stanley A. Plotkin, "Chimpanzees and Journalists," *Vaccine* 22 (2004): 1829–30. Hooper's rebuttal to this allegation can be read on his website: "The Allegation That *The River* Has Damaged Modern Attempts to Eradicate Polio," *AIDS Origins* (blog), October 15, 2004, http://www.aidsorigins.com/allegation-river-has-damaged-modern-attempts-eradicate-polio.

panzee to a single human.[34] Others have investigated the sociopolitical and environmental conditions in early twentieth-century Africa that may have contributed to the early expansion of HIV.[35]

The Origins of AIDS (2011)—a substantial contribution to the discussion from Jacques Pepin, a microbiologist and infectious disease specialist—offers a detailed contextualization of the colonial environment of central Africa in the first half of the twentieth century and argues for the plausibility of the "cut hunter" theory. Pepin presents compelling evidence for a previously little-known outbreak of disease suggestive of AIDS in a railway camp in French Equatorial Africa in the 1920s and early 1930s. Building on computer estimations that have dated the crossover event to the first decades of the twentieth century, he takes "1921" as a date for argument's sake. Around this time, he proposes, an unknown individual—"the true 'patient zero,'" he writes—came in contact with the blood of a chimpanzee infected with a simian immunodeficiency virus; Pepin suggests that sixty million people in the world today can trace their infections from this individual.[36] Pepin also provides useful historical evidence to demonstrate the close trade and employment ties linking the colonial territories of French Equatorial Africa and the Belgian Congo near the towns of Brazzaville and Léopoldville. Here, an

34. Michael Worobey et al., "Direct Evidence of Extensive Diversity of HIV-1 in Kinshasa by 1960," *Nature* 455, no. 2 (2008): 661–64. By holding as a constant the rate at which a virus mutates, they argue that this "relaxed molecular clock" method allows researchers to estimate backward to the time of the initial crossover event, to a virus from which all subsidiary strains began mutating away. Critics of this approach, of which Hooper is again one of the most vocal, contend that such a method cannot work with a virus like HIV. The virus evolves four to ten times as much through recombination—when an individual is infected with two or more strains of HIV and the viruses swap genetic information with each other—as it does through mutation. The relaxed molecular clock method, these critics contend, cannot control for this recombination. See Hooper, "Michael Worobey's Wobbly Research into the Early History of HIV," *AIDS Origins* (blog), March 19, 2008, http://www.aidsorigins.com/michael-worobey-wobbly-research-early-history-hiv; Simon Wain-Hobson et al., "Network Analysis of Human and Simian Immunodeficiency Virus Sequence Sets Reveals Massive Recombination Resulting in Shorter Pathways," *Journal of General Virology* 84, no. 4 (2003): 885–95.

35. For example, Tamara Giles-Vernick et al., "Social History, Biology, and the Emergence of HIV in Colonial Africa," *Journal of African History* 54 (2013): 11–30.

36. Jacques Pepin, *The Origins of AIDS* (Cambridge: Cambridge University Press, 2011), 1–58, "patient zero" quotation at 40.

unknowingly infected individual could have brought HIV from one colonial region to another relatively easily on a one-hour boat ride. He also
contends that iatrogenic infections—unintentional HIV transmission by
doctors reusing unsterilized needles—are likely to have played a significant role in the rise of HIV in Africa in the early to mid-twentieth century (though not in the present day).[37]

Pepin draws on recent studies to conclude that the virus traveled from
central Africa to Haiti during the 1960s, in the body of one among several thousand Haitian workers who were recruited to work in Zaire during that decade and who later returned to their home country.[38] He suggests the possibility that high-volume blood plasma collection in Haiti
provided an efficient means of transmitting the newly introduced virus
to many Haitians. From there, through the transnational blood industry and sexual liaisons between American homosexual travelers and infected Haitian men, the same subtype of HIV made its way from Haiti
into North America by the early 1970s. There it spread silently through
populations of injecting drug users, men who had sex with other men,
and the recipients of blood products, before coming to the attention of
investigators when these infected individuals fell sick up to ten years
later.[39] From the vantage point of 2011, Pepin is able to place "the case
of the Air Canada flight attendant, the so-called 'patient zero,'" at the
very end of his account. He serves as a highly visible figure, emblematic of the disease's amplification and rapid spread in the 1970s through
North America's gay communities, but not a unique player in this overall global diffusion.[40] North American readers did not share the benefit
of this synthesis in 1987, when newspapers reported the identification of
a Canadian flight attendant as "Patient Zero" for an epidemic thought
then to have begun in the late 1970s. "Patient Zero" would therefore, by
virtue of his transatlantic travels, offer the simple solution to Americans
asking the question, "How did AIDS arrive here?"[41]

37. Ibid., 3–4.
38. Ibid., 187–90.
39. Ibid., 231–33.
40. Ibid., 234.
41. Embellishing Randy Shilts's account, media accounts hypothesized that the flight
attendant had been infected with the virus during sexual encounters with "Africans" in
Europe; see, for example, "Canadian Said to Have Had Key Role in Spread of AIDS,"
New York Times, October 7, 1987, B7.

HIV/AIDS Histories

Following a few questions and an announcement apologizing for the need to reschedule a talk by the NCI scientist Robert Gallo, Curran took the microphone. He began his presentation with the ominous note that "we are in the first couple years of the recognition of a disease that's going to probably be with us forever. You will hear a lot about this over the next decade or so I think."[42]

* * *

The bulk of this book is concerned with the early North American AIDS epidemic, roughly between 1981 and 1996.[43] The beginning of this period is marked by the first organized recognition of the emergence of a possibly new disease and the growing awareness of the problem's scale and severity. The numbers of dying patients intensified year by year during this time—dozens, hundreds, and eventually thousands—against an initial backdrop of governmental silence, widespread homophobia, and apparent apathy. To fill this void, a remarkable patchwork of community-based voluntary service organizations sprang up in lesbian and gay communities across North America to respond to the needs of the sick and dying.[44] Mounting anger among these communities gave rise, from 1987 onward, to direct action groups such as the AIDS Coalition to Unleash Power (ACT UP). These activists succeeded in challenging the view that AIDS was universally fatal and in changing the contours of treatment access.[45] The health circumstances of most people with AIDS did

42. "NCAB Meeting," 15–16.

43. Drawing upon UNAIDS categorizations, this book defines *North America* as Canada and the United States. Within this official categorization system, Mexico is grouped with Latin America, a separation which is obviously arbitrary. As will be demonstrated in chapter 2, there is a long history of cross border flow of sexually transmitted diseases between Mexico and the United States. Indeed, political borders have never halted the movement of populations and diseases.

44. When compared with later decades, individuals who identified as bisexual and as transgender or transsexual were less frequently highlighted as distinctive community members during this period. In a bid to strike a balance between historically sensitive terminology and recognition of these often more marginalized individuals, in this book I will refer to both "lesbian and gay communities" and "LGBT individuals."

45. Deborah B. Gould, *Moving Politics: Emotion and ACT UP's Fight against AIDS*

not substantially improve, however, until the development of treatment regimens that made use of several antiretroviral drugs simultaneously. This advance, known as *combination therapy* or *highly active antiretroviral therapy* (HAART), was publicly heralded at the 1996 International AIDS Conference in Vancouver. From this point on, the character of the epidemic, in resource-rich countries at least, changed irrevocably. With HAART, many patients who had previously been near death experienced the "Lazarus effect," restored to nearly full health like the biblical character said to have been resurrected through a miracle of Jesus.[46] This is not to suggest that this breakthrough, brought about through the work of patient activism and scientific research, was a panacea. Side effects from antiretrovirals, divisions in the highly affected gay communities between HIV-positive and -negative individuals, and shifts in activism toward gay marriage and away from community involvement in health have all left many survivors doubting the "miracle" of their extended lives.[47] The point to be made, rather, is that the pre-HAART era of the epidemic was substantially different from the period that followed in the United States and Canada, and this book's chronological focus reflects this difference.[48]

Within this early period of the epidemic, the three years from the spring of 1981 to the spring of 1984 are of particular historical interest.

(Chicago: University of Chicago Press, 2009), 55–175; *United in Anger: A History of ACT UP* (New York: United in Anger, 2012), documentary film directed by Jim Hubbard and produced by Jim Hubbard and Sarah Schulman; the director kindly provided me with a review copy of this ninety-three-minute film via online streaming prior to its release on DVD in 2014.

46. Jason Szabo, "Re-Birthing Pains: Protease Inhibitors, The 'Lazarus Syndrome,' and the Transformation of the Acquired Immunodeficiency Syndrome" (paper presented at the 82nd annual meeting of the American Association for the History of Medicine, Cleveland, OH, April 26, 2009); John 11:1.

47. See, for example, George Chauncey, *Why Marriage? The History Shaping Today's Debate over Gay Equality* (New York: Basic Books, 2004); Rupert Whitaker, "Thirty Years of AIDS: Triumphs, Failures, and the Unlearned Lessons," lecture at King's College, London, November 3, 2011, podcast, MP3 file, 49:10, http://podcast.ulcc .ac.uk/accounts/kings/Humanities_and_Health/3_11_2011_Rupert_Whitaker_Triumphs _failures_and_unlearned_lessons.mp3.

48. This periodization is borne out in Ronald Bayer and Gerald M. Oppenheimer, *AIDS Doctors: Voices from the Epidemic: An Oral History* (Oxford: Oxford University Press, 2000), 226–33. More recently, one of the physicians interviewed by Bayer and Oppenheimer referred to the pre-1996 years as "the hysterical old days of AIDS": Abigail Zuger, "With AIDS, Time to Get beyond Blame," *New York Times*, April 19, 2010, D6.

They span the time separating the earliest concerted efforts by physicians and epidemiologists to identify and investigate the problem, and they include the widely reported discovery of a virus by a team of NIH scientists led by Gallo.[49] While discussions and debates over the cause of AIDS would smolder on after this time, these disputes were gradually exiled to the edges of orthodoxy. Before the spring of 1984, there had been a multitude of theories about how AIDS was caused and much debate about the consequences for the gay community. After May 1984, the scientific consensus that AIDS was caused by a virus legitimated the greater involvement of the scientific and medical establishment, and it downplayed the importance of the epidemiological research that had played an important part in the earliest phase of the epidemic.[50] It also paved the way for a more generalized acceptance—or "blackboxing"—of the idea that the condition was caused by a single virus, though there would be continued, limited resistance to this dominant view from a small minority of dissenters.[51]

Historians and other observers examined the period from 1981 to 1996 in evolving waves of coverage. Some initially attempted to draw lessons from the past—for example, past responses to plague or syphilis in North America or Western Europe—to interpret the unexpected arrival of a deadly new epidemic in resource-rich countries in the late twentieth

49. At the time, Gallo's discovery of the virus drew the most media attention in North America, notwithstanding the isolation of a virus by a team of French scientists at the Pasteur Institute in Paris in 1983. Later, after many years of dispute, the French team would be widely acknowledged as having priority for the discovery, a view which was bolstered in 2008 when Françoise Barré-Sinoussi and Luc Montagnier were awarded a Nobel Prize for their work. In her recent book on three decades of AIDS, Victoria Harden traces to Shilts's book what she describes as the "character assassination" of Gallo; see Harden, *AIDS at 30: A History* (Dulles, VA: Potomac Books, 2012), 170.

50. Gerald M. Oppenheimer, "In the Eye of the Storm: The Epidemiological Construction of AIDS," in Fee and Fox, *AIDS: The Burdens of History*, 284–86.

51. Epstein, *Impure Science*, 26–31. One thread of dissent, HIV denialism, downplayed the role of HIV, emphasizing instead the importance of cofactors in individuals who developed AIDS. From 1987 onward, Peter Duesberg, a biochemist and vocal minority protester in studies about the etiology of AIDS, would repeatedly challenge the dominant view that HIV caused AIDS; Epstein, *Impure Science*, 105–78. Denialism took a more political, anti-Western, and ultimately tragic shape when South African president Thabo Mbeki drew on Duesberg's ideas to resist the considerable evidence that AIDS was caused by a virus that could be treated with antiretroviral therapy; Nattrass, *AIDS Conspiracy*, 77–104.

century.[52] Gradually, this "apocalyptic" coverage yielded to a more nor-
malized approach, mirroring a more routinized medical response to
AIDS, which by the early 1990s began to assume the characteristics of a
more chronic condition.[53] Some academic historians struggled with the
challenge of writing dispassionately about contemporary events, particularly when their interpretations faced angry resistance from more activist observers, for whom these events were frequently conflicts with mortal consequences.[54]

The earliest of the AIDS histories, *And the Band Played On*, a powerful chronicle written by the San Francisco–based journalist Randy
Shilts, remains one of the most cited accounts of the American experience and continues to shape historical interpretations of the first
five years of the epidemic. In 2007, a *USA Today* editors' choice article listed the bestseller, alongside Stephen Hawking's *A Brief History of
Time* and Salman Rushdie's *The Satanic Verses*, as one of the most influential books of the past quarter century.[55] The Library of Congress
included the book in its 2012 exhibition entitled "Books that Shaped
America," seeing it as having "a profound effect on American life."[56] By
the time Shilts died of AIDS in 1994, his book had been translated into
seven languages and released in sixteen countries.[57] There is no question that Shilts saw himself as writing history, and the impact of the book

52. For example, Robert M. Swenson, "Plagues, History, and AIDS," *American
Scholar* 57, no. 2 (Spring 1988): 183–200; Guenter B. Risse, "Epidemics and History: Ecological Perspectives and Social Responses," in Fee and Fox, *AIDS: Burdens of History*,
33–66.

53. For a sense of this shift, compare the titles and contents of two edited volumes
of historical essays by Elizabeth Fee and Daniel M. Fox: *AIDS: The Burdens of History*
(Berkeley: University of California Press, 1988) and *AIDS: The Making of a Chronic Disease* (Berkeley: University of California Press, 1992).

54. Virginia Berridge and Philip Strong, "AIDS and the Relevance of History," *Social
History of Medicine* 4, no. 1 (1991): 129–38; Virginia Berridge, "The History of AIDS,"
AIDS 7, Suppl. 1 (1993): S243–48. See also Howard Markel, "Journals of the Plague Years:
Documenting the History of the AIDS Epidemic in the United States," *American Journal
of Public Health* 91, no. 7 (2001): 1025–28.

55. "The Most Memorable Books of the Last 25 Years," *USA Today*, April 9, 2007,
http://www.usatoday.com/life/top25-books.htm.

56. *Books That Shaped America* (Washington, DC: Library of Congress, June 25,
2012), exhibition catalog, https://www.loc.gov/exhibits/books-that-shaped-america/overview
.html.

57. Biography of Randy Shilts, n.d., p. 1, Randy's Bio, Carton 2/5, Linda Alband Collection of Randy Shilts Materials (hereafter Alband Collection), 2003–09, accretion 1 of 2,

and of its construction of "Patient Zero" on popular consciousness was significant.[58]

Other historians would draw on Shilts's pioneering work. Mirko Grmek, a Croatian-French physician and historian, wrote his *History of AIDS* (1990), a scholarly account of the epidemic, in the middle of the first phase of the crisis. Grmek sought to place the pandemic in a long-term ecological context of disease environments and emergence. Grmek spoke with interest about the CDC's Los Angeles cluster study and of Gaétan Dugas, seeing the flight attendant as "both an example and a caricature." Though he expressed skepticism about whether Dugas had brought the disease to the United States, Grmek wrote that the flight attendant had "sown the disease and death all along his route, at the rate of about 250 partners per year." Citing only Shilts's book as a source, the historian surmised of Dugas that "a kind of deaf rage against fate had seized him, a desire for vengeance. In a medical interview, he had shamelessly declared, 'I've got it; they can get it too.' Every historian of disease knows that such an attitude of vengeance, or at least of recklessness, had contributed in other times to the spread of tuberculosis and syphilis."[59] This book examines some of the historical precedents to this story to question Grmek's straightforward suggestion that deliberate disease spreading played a significant role in earlier epidemics.

Another historian, Peter Baldwin, later undertook an impressive comparative analysis of the public health responses to AIDS in five resource-rich countries: the United States, Britain, France, Germany, and Sweden. In *Disease and Democracy*, Baldwin argued that the actions taken by different countries could not be predicted based on their politics but rather depended on paths taken in responding to epidemic disease in previous centuries. Dugas garners two mentions in Baldwin's piece, references which point to a weakness of this otherwise very strong work. Baldwin relied—of necessity, given the broad scope of his

---

San Francisco Gay, Lesbian, Bisexual, Transgender Historical Society. Alband was Shilts's business manager during the last five years of Shilts's life.

58. Said one oral historian of Shilts's history: "Like every author of an AIDS book, I read *And the Band Played On* first"; see Benjamin Heim Shepard, *White Nights and Ascending Shadows: An Oral History of the San Francisco AIDS Epidemic* (London: Cassell, 1997), 250.

59. Mirko D. Grmek, *History of AIDS: Emergence and Origin of a Modern Pandemic*, trans. Russell C. Maulitz and Jacalyn Duffin (Princeton, NJ: Princeton University Press, 1990), 18–19.

project—on published materials and, like Grmek, based his assessment of Dugas on Shilts's book. Baldwin's first description of Dugas—"the epidemic's Typhoid Marvin . . . the spectacularly promiscuous and conscienceless airline steward who disseminated HIV transcontinentally"— served for the author as one example of "cases that most would agree deserved censure." The second reference was to suggest that "knowledge of [one's] serostatus appeared to have an ambiguous effect. Devil-may-care conduct was not unheard of. Gaetan Dugas, the French Canadian airplane steward immortalized by Randy Shilts as Patient Zero in *And the Band Played On,* refused to change his globally transmissive behavior or to warn his partners."[60] This book will demonstrate the tenuous nature of these recirculated claims.

The chapters that follow interweave the development and transmission of ideas about AIDS across North America. This transnational approach is partly in response to a tendency in the existing historiography to focus on the United States at the expense of attention to the Canadian experience.[61] Despite the widely noted divergences in their health-

---

60. Peter Baldwin, *Disease and Democracy: The Industrialized World Faces AIDS* (Berkeley: University of California Press, 2005), 90, 127. Dugas did not have the benefit of a blood antibody test to learn his serostatus, as this diagnostic tool was not developed until after his death.

61. Scant work on the history of the AIDS epidemic in Canada exists, a lacuna noted by several observers: Derek G. Steele, "The Evolution of the Canadian AIDS Society: A Social Movement Organization as Network, Coalition and Umbrella Organization" (DPhil thesis, McGill University, 2000), 27; Mark L. Robertson, "An Annotated Chronology of the History of AIDS in Toronto: The First Five Years, 1981–1986," *Canadian Bulletin of Medical History* 22, no. 2 (2005): 314. Jacalyn Duffin's concise 1994 article is one of the few offerings from a historian: "AIDS, Memory and the History of Medicine: Musings on the Canadian Response," *Genitourinary Medicine* 70, no. 1 (1994): 64–69. One of the most useful and comprehensive accounts is Ivan Emke, "Speaking of AIDS in Canada: The Texts and Contexts of Official, Counter-Cultural and Mass Media Discourses Surrounding AIDS" (DPhil thesis, Carleton University, 1991). Political scientists have provided an analysis of the limitations of the federal government's response and outlined the reactions in the country's three largest cities: Vancouver, Toronto, and Montreal: David M. Rayside and Evert A. Lindquist, "Canada: Community Activism, Federalism, and the New Politics of Disease," in *AIDS in the Industrialized Democracies: Passions, Politics, and Policies,* ed. Ronald Bayer and David L. Kirp (New Brunswick, NJ: Rutgers University Press, 1992), 49–98. The journalist Ann Silversides's biography of AIDS activist Michael Lynch remains the best published overview of the early Canadian response, providing a remarkably detailed description of the slow development of policy and of the rise of community-based AIDS organizations and patient advocacy. Silversides's work focuses on Toronto, at times

care systems—predominantly privately funded in the United States versus a primarily publicly funded system in Canada from the late-1960s onward—a comparative approach reveals some striking similarities. In both Canada and the United States, for example, federal officials were slow to enact a public response. US President Ronald Reagan, whose public silence over the disease lasted until 1987, was heavily criticized for his lack of leadership on the issue. Although Canada's minister of health appointed an advisory board to offer guidance on the epidemic in 1983, the country would not develop a federal policy until 1990. Canadian Prime Minister Brian Mulroney did not publicly discuss the disease until his opening speech at the 1989 World AIDS Conference in Montreal, whereupon he was greeted by activists from ACT UP and the Canadian group AIDS Action Now! shouting "Silence equals death!"[62] Both countries experienced early cases in Haitian immigrants, before the epidemic shifted to predominantly affect gay and bisexual men.[63] Early community-based organizations shared information about the disease and response strategies between cities; later, the work of treatment activists flowed across the shared border. One of the contributions of this study, therefore, is to more effectively blend disparate threads of previously separated national histories, leading to not just a Canadian

---

at the expense of local developments elsewhere in Canada: Ann Silversides, *AIDS Activist: Michael Lynch and the Politics of Community* (Toronto: Between the Lines, 2003). Indeed, much of the scholarship on AIDS in Canada has been shaped either by a regional or city focus, or offered through the retrospective accounts of health-care professionals; looking at Vancouver: Michael P. Brown, *RePlacing Citizenship: AIDS Activism and Radical Democracy* (London: Guilford Press, 1997); focusing on Montreal: René Lavoie, "Deux solitudes: les organismes sida et la communauté gaie," in *Sortir de l'ombre: histoires des communautés lesbienne et gaie de Montréal,* ed. Irène Demczuk and Frank W. Remiggi (Montreal: VLB Éditeur, 1998), 337–62; for Quebec more generally: Carole Graveline, Jean Robert, and Réjean Thomas, *Les préjugés plus forts que la mort: le sida au Québec* (Montreal: VLB Éditeur, 1998). It would not be until the final report of the Krever Commission's inquiry into the safety of the Canadian blood system was released in 1997 that a national history of AIDS was published. Even then, the commission's terms of reference meant this history focused primarily on how HIV had entered and spread throughout the country's blood supply. As will be seen in chapter 5, this absence of a Canadian history of the epidemic influenced a gay coalition's decision to seek standing at the Krever inquiry.

62. Michelle Lalonde and Andre Picard, "AIDS Activists Disrupt Opening of Conference," *Globe and Mail* [Toronto], June 5, 1989, A1, A5.

63. See, for example, Grégoire E. Noel, "Another Case of AIDS in the Pre-AIDS Era," *Reviews of Infectious Diseases* 10, no. 3 (1988): 668–69.

or a US history of "Patient Zero" and the AIDS epidemic but a North American one.

Regional Differences and Transnational Sex

With opening statements completed at the meeting, Curran quickly got to the main topics of his presentation: surveillance and epidemiological research. He summarized the CDC's involvement with the epidemic, stemming from the recognition of an increase in 1980 of requests for pentamidine—a drug stocked at the CDC to treat the rare PCP—and provided a list of the life-threatening opportunistic infections the CDC's Task Force had since found in AIDS patients. Curran covered the unusually high frequency of AIDS cases in New York—"about 97 percent of the cases reported in the entire world are in the United States and half of them are in New York City"—and offered a summary of the CDC's case control study and its findings. The study had found significantly higher sexual activity and amyl nitrite drug usage among the cases than the controls. Curran noted that 75 percent of the reported cases were in gay or bisexual men, and he suggested, in words that are important to this book, that there was a variation in the responses to the disease based on location. "In Toronto," he noted dryly, "they think this is a syndrome that's been made up by somebody else. In New York City they really really believe it."[64]

*   *   *

In her book *Sex and Germs* (1985), the community activist and cultural critic Cindy Patton outlined homophobic ideas about sexuality that were present in the scientific treatment of AIDS and urged scientists to "reorient their assumptions that gay men represent a homogeneous population." She wrote that "each city where AIDS appears has different gay community patterns and histories, sexual mores, and even sexual practices, with differing levels of gay health care and possibly different opportunistic disease pools which affect the secondary disease patterns in AIDS."[65] Patton argued that attention to the regional vari-

64. "NCAB Meeting," 15–34, quotation at 33–34.
65. Patton, *Sex and Germs*, 26.

ations in gay communities might reveal unexpected information about the disease. One could extend her point about regional variation to the manner in which different gay communities responded to the arrival of AIDS. Curran's seemingly glib remark, about the disbelief about AIDS in Toronto's gay community, is almost certainly a reference to an article written by Toronto-based activist Michael Lynch and published a month before the NCAB meeting in the November 1982 issue of the *Body Politic*, a gay Canadian left-wing monthly newspaper with a circulation spanning North America. The article urged gay men to be suspicious of any attempts to link homosexuality to disease for fear that it would represent an undesirable return to an earlier era of medical control over sexuality.[66]

During the 1970s and 1980s, struggles for gay and lesbian equality gained a new visibility. As the authors of an amicus brief submitted for the 2003 US Supreme Court decision in *Lawrence v. Texas* noted, substantial gains were made in terms of social acceptance of homosexuals after the delisting of homosexuality as a mental disorder by the American Psychiatric Association (APA) in 1973, and particularly since the 1986 sodomy case of *Bowers v. Hardwick*. Religious attitudes changed substantially, particularly within mainstream American Protestant denominations. The federal government implemented changes to prevent discrimination in the federal workforce on the basis of sexual orientation, and many companies and several states followed suit. A growing mainstream interest in gay issues meant that the media gave increasing coverage to these matters.[67]

These increasing levels of struggle and awareness did not, however, result in immediate and lasting change; indeed, they produced resistance in many quarters. Widespread discrimination and antipathy toward lesbian, gay, bisexual, and transgender/transsexual (LGBT) individuals was common and continued across much of Canada and the United States, sustained by medical and scientific discourse and an expansive web of antihomosexual laws. Activists' gains were accompanied by setbacks. Although homosexuality was eliminated—after a bitter

66. Michael Lynch, "Living with Kaposi's," *Body Politic* 88 (November 1982): 31–37. For Lynch's preparation of this article, see Silversides, *AIDS Activist*, 21–23.

67. George Chauncey, "'What Gay Studies Taught the Court': The Historians' Amicus Brief in *Lawrence v. Texas*," *GLQ: A Journal of Lesbian and Gay Studies* 10, no. 3 (2004): 509–38.

dispute—from the American Psychiatric Association's official list of mental disorders in 1973, the condition of gender identity disorder was added in 1980.[68] During the 1970s, a number of American states introduced specifically antihomosexual sodomy laws, a move that can be viewed not only as a response to gay liberation efforts but also as evidence of a wide level of social support for this discrimination.[69] Between 1973 and 1994, two-thirds to three-quarters of American respondents agreed with the statement that sexual relations between two adults of the same sex were always wrong. These results peaked at 78 percent in agreement in 1991, before they began a gradual but lasting downward trend. Evidently, during the period under study, homophobic ideas and attitudes were widespread.[70]

In view of the conflicts over sexuality that had emerged in the 1970s—both socially with Anita Bryant, the conservative American social reformer, and medically with the delisting of homosexuality—there was a particular suspicion held by many LGBT people about the intrusion of the state into matters of sexuality. In 1981, gay Torontonians rioted in furious response to a police invasion of the city's four main bathhouses. Nearly three hundred men frequenting the premises were arrested, and some of these individuals forced to undergo testing for sexually transmitted infections. Medical experts had for decades pathologized gays and lesbians; within this context, knowledge claims about a disease seemingly related to sexuality were seen as extremely problematic.[71] Since the

68. Joanne Meyerowitz, *How Sex Changed: A History of Transsexuality in the United States* (London: Harvard University Press, 2002), 255.

69. Chauncey, "Gay Studies," 518.

70. Karlyn Bowman, Andrew Rugg, and Jennifer Marsico, *Polls on Attitudes on Homosexuality & Gay Marriage* (Washington, DC: American Enterprise Institute for Public Policy Research, 2013), 4, http://www.aei.org/files/2013/03/21/-polls-on-attitudes-on-homosexuality-gay-marriage_151640318614.pdf. See also Lisa Duggan and Nan D. Hunter, *Sex Wars: Sexual Dissent and Political Culture* (London: Routledge, 1995).

71. "Medical Caution and Political Judgment," *Body Politic* [Toronto], May 1983, 8. Suspicion of medical truth claims was certainly not limited to North American gay men at this time. By the mid-1970s, a number of influential authors, including Thomas Szasz, Erving Goffman, Michel Foucault, and Ivan Illich, had mounted a sustained critique on the authority of medical knowledge and its extensive reach. See, for example, Thomas Szasz, *The Myth of Mental Illness: Foundations of a Theory of Personal Conduct* (New York: Dell, 1961); Erving Goffman, *Asylums: Essays on the Social Situation of Mental Patients and Other Inmates* (Garden City, NY: Anchor Books, 1961); Michel Foucault, *Madness and Civilization,* trans. Richard Howard (New York: Pantheon Books, 1965); Michel Fou-

goal of free sexual expression—unencumbered by intrusions of the state, the church, and medicine—had been a key driver of lesbian and gay liberation in the 1970s, it often took personal experience of the devastation caused by AIDS for many LGBT individuals to even begin thinking of compromising any aspect of their hard-won sexual rights.[72]

Between 1981 and 1984, the terrain of accepted knowledge was very uneven and fiercely contested, not simply between scientists and activists but also among activists in lesbian and gay communities themselves. Many of the changes suggested out of concern for safety were radical in the context of a sexual revolution that had been strongly under way since the early 1970s. Toronto, to return to Curran's remark that singled out that city, was not hard-hit by AIDS until early 1983, and it would take several months for its gay community to develop an organized response, in the absence of action by public health authorities.[73] The delayed visibility of the syndrome in Toronto combined with the recently reinvigorated activism against sexual regulation to produce discussions that differed substantially from those in New York or San Francisco, cities with different gay community formulations, different histories, and earlier dates of epidemic emergence. Individuals who traveled between these cities would encounter strikingly different local responses and attitudes. Bearing this uneven terrain in mind, this book draws attention to the problem of knowledge dissemination, contestation, and uptake in a time of change, as well as the problem of assuming a homogeneous culture of reception.

The emergence of AIDS occurred in parallel with an increase in scholarship investigating the history of sexuality. Following Michel Foucault's field-shaping work in the late 1970s, historians, sociologists, and journalists have undertaken a large number of projects in this area, with a particular focus on the United States, examining the rise of modern gay and lesbian communities and questioning a simple trajectory from repression to sexual liberation.[74] Much of this work has focused on

cault, *The Birth of the Clinic: An Archaeology of Medical Perception,* trans. A. M. Sheridan Smith (New York: Pantheon Books, 1973); Ivan Illich, *Medical Nemesis: The Expropriation of Health* (London: Calder and Boyars, 1975).

72. Gary Kinsman, *The Regulation of Desire: Homo and Hetero Sexualities,* 2nd ed. (Montreal: Black Rose Books, 1996), 288–329; Tom Warner, *Never Going Back: A History of Queer Activism in Canada* (Toronto: University of Toronto Press, 2002), 61–164.

73. Silversides, *AIDS Activist,* 37–61.

74. Michel Foucault, *The Will to Knowledge,* vol. 1 of *The History of Sexuality,* trans.

metropolitan areas, both by tracing the development of lesbian and gay communities within individual cities and by examining the assumption that networks of same-sex attraction depended on urban concentrations of like-minded individuals.[75] Historians have explored attempts to medicalize and pathologize homosexuality, as well as efforts to challenge this process.[76] Increased attention to sexuality led to histories of sexually transmitted diseases (STDs), in both Canada and the United States, which offered overviews of social and medical responses to the problem from the nineteenth century onward, though these accounts have often paid little notice to the particular linkages of same-sex contacts with venereal disease (VD).[77]

Historians have increasingly begun to consider matters of sexuality

---

Robert Hurley (1978; repr., London: Penguin, 1998); John D'Emilio, *Sexual Politics, Sexual Communities: The Making of a Homosexual Minority in the United States, 1940–1970* (Chicago: University of Chicago Press, 1983); John D'Emilio and Estelle B. Freedman, *Intimate Matters: A History of Sexuality in America*, 2nd ed. (New York: Harper & Row, 1997).

75. For example, Elizabeth Lapovsky Kennedy and Madeline D. Davis, *Boots of Leather, Slippers of Gold: The History of a Lesbian Community* (New York: Routledge, 1993); Esther Newton, *Cherry Grove, Fire Island: Sixty Years in America's First Gay and Lesbian Town* (Boston: Beacon, 1993); George Chauncey, *Gay New York: Gender, Urban Culture, and the Making of the Gay Male World, 1890–1940* (New York: Basic Books, 1994); Nan Alamilla Boyd, *Wide-Open Town: A History of Queer San Francisco to 1965* (Berkeley: University of California Press, 2003); Marc Stein, *City of Sisterly and Brotherly Loves: Lesbian and Gay Philadelphia, 1945–72* (Philadelphia: Temple University Press, 2004); Lilian Faderman and Stuart Timmons, *Gay L.A.: A History of Sexual Outlaws, Power Politics, and Lipstick Lesbians* (New York: Basic Books, 2006). For a review of this literature, which sees much of it as examples of local studies responding to the national focus of John D'Emilio, see Marc Stein, "Theoretical Politics, Local Communities: The Making of U.S. LGBT Historiography," *GLQ: A Journal of Lesbian and Gay Studies* 11, no. 4 (2005): 605–25.

76. Jennifer Terry, *An American Obsession: Science, Medicine and Homosexuality in Modern Society* (London: University of Chicago Press, 1999); Henry L. Minton, *Departing from Deviance: A History of Homosexual Rights and Emancipatory Science in America* (London: University of Chicago Press, 2002).

77. Allan M. Brandt, *No Magic Bullet: A Social History of Venereal Disease in the United States since 1880*, expanded ed. (Oxford: Oxford University Press, 1987); Jay Cassel, *The Secret Plague: Venereal Disease in Canada, 1838–1939* (London: University of Toronto Press, 1987); Jay Cassel, "Private Acts and Public Actions: The Canadian Response to the Problem of Sexually Transmitted Disease in the Twentieth Century," *Transactions of the Royal Society of Canada* 4 (1989): 305–28. While the term *sexually transmitted infections* (STIs) now appears to be preferred, this book will make use of the historically ap-

from a transnational perspective. "Sexual behavior," wrote one historian in 2009, "is fundamentally about interconnection, and it is not unusual for sexual actors to transgress the boundaries constructed to constrain them."[78] A decade earlier, two fellow historians argued that "it is impossible to understand the sexual history of New York, Rio de Janeiro, San Juan, and other cities in the Americas without coming to terms with the implications of such transnational movements and the tremendous translocal mobility of every city's residents."[79] National boundaries did not constrain the AIDS epidemic. They did not halt the silent spread of HIV through migration movements or the flow of blood products. Nor did they limit Gaétan Dugas and other unnamed young gay men before and after him as international residents and lovers, unaware of a viral passenger they brought with them on their sexual travels. For these reasons, the importance of adopting a transnational approach is clear. A historical investigation of the "Patient Zero" story focusing solely on one country would inevitably yield an incomplete and unsatisfactory analysis.

The Limits of Public Health

Near the end of his presentation, Curran summarized a study undertaken earlier that year in Los Angeles that supported "the postulate that this might be a sexually transmitted etiology among homosexual men."[80] He highlighted "one case outside of California who had had direct sexual contact with four cases in Los Angeles, none of whom knew each other and were separated by some 75 miles in terms of their living residence." He went on to reinforce his point: "Further interview of this out of California case, who has lived now in two countries and four different states, we found that we were able to get a list of some 72 sexual partners whose names he had, out of a number of 750 that he claimed to have had during

---

propriate terms: *venereal disease* (VD) until the 1970s and *sexually transmitted diseases* (STDs) in the 1980s and 1990s.

78. Joanne Meyerowitz, "*AHR Forum:* Transnational Sex and U.S. History," *American Historical Review* 114, no. 5 (2009): 1274; see also Margot Canaday's introduction to this forum, pp. 1250–57.

79. Elizabeth A. Povinelli and George Chauncey, "Thinking Sexuality Transnationally," *GLQ: A Journal of Lesbian and Gay Studies* 5, no. 4 (1999): 440.

80. "NCAB Meeting," 28.

the past three years. He is a living man with Kaposi's sarcoma. He is still out there."[81] Curran pointed out that "five of the patients that he had sexual contact with that developed illness were during 1980," between nine and twenty-two months before they developed symptoms. Although he suggested that it was a "very loose figure," he concluded that the average time period "between contact and onset of illness is about 14 months."[82]

Curran's mention of the cluster study and the "out of California case," the individual whom his colleagues at the CDC had already begun calling "Patient O," obviously made a significant impact on the gathering. Several minutes later, after Curran had moved on from the Los Angeles cluster study and was considering the transmission patterns in IV drug users and hemophiliacs, there was an interruption from the board panel, which bears reprinting here at length:

> MS. KUSHNER: May I ask if the gentleman with several hundred fifty partners is still out there loose or has he been put away? I mean really, is there no recourse?
>
> DR. CURRAN: We're dealing with a hypothesis that this is a transmissible agent. It's been recommended to him that he (laughter) that he (laughter) [sic] not have any sexual partners. It was recommended that he go into seclusion.
>
> MS. KUSHNER: But, there's no legal, nothing that CDC can do in a case like this?
>
> DR. CURRAN: Well, the country's been fairly, this is a philosophical remark, but I think the country's been fairly conservative about making recommendations towards people's personal lives. What do we tell surgeons who are hepatitis B surface antigen and E antigen positive, or dentists who are hepatitis B surface antigen E antigen positive? And I've got to clean my teeth, I'll tell you.
>
> MS. KUSHNER: People with TB have to go to homes in the state of Maryland.
>
> DR. CURRAN: Well, there's no definite test for this disease and there probably are many people who may be carriers of it and it's very difficult to—We'll be talking about prevention recommendations later.[83]

81. Ibid., 29. Curran's comments suggest that he was aware that Dugas had lived in Quebec, Ontario, New York, and California.

82. Ibid.

83. "NCAB Meeting," 31–33. The typist's interjections are in rounded parentheses; mine are in square brackets. For more on homophobia at the NIH, see Altman, *AIDS in*

Curran had captured the attention of Rose Kushner, one of the advisory board's public representatives. On the basis of her advocacy work for women with breast cancer, she had been nominated to the board by President Jimmy Carter in 1980 for a six-year term.[84] It is quite likely that Kushner would have presented herself, in a high-level scientific environment such as the NCI, as a vox populi; as a result, her comments with regard to isolation offer an early indication of what one aspect of the wider public reception of the "Patient Zero" story would later be.[85] Kushner's own position on the committee, a result of late twentieth-century developments in health activism by patients, did not appear to instill her with any particular sympathy for the patient under discussion. However, the social developments that brought advocates like her—though often not gay men—to the table will be an important theme running through this book, as the patient-rights movement would unsettle long-standing patriarchal assumptions on the part of physicians.

The laughter at the NCAB meeting, elicited by the number of sexual partners reported by the "Out of California" case, suggests the positions of disdain, distance, and disbelief from which many members of the scientific community and the wider public viewed the behavior and practices of the homosexual men under study during this period.[86] It tes-

---

the Mind of America, 49. Curran's remark about dentists was prescient, given the intense debates surrounding this profession and the risk of transmitting HIV in the late 1980s. See, for example, Wald, Contagious, 251–54.

84. Barron H. Lerner, "Ill Patient, Public Activist: Rose Kushner's Attack on Breast Cancer Chemotherapy," Bulletin of the History of Medicine 81, no. 1 (2007): 227. A vocal critic of the medical establishment, and well-known for her efforts to empower women in the decision-making process for their treatments, Kushner had a reputation for being abrasive, acknowledging in an interview earlier that year that some people in the government's cancer research community considered her "an angry, hateful witch"; see Sandy Rovner, "Healthtalk: For Everywoman," Washington Post, September 12, 1980, F5.

85. Kushner appears to have been mistaken with regard to the institutional isolation of contemporary tuberculosis (TB) patients. Although convalescence in sanatoriums was certainly part of the treatment for tuberculosis during Kushner's lifetime, the rise of successful drug treatments meant that such isolation was—temporarily, before the rise in HIV-related drug-resistant TB—largely a thing of the past in Maryland and across the nation, as a series of Washington Post articles had recently highlighted. See Sandra R. Gregg, "City's TB Clinic Survives by Borrowing Everything," Washington Post, May 25, 1981, B1; Leslie Berger, "Nurse Battles City's TB Cases with Cunning Detective Work," Washington Post, August 11, 1982, sec. District Weekly, DC1.

86. See also Jon Cohen, Shots in the Dark: The Wayward Search for an AIDS Vaccine (New York: W. W. Norton, 2001), 3–15.

tifies to the differences in sexual norms between the scientific and medical communities and the "sub-population" of the gay community under investigation, differences which would hamper communication between and among these groups.[87] Kushner's remarks and the laughter Curran's response elicited also express an acute uneasiness about the mobile nature of the perceived threat and point to a classic public health dilemma: How to balance the liberty of a sick individual against the community's presumed right to health?[88] The story of "Patient Zero" would engender strong views in this debate and raise questions about the role of criminal law in resolving this conflict. It would also test the limits of how far and how widely public health officials might be expected to share information in the jet age, when individuals with transmissible disease might swiftly and easily move between public health jurisdictions.

Writing a "Patient's View" History

"He is a living man with Kaposi's sarcoma. He is still out there." With these rather ominous words, Curran encapsulated the ambiguity and fear surrounding Dugas, the man at the center of the "Patient Zero" narrative. He was a patient who had not died quickly, who was still at large,

---

87. With the words *"Holy mackerel,"* Richard Mathias—a physician who worked during the early 1980s as a consultant epidemiologist for British Columbia's Ministry of Health— later summed up the astonished response he shared with his heterosexual colleagues upon learning how many partners this individual had reported. For him their surprise reflected how little they knew at the time about the sexual behaviors of the gay men they were studying. He also suggested that, in retrospect, researchers' early hypotheses were too often underpinned by a desire to establish a notional safe distance between their own behaviors and those of the gay men deemed at risk of developing AIDS; Richard Mathias, interview with author, Vancouver, August 28, 2007, recording C1491/16, tape 1, sides A and B, British Library Sound Archive, London (hereafter cited as BLSA); emphasis on recording. All such interviews are part of Richard A. McKay, 2007 and 2008, Imagining Patient Zero: Interviews about the History of the North American AIDS Epidemic, © Richard A. McKay and The British Library, Reference C1491. A full list of interviewees appears in the appendix at the back of this book. All the recordings are archived in the BLSA as part of the Oral History collections and can be accessed at the British Library, subject to any access restrictions requested by interviewees and the author.

88. See Judith Walzer Leavitt's exemplary work on this complex question, explored through the life of "Typhoid Mary" Mallon: *Typhoid Mary: Captive to the Public's Health* (Boston: Beacon Press, 1996).

and whose medical condition was becoming understood to be much more dangerous than originally suspected. His case and initial cooperation with researchers offered suggestive evidence to support an emerging consensus that AIDS was caused by a transmissible agent, and yet there were not sufficient data to convince him to change his behavior. While Curran would go on to say that this man was simply one of many who might be "carriers," the fact that he had been singled out for mention, and was "still out there," undercut this notion.

At the heart of this book is the experience of a gay man, one of the earliest persons identified with AIDS in North America, whose own voice has been silenced by particularly successful retellings of his story, versions which are "still out there." This book grounds the evocative ideas of origins, carriers, and disease spreading with an account of this man's life and experience. Such an effort draws on a body of work in the subfield of medical history that emphasizes the importance of considering "the patient's view." Epitomized by a 1985 article by Roy Porter that extended the ambitions of 1960s and 1970s social history, this trend sought to examine the physician–patient encounter from the patient's perspective and urged historians to overcome the methodological challenges posed by the bulk of the records documenting these encounters being written by practitioners.[89] Porter has been criticized for focusing too much on the doctor–patient relationship, at the expense of such other individuals as nurses, technicians, and carers, who often play roles in the medical encounter.[90] Bearing this criticism in mind, the book attempts to draw on a wider variety of sources, including Dugas's friends, colleagues, and health workers, in an attempt to provide a richer social depiction of the early AIDS epidemic.

Guided by the work of queer, transnational, and medical historians, *Patient Zero* blends archival research with oral history methods to articulate and analyze previously marginalized historical accounts. It incorporates evidence of a popular story's transmission and reception beyond American borders and actively addresses the challenge of locating the patient's view in a historical record largely constructed by health-care

89. Roy Porter, "The Patient's View: Doing Medical History from Below," *Theory and Society* 14, no. 2 (1985): 175–98. For an example of patient's view history for "Typhoid Mary" Mallon, see Leavitt, *Typhoid Mary*, 162–201.

90. Flurin Condrau, "The Patient's View Meets the Clinical Gaze," *Social History of Medicine* 20, no. 3 (2007): 533–34.

workers. To counterbalance an abundance of accounts from physicians and public health workers in the dominant narrative of the early AIDS epidemic, I made a concerted effort to interview those identifying themselves as LGBT individuals, people living with HIV/AIDS, and acquaintances and coworkers of Dugas, using a combination of targeted and chain-referral sampling. Research in LGBT and queer history has relied heavily on the use of oral history interviewing, with many practitioners aiming to address the manner in which these individuals have been systematically excluded from large parts of the published record.[91] These reminiscences were supplemented by interviews with key AIDS physicians, public health workers, and the commissioner of the public inquiry into the Canadian blood system. The book assembles primary source material from public and private archives from across the United States and Canada. Records of the CDC's AIDS Task Force were examined to chart the evolution and consequences of the Los Angeles cluster study that focused on the flight attendant. In addition, I analyzed Shilts's personal and professional papers—particularly the interview notes from which he built his characterization of Dugas and the extensive press coverage generated by *Band*—as well as records from community-based AIDS organizations in New York, San Francisco, Toronto, and Vancouver, and gay periodicals from across North America.[92]

The process of recovering, organizing, and presenting these varied and far-flung sources—laborious and time-consuming in its own right— also presented some challenging ethical quandaries for a historian to puzzle through, most relating to posthumous confidentiality. To what ex-

91. John Howard, *Men Like That: A Southern Queer History* (London: University of Chicago Press, 1999), 12–13; Nan Alamilla Boyd, 'Who Is the Subject? Queer Theory Meets Oral History,' *Journal of the History of Sexuality* 17, no. 2 (2008): 177–89. This is a well-established methodology in the history of medicine as well; see Nancy Tomes, "Oral History in the History of Medicine," *Journal of American History* 78, no. 2 (1991), 607–17; Paul Thompson and Rob Perks, *An Introduction to the Use of Oral History in the History of Medicine* (London: National Life Story Collection, 1993). Of course, Randy Shilts was himself an author whose work was primarily based on oral testimony.

92. The reporter's interview notes form part of a large collection of his personal and professional papers, bequeathed to the San Francisco Public Library after his death from AIDS in 1994. The collection holds drafts for virtually all his writing, including journals, early college compositions, reporting for the *Advocate* and *San Francisco Chronicle*, and research materials for his three books; Randy Shilts Papers (GLC 43), LGBTQIA Center, SFPL (hereafter cited as Shilts Papers). All quotations from Shilts's unpublished work appear with permission given by the Shilts Literary Trust.

tent ought information shared by Dugas on his medical journey be held in confidence after his death? And, on a related note, if journalists bequeath their records to public archives, as Shilts and others have done, should the confidence they provided to their sources during their lifetimes extend beyond the grave?

The second question may be easier to resolve than the first. Reporters' privilege—the right for journalists to refuse to testify in legal proceedings to protect their anonymous sources—exists for a number of reasons: to maintain the focus of a news organization's staff and resources on news gathering instead of responding to subpoenas; to protect journalists' sources from retribution or embarrassment; and to clearly separate a free press from the government.[93] Current legislation in the United States focuses chiefly on preventing living journalists from being forced to identify their sources during their lifetimes and pays little explicit attention to any long-term duties of confidence.[94] This is not to suggest that no one has contemplated the problems associated with posthumous confidentiality. In the forceful words of a British journalist and media scholar, "Protecting a source is without qualification. It should never be given up—not to the editor or proprietor; not even after death. Journalists should never identify confidential sources on any traceable record, without the knowledge and permission of their informant."[95] By contrast, when an American reporter raised the alarm about federal agents hunting for information about decades-old unauthorized disclosures, his questions balanced concerns about deterring future sources with the broader protection of the historical record. Would the agents, seeking access to a recently deceased journalist's files before they were catalogued for archival use, rob historians of the fullest possible historical documentation and deprive the public of their right to learn about the historical past?[96] These examples may indicate a need for reporters to reflect carefully on whether they wish to deposit their papers for

93. Reporters Committee for Freedom of the Press, *The First Amendment Handbook*, 7th ed. (Arlington, VA: Reporters Committee for Freedom of the Press, 2011), http://www .rcfp.org/rcfp/orders/docs/FAHB.pdf.

94. I have drawn this conclusion from a review of material posted on the Reporters Committee for Freedom of the Press website, http://www.rcfp.org.

95. Tim Crook, "Don't Attack Gilligan for Doing His Job," letter to the editor, *Guardian* [London], September 9, 2003, https://www.theguardian.com/media/2003/sep/10/bbc .guardianletters.

96. Mark Feldstein, "Not after Reporters . . . Just Their Sources," *News Media and*

posterity. If they proceed, do they have a responsibility to protect the identities of their sources and, if so, for how long? With regard to individuals named in Shilts's publicly available records, my own approach was a pragmatic one. Since this reporter recorded in his notes whether a source wished to be identified or not, it was possible for me to employ pseudonyms for these individuals in my own book.

Returning to the initial question about Dugas's medical information, it is tempting, at first, to respond that it should remain confidential in its entirety. To begin with, this stance accords with current ethical guidance promoted in codes of medical and public health ethics: confidentiality is a fundamental value, and patients' information should remain secret even after they die.[97] Health professionals work hard every day to preserve the public's trust in this confidentiality when they discuss individual cases, removing personal identifiers and using pseudonyms as a form of protective code.

Yet at the heart of this book is a story of how one such code was broken. In many ways the story of Gaétan Dugas as "Patient Zero" is a perfect example of both the dangers of unauthorized disclosure of confidential information and the complexity of documenting this history. It also draws focus to contradictory tensions at play in the 1980s, between patients wishing to preserve their privacy yet facing an increasing political imperative to render their private struggles more visible to bring attention to a condition that many refused to see. In 1987 Randy Shilts publicly identified Dugas, four years after the man's death, relaying information about his having contracted and transmitted STIs and HIV and intimating that he was deliberately trying to spread disease. The journalist did so in part to focus national attention on the epidemic. When these stories were widely repeated in subsequent reporting—reaching millions of readers and television viewers within weeks—Dugas was explicitly blamed for starting a continental epidemic and reached an almost unparalleled posthumous notoriety.

Dugas's example points to the challenges of anonymizing unusual

the Law 30, no. 2 (Summer 2006), http://www.rcfp.org/browse-media-law-resources/news -media-law/news-media-and-law-summer-2006/not-after-reporters-just-th.

97. See, for example, General Medical Council, Confidentiality, October 12, 2009, http://www.gmc-uk.org/static/documents/content/Confidentiality_-_English_1015.pdf; and Lisa M. Lee and Christina Zarowsky, "Foundational Values for Public Health," Public Health Reviews 36, no. 2 (2015): 1–9.

cases. He had a rare, distinctive, and at times visible condition. He traveled widely, actively participated in numerous communities, and interacted with many sexual contacts and health workers. When interviewed by CDC researchers, he agreed for his name to be shared with other researchers as part of their investigations, and his example was much discussed among health professionals. Though there is no evidence his name was used publicly, personal identifiers linked to his case were shared within sufficiently small communities of early cases and health workers. In essence, the clues were there to be tied together, waiting for a reporter to decide that it was in the public interest to name names.

In addition to affecting forever the reputations of a dead man and his surviving family members, Shilts's actions threw up difficulties for any conscientious historian wishing to understand how this story had developed. By revealing "Patient 0" to be Dugas, sensitive information which researchers had released publicly in coded terms before 1987 became instantly linked to him. Internal CDC documents referring to individuals by pseudonyms, which might otherwise have been shared relatively securely to provide additional contextual details about the cluster study, now risked further disclosures about a now-identifiable "Patient 0." Taking a hard line on confidentiality might mean preventing all unpublished material that related to this man and the process by which he became known as "Patient 0," even if it was encoded, to remain forever closed to historians and the public.

However, problems with this approach become readily apparent. Is it not akin to shutting the barn door after the horses have escaped? If anyone questioned, as many did, the way by which this individual took on a role of importance in the history, crucial information for understanding and critiquing this process would be lost. If his family wondered, as they did in 1987, whether his identity had been disclosed through the leaking of confidential hospital medical files, their questions would remain unanswered. Although the official stance of the CDC for years was to neither confirm nor deny the identity of this individual, newspaper interviews from both individual CDC investigators and Shilts confirmed that the code had been breached.[98] Was Dugas now a public figure, permitting some of his physicians to speak publicly about their interactions

---

98. "'First AIDS Patient' Story Dismissed," *Gazette* [Montreal], October 17, 1987, A3; Duncan Campbell, "Shilts Theory Is Nonsense!" *Capital Gay*, March 4, 1988, 1, 4; Duncan Campbell, "An End to the Silence," *New Statesman*, March 4, 1988, 22–23. According to a

with him? As readers will see, some doctors would denounce him as a sociopath or use his actions as a way of justifying their own ethically dubious behavior. Or were other doctors, who revealed confidential details about him when speaking more cautiously in his defense, relying on the fact that much time had passed since his death and that far more damning accusations had long been in the public domain? Or, perhaps, were they abiding by another long-standing guideline for medical conduct: if in doubt, choose a course of action that will benefit the patient or protect his interests?[99] If so, do a patient's interests extend to the afterlife? Historians of medicine have adopted a number of approaches to this question when dealing with patients whose names are not already widely known. Many have taken steps to disguise individuals' identities; others, however, have justified identifying patients on the basis of giving them voice and agency and viewing anonymization as risking the perpetuation of stigma and marginalization.[100] In practice, it seems that historians' decisions on how to proceed are rooted in the complex specificities of their source material.[101]

One is on firmer ground when one recognizes the privacy interests of surviving relatives and those who had a relationship with the deceased patient.[102] Learning early in my research about the scrutiny Dugas's family had faced in the media, I wished initially not to disturb them at all. When it became apparent that my project had grown beyond a master's dissertation, it occurred to me that by not alerting them to my research, I might unintentionally re-create the circumstances of their shock at the

---

letter Campbell sent to Bill Darrow in March 1988, he based his claim about death threats faced by the Dugas family on reports in the British press; William W. Darrow Papers, Miami.

99. Gerald L. Higgins, "The History of Confidentiality in Medicine: The Physician–Patient Relationship," *Canadian Family Physician* 35 (April 1989): 921–26, 14.

100. David Wright and Renée Saucier, "Madness in the Archives: Anonymity, Ethics, and Mental Health History Research," *Journal of the Canadian Historical Association* 23, no. 2 (2012): 65–90.

101. Susan C. Lawrence, *Privacy and the Past: Research, Law, Archives, Ethics* (New Brunswick, NJ: Rutgers University Press, 2016), 89–114.

102. In 2013, the Final Rule for the Health Insurance Portability and Accountability Act (HIPAA) suggested that, in most cases, fifty years struck the right balance between these privacy concerns and wider interests; US Department of Health and Human Services, "Modifications to the HIPAA Privacy, Security, Enforcement, and Breach Notification Rules under the Health Information Technology for Economic and Clinical Health Act and the Genetic Information Nondiscrimination Act; Other Modifications to the HIPAA Rules; Final Rule," *Federal Register* 78, no. 17 (2013): 5613–14.

1987 revelations, about which they had received no prior consultation from Shilts or his publisher. After seeking guidance from senior historians, I sent a letter in 2008 explaining my research project and inquiring whether the family wished to participate. A polite, brief, and firm answer to a follow-up inquiry two months later made the family's position of noninvolvement clear. This respectful distance remained in place until an article I wrote was accepted for publication in 2013. In it I quoted extensively from a letter shared with me by one of Dugas's former lovers, one of the few known surviving documents in the flight attendant's hand. Copyright law requires permission from a letter's author or his or her heirs to reproduce more than a few words from such a document. I paid for my article to be professionally translated into French and sent it to the family, along with a copy of the letter and a photograph of Dugas from his former lover. From that point, a series of letters and phone calls with Dugas's surviving family members established a cautious and cordial relationship. They eventually granted permission for me to publish quotations from Dugas's letter and photographs of him, reaffirmed their clear wishes to remain undisturbed by journalists, and expressed gratitude at the possibility of rehabilitating their younger brother's memory.

Discussing this material more than thirty years after his death brings with it some challenging decisions about disclosure. Ultimately, given the highly unusual circumstances of Dugas's case, it seems very unlikely that my discussion of his confidential information risks weakening the prevailing commitment of historians to preserve patient confidentiality. Furthermore, given the monumental damage Dugas's reputation suffered in 1987, it seems highly unlikely that any additional release of information could worsen his posthumous memory or create deeper intrusions into the family's privacy, although, there remains the possibility of drawing continued attention to a controversy that they would prefer to leave to rest. There is, on the other hand, a much stronger likelihood that articulating this history will—without removing all traces of bad feeling—promote greater understanding and allow the chance for his surviving family members, friends, and lovers to achieve some sense of closure. Bearing this in mind, I have attempted to observe a respectful distance of the family's domestic sphere, exercised restraint over details that might be deemed prurient, and granted the family veto rights over certain stories and the reproduction of personal images.

Who gets to name? How do they see the world? How do they represent what they see? To whom? A resolute belief in the importance of these questions and the impact they have on the practices of making science and writing history moves me to place myself, as this book's author, more explicitly into the frame. Like all other knowledge creators, I bring to this book my own subjectivity, a particular worldview shaped by my own historically situated experiences, which in turn has influenced—at some levels consciously, and at other levels less so—the history I have written. [103] As a white, middle-class teenager coming of age in the 1990s in a suburban city near Vancouver, Canada, my understanding of sexual contact was always informed with an awareness of the risks of HIV and other sexually transmissible diseases. Less clear to me, at that time, was my own sexuality, which, by the time that I neared the completion of my undergraduate degree at the University of British Columbia, was urgently pressing me to acknowledge that I was attracted to other men. Though remaining closeted to friends, colleagues, and family members, I began a sexual relationship with a handsome male graduate student I met at one of Vancouver's few gay night clubs. Shortly thereafter, having imbibed the message that responsible sexual health rested upon regular testing for STDs, we went together for what I had assumed to be a regular checkup at a local community-based gay health clinic. My assumption proved to be incorrect when the results returned: the community nurse, after asking whether I thought that I might, in fact, be HIV-positive, informed me that the test indicated that I had contracted HIV. My new partner tested negative.

Three very stressful months of further tests and much waiting eventually confirmed that I had been the recipient of a false-positive diagnosis. My initial result, an indeterminate combination of a positive screening test and a negative confirmation test, raised the possibility that I had been recently infected and had not created enough antibodies to be read by the confirmation test. As time and further testing proved, a far less likely scenario had occurred. I was one of a very small percentage of individuals whose blood cross-reacted with the highly sensitive ELISA screening test. Though I had not been exposed to HIV, my blood yielded a falsely positive test result.

This experience, at the age of twenty-two, was profoundly transfor-

---

103. For a call to historians to be aware of "our own historicity" and to embrace more self-reflexive modes of practice, see Roger Cooter with Claudia Stein, *Writing History in the Age of Biomedicine* (New Haven, CT: Yale University Press, 2013), x.

mational on a personal level. At the time of my diagnosis—despite it taking place in the same city where only a few years earlier the announcement of new therapy regimes had heralded a transformation of the disease—my mind conjured up older and more resilient notions: HIV leading to early death, infection with the virus as a consequence of gay sex. Spending several months thinking of myself as HIV-positive sensitized me to fears of dying young and social rejection, to a sense of self-pollution, and to a radically diminished sense of self-worth. Though in retrospect I can see that I faced these challenges from a position of relative social and economic privilege, the experience often seemed overwhelming at the time. It shattered my previously untroubled confidence in scientific progress and medical authority and introduced a far more critical engagement with the media's representations of disease. Not long after this experience, I read *And the Band Played On* for the first time and became transfixed by Shilts's accounts of the 1980s medical and social struggles that forged subsequent understandings of the disease. I was also seduced by his dark depiction of the flight attendant who had spent the last year of his life in my hometown. The sixteen years in between this triggering personal incident and my completion of my own book have seen me relocate to the United Kingdom for further study and research, with a significant amount of that time spent grappling with the multifaceted story of "Patient Zero." A commitment to exposing the ways in which knowledge is created—particularly in a work that uses biography as a contextualizing explanatory tool—means that it is important that readers be aware of this background. No scientific or historical account is neutral, nor any author objective, though these caveats do not foreclose a rigorous commitment to honesty and truth.

The idea of "Patient Zero" developed as part of an ongoing process in which scientific research was imagined, represented, and shaped through words, stories, and images that carried a legacy of cultural assumptions about disease, origins, and sexuality. As this book demonstrates, this idea was disseminated and sustained by four key trends: a broad societal need to imagine and then seek a simple explanation and source for complex patterns of contagion; the unintended consequences of hypotheses and decisions made by scientific and medical researchers who investigated the epidemic; tense divisions within the affected gay communities, where one response to the intense blame from without was to assign blame within; and a sensation-seeking media culture. Many during this period—individuals and groups, gay and straight—found that the idea of "Patient Zero" offered them something useful: something to explain with, to entice with, or to fight against. In its perceived utility, widespread flexibility, and remarkable longevity, the tale of "Patient Zero" has played an important part in shaping the scientific and popular understandings of the North American HIV/AIDS epidemic and later disease outbreaks. In this regard one could also say that, in many ways, *he is still out there.*

Readers interested in the long historical background to these trends should continue to chapter 1 for a detailed examination of the constituent parts of the "Patient Zero" story, one which helps explain the full power of their eventual combination. Those more keen to learn about the CDC's early AIDS research and the mid-twentieth-century forces shaping it might prefer to proceed directly to chapter 2. Chapters 3 and 4 offer a detailed examination of the process by which Randy Shilts came to write *And the Band Played On* and how the book was promoted and received by audiences across North America in the late 1980s. The book's final pair of chapters pay particular attention to the Canadian side of this history. Chapter 5 draws an extended comparison between the production of John Greyson's musical film *Zero Patience* (1993) and the curious resilience of interest in Gaétan Dugas's role as "Patient Zero" during the 1990s in a commission of inquiry investigating the country's blood system. Chapter 6 pays close attention to the lived experience of Dugas, seeking to counterbalance the sensational coverage the flight attendant's life received in *And the Band Played On* and subsequent reports.

The Los Angeles cluster study and its "Patient 0" were significant in the early 1980s for making sense of how some of the earliest then recognized cases of AIDS fit together and for demonstrating the hypothesis that the condition was caused by a sexually transmissible agent. This explanation, in turn, was key to focusing research and resources in the years that followed. When it was resurrected, rechristened, and redistributed in 1987, the story of "Patient Zero" was essential, to many observers, for understanding how AIDS had arrived in North America and, to some, for deciding whom to blame, despite the many questions which had begun to unsettle the hypotheses that held the threads of the story together. Rewriting the by-then widely accepted and understood definition of "Patient Zero" would have meant unsettling that certainty and opening the door to a world of far greater complexity. In many ways and in many settings—in public health, in the media, and in wider public consciousness—"Patient Zero" was a foundational idea in the making of the North American AIDS epidemic. It is my hope that the history I relate in the following pages will prevent this idea from being applied uncritically to future disease outbreaks.

CHAPTER ONE

What Came Before Zero?

In a book about AIDS first published in 1984, Dr. Alvin Friedman-Kien, a New York dermatologist and virologist, reminisced about attempts that he and his colleague, Dr. Linda Laubenstein, had made in 1981 to locate an individual of interest to their investigations of the new disorder:

> One of these men, who had died, had had sex with a man who had KS, and who traveled a lot for a Canadian company. Call him Erik. Someone else also knew that Erik had lived in a house on Fire Island where three men had died. So I said, "We've got to get hold of him." Linda said she'd tried to reach him but he'd moved. . . . Then I was asked by Marc Conant and Bob Bolan to go out to the first meeting of the Physicians for Human Rights in San Francisco [in June]. . . . I went out, gave my talk, then sat down to listen to some of the other talks. A doctor came over to me and said, "I have a date tonight with a Canadian who has Kaposi's sarcoma. Do you think it's okay for me to go to bed with him?" I just stared at him, then said, "Is it a man named Erik?" "Yes," he said, "do you know him? Isn't he a beauty!" I almost fell off my seat. I said, "Could you do me a favor? Give him my hotel number and tell him to call me. Or, if he can't do that, to contact me in New York in my office." I went back to the hotel and called Linda and said, "Linda, I've located our Typhoid Mary."[1]

1. Ann Giudici Fettner and William A. Check, *The Truth about AIDS*, rev. ed. (New York: Henry Holt, 1985), 85. Crimp cites this recollection in "How to Have Promiscuity in an Epidemic," in Crimp, *AIDS*, 245. The Bay Area Physicians for Human Rights conference, which coincided with the San Francisco Gay Freedom Day Parade, drew gay physicians from across North America. See also Silversides, *AIDS Activist*, 16–17.

For Friedman-Kien, the label of "Typhoid Mary"—the name bestowed upon an ill-fortuned Irish American cook whose story will be retold later in this chapter—summed up his view that this individual was spreading disease to his sexual partners. Laubenstein would echo her professional partner's tone when she spoke with a San Francisco journalist in 1986. In the reporter's notes for the interview, roughly scribbled as he tried to keep up with Laubenstein's words, this man was described as a "vector of disease." The importance that he would come to signify to epidemiologists was also suggested by Laubenstein's remark that his "'little bl[ac]k book' wasn't little." When the journalist in question, Randy Shilts, published *And the Band Played On* in 1987, he identified "Erik" as Gaétan Dugas, a French Canadian flight attendant whom investigators at the US Centers for Disease Control (CDC) had previously labeled as "Patient 0."[2]

A collection of oral history interviews published in 2000 featured the reminiscences of physicians who had played significant roles in the American epidemic over the previous twenty years. By this time, Laubenstein had died, but once again Friedman-Kien gave an interview, and again he spoke of Dugas, the only patient to be identified by his full name in that book. Time had not dulled the physician's recollection, nor his earlier view that Dugas was sowing disease. Once again, he invoked one of the more negative images associated with "Typhoid Mary": "While he was in New York, he would go to gay bathhouses and have unprotected sex with a variety of people despite the fact that we warned him against it. I once caught him coming out of a gay bathhouse, and I stopped the car and said, 'What are you doing there?' And he said, 'In the dark nobody sees my spots.' He was a real sociopath. At which point I told a colleague the story. She was enchanted with him, as most people were. I stopped seeing him, I was just so angry."[3] This pair of recollections from Friedman-Kien indicate the breadth of feelings aroused by his interactions with this individual between 1981 and 1982. On the one

2. "Dr. Linda," interview notes, 1986, p. 2, folder 10, box 34, Shilts Papers. Shilts's underlined photocopy of the chapter discussing "Erik" in Fettner and Check's book can be found in folder 23, box 34, Shilts Papers.

3. Bayer and Oppenheimer, *AIDS Doctors*, 61. Leavitt describes a pervasive mid-twentieth-century characterization of "Typhoid Mary" as "a person to be feared and shunned, someone who carries contagion inside her body and uses it to harm people around her." She also draws an explicit comparison between the experiences of Mallon and Dugas; Leavitt, *Typhoid Mary*, 203, 234–38.

hand, he describes his excitement of tracking down an elusive patient who might offer insight into a mysterious condition. On the other, he reports feeling such anger and disgust with the patient's behavior that he ultimately withdrew his services. Friedman-Kien's telling use of the term "Typhoid Mary" indicates the way in which historical narratives about epidemics and the characters featured in them subtly shaped the mindsets of those responding to AIDS. It also demonstrates the importance of being aware of these older histories to comprehend the full communicative force summoned by the story of Gaétan Dugas as "Patient Zero."

A long history of prejudice, fear, and blame directed toward suspected disease carriers preceded AIDS, and the cultural weight of these past occasions contributed palpably to responses to this epidemic on its emergence in the late twentieth century.[4] This chapter provides an overview of this general history and of the key ideas and precedents that animated the story of the flight attendant and the labels "Patient O," "Patient 0," and "Patient Zero" as their use spread from the 1980s onward. This *longue durée* approach treads lightly over several hundred years of events and ideas in Western Europe and North America from the late medieval period to the twentieth century.[5] Historians tend to be wary of drawing examples from different periods to illustrate an argument, since doing so risks severing the incidents from the original interpretive frameworks that imbued them with meaning. However, as the following pages suggest, other observers have been less concerned about original context when reappropriating and recirculating older ideas, thus it seems justifiable to cast a wide net in this instance.

Five themes emerge in this overview which inform the chapters that

4. As Michael Willrich explains in his account of late nineteenth- and early twentieth-century responses to smallpox in the United States, "The age of AIDS did not invent the notion of 'Patient Zero.'" See Willrich, *Pox: An American History* (New York: Penguin, 2011), 18.

5. This geographic focus is not to suggest that cultural narratives from other parts of the world did not shape how North Americans made sense of the AIDS epidemic during this period. Rather, on occasions when history seemed relevant to contemporary observers and policy makers, they seem generally to have paid more attention to American and European precedents. See, for example, the testimony and materials submitted for the "Epidemics of the Past, Implications for the Future" panel before the Presidential Commission on the Human Immunodeficiency Virus Epidemic, April 5, 1988, National Commission on Acquired Immune Deficiency Syndrome Records 1983–1994, MS C 544, History of Medicine Division, Archives and Modern Manuscripts Collection, National Library of Medicine, Bethesda, MD (hereafter cited as NCAIDS Records).

follow: plague as divine punishment and the linked rise of scapegoating; fascination with the origins and spread of disease; recurrent fears about deliberate disease spreading; dangerous beauty coupled with defilement and sexual activity; and the challenges posed by healthy disease carriers. In some cases, the incidents to follow—such as the stories of well poisoning and of "Typhoid Mary" Mallon—were well known to participants responding to AIDS in the 1980s and 1990s. Others, such as the tale of the most beautiful fifteenth-century Italian prostitute said to have generated the "French Disease," were less widely circulated and have only more recently been examined by historians. Nonetheless, they are all included to demonstrate the long history underpinning the impulses to trace contagion, harbor suspicion, and lay blame in times of epidemic. An epigraph from Randy Shilts's popular book introduces each theme, demonstrating how *And the Band Played On* both was embedded in and contributed to this intertexual history of epidemics.

Plague as Divine Punishment and the Rise of Scapegoating

"Maybe Falwell is right," said Gaetan. "Maybe we are being punished."[6]

When Moral Majority leader Jerry Falwell expounded his view in July 1983 that diseases such as AIDS were a "definite form of the judgment of God upon a society," he was certainly not pronouncing a new view. Nor was it unprecedented for him to suggest that it was "perverted" homosexual behavior that had incited this "spanking" from God. Falwell's viewpoint, that AIDS was a "gay plague," echoed the published opinions of Republican speechwriter and senior advisor Patrick Buchanan and other social conservatives in the spring and summer of 1983. The explanation was consistent with many centuries of blaming socially disadvantaged groups for the appearance of epidemic disease.[7] During these centuries, first in Europe and later in North America, those whose

6. Shilts, *Band*, 348.

7. Sue Cross, "Jerry Falwell Calls AIDS a 'Gay Plague,'" *Washington Post*, July 6, 1983, B3. A survey undertaken in August 1985 indicated that 11 percent of Americans agreed with the statement that AIDS was God's punishment against homosexuals for their way of life; see Victor Cohn, "Poll Shows Widespread Awareness, Misguided Fears About Disease," *Washington Post*, September 4, 1985, H7; Steven Seidman, "Transfiguring Sexual Identity: AIDS and the Contemporary Construction of Homosexuality," *Social Text* 19–20

religious, social, and sexual behavior did not meet the prescribed standards of their communities were repeatedly accused of incurring divine wrath. For many people who made such judgments, notions of contagion revealed a clear and unbreakable link between an individual's moral choices and wider communal responsibility.[8]

In Western Europe from the eleventh century onward, a trend developed in which various minority groups—"lepers," Jews, heretics, and sodomites—were repeatedly cast as enemies of the state, to the point that such scapegoating became a permanent cultural fixture of that part of the world. Collectively, societies would come to the consensus that a particular named group was to blame for certain social ills. The members of this group were then systematically excluded from society and faced the loss of their civil rights and, too frequently, the risk of being put to death.[9] These categorized groups might be blamed for specific acts or occurences, or for generic, transferable threats and conspiracies. Though in some cases a rumor or conspiracy might initially be linked to a specific historical event, these explanations often evolved over time, serving as adaptable answers for later generations to make sense of new situations of collective hardship.

In 1321, communities in France and several other Christian countries blamed and in many cases executed individuals marked by leprosy for an elaborate plot—involving shadowy foreign powers, secret meetings, and deadly powders—to poison local water sources.[10] A generation later, this conspiracy was recycled with Jews as the chief villains when Europe was overcome by the Black Death, reportedly following the arrival in Sicily of twelve plague-infected Genoese ships from Constantinople in 1347.[11] At that time, it was widely understood that there could be a separation

---

(Autumn 1988): 187–205. The writing of Buchanan, an established political figure and future presidential candidate, carried a large influence.

8. Margaret Pelling, "The Meaning of Contagion: Reproduction, Medicine and Metaphor," in *Contagion: Historical and Cultural Studies*, ed. Alison Bashford and Claire Hooker (London: Routledge, 2001), 17.

9. R. I. Moore, *The Formation of a Persecuting Society: Authority and Deviance in Western Europe, 950–1250*, 2nd ed. (Oxford: Blackwell, 2007), 93.

10. Carlo L. Ginzburg, *Ecstasies: Deciphering the Witches' Sabbath*, trans. Raymond Rosenthal (New York: Pantheon Books, 1991), 33–35.

11. Ibid., 63. Historians themselves frequently attempt to trace the source of epidemics in the past. As William Coleman writes, the arrival of a ship is a datable event; see W. Coleman, *Yellow Fever in the North: The Methods of Early Epidemiology* (Madison: University of Wisconsin Press, 1987), 109.

between the underlying cause of plague—for example, the position of the stars or contaminated air and waters—and the more immediate reason for its spread, such as interpersonal contact. Given the vigorously anti-Jewish attitudes of the time and the devastation of the plague, it is, lamentably, not difficult to imagine how the two theories could have combined into the popular view that the Jews were contaminating well water with poison to spread the pestilence.[12]

Such water-based plague anxieties date to ancient times. In his account of the fifth century BCE Peloponnesian war, the Greek historian Thucydides discussed the sudden appearance of a deadly outbreak during the conflict's second year. Though he left speculation about the plague's origins and causes to other writers, he recorded a story told by residents of the Piraeus, the port district on the outskirts of Athens that was first struck by the pestilence shortly after the Peloponnesians invaded. The residents maintained that their enemies had poisoned the water reservoirs. For an arid region where drinking water was precious and often associated with divine beneficence, the accusation of poisoning a communally shared source of life conveys the compounded horror, fear, and disgust aroused by the double devastation of invasion and plague. The fact that the disease had not seemed to affect the Peloponnesian peninsula to a degree worth recording would only have added to their opponents' presumed culpability.[13] Thucydides's work was not widely available in Europe when these stories of well poisoning later recirculated. However, other ancient writers including Seneca, whose moral essays did influence medieval thinkers, particularly from the mid-thirteenth century onward, also wrote "of springs defiled by poison, of plague the hand of man has made . . . and secret plots for regal power and for subversion of the state."[14]

During the late medieval and early modern period, differences of

12. Ginzburg, *Ecstasies*, 64. For more about the classification of causes into primary, proximate, and predisposing categories, see Pelling, "Meaning of Contagion," 17–19; Vivian Nutton, "The Seeds of Disease: An Explanation of Contagion and Infection from the Greeks to the Renaissance," *Medical History* 27, no. 1 (1983): 4–5; and Epstein, *Impure Science*, 53.

13. Robert B. Strassler, ed. *The Landmark Thucydides: A Comprehensive Guide to the Peloponnesian War* (New York: Touchstone, 1996), 118–21; Ellen Churchill Semple, "Domestic and Municipal Waterworks in Ancient Mediterranean Lands," *Geographic Review* 21, no. 3 (1931): 466–74.

14. Seneca, *De Ira* [*On Anger*] 2.9.3, in *Seneca: Moral Essays*, vol. 1, trans. John W.

background and class also shaped perceptions, with travelers and the poor frequently featuring in accounts of plague spreading. In some northern areas of early modern Italy, for example, these marginalized groups replaced the Jews or witches who normally featured in such stories. Wealthier members of society worried that graveyard workers, a group which tended to draw vagrants and criminals in times of pestilence, might attempt to prolong epidemics. Some feared they had ready access to deadly matter drawn from bodies and clothing, which they could surreptitiously scatter throughout unsuspecting neighborhoods.[15] Similarly, impoverished linen washers in early sixteenth-century Geneva were accused of deliberately spreading plague-infected ointment in the houses they cleaned in order to kill the inhabitants and then steal their possessions.[16] Travelers also implicated local prostitutes in social condemnation. Even before brothels became associated in the late fifteenth century with the spread of the great pox, or the "French Disease"—a sexually transmitted affliction now commonly thought to be syphilis—they faced punitive sanctions in times of plague. It remains unclear whether these sexual sites drew condemnation more for their indiscriminate welcoming of strangers or for encouraging divine displeasure to fall on a society that permitted fornication.[17]

At times, early modern Europeans grouped sodomites with prostitutes as moral offenders to be marked as different and expelled from the community along with other types of corrupt matter in times of disease.[18] Indeed, historical evidence suggests that in northern Italy both

Basore (London: William Heinemann, 1928), 183–85; L. D. Reynolds, "The Medieval Tradition of Seneca's *Dialogues*," *Classical Quarterly* 18, no. 2 (1968): 355–72.

15. Brian Pullan, "Plague and Perceptions of the Poor in Early Modern Italy," in *Epidemics and Ideas: Essays on the Historical Perception of Pestilence*, ed. Terrence Ranger and Paul Slack (Cambridge: Cambridge University Press, 1992), 118.

16. William G. Naphy, "Plague-Spreading and a Magisterially Controlled Fear," in *Studies in Early Modern European History*, ed. William G. Naphy and Penny Roberts (Manchester, UK: Manchester University Press, 1997), 28–29. See also Naphy, *Plagues, Poisons, and Potions: Plague-Spreading Conspiracies in the Western Alps, c. 1530–1640* (Manchester, UK: Manchester University Press, 2002).

17. Pullan, "Plague and Perceptions," 113. On the importance of strangers to origin stories for infectious diseases, see Anne Kveim Lie, "Origin Stories and the Norwegian Radesyge," *Social History of Medicine* 20, no. 3 (2007): 571–73; and Wald, *Contagious*, 22–23.

18. Ann G. Carmichael, *Plague and the Poor in Renaissance Florence* (Cambridge:

prostitutes and sodomites joined Jews in being required to wear yellow to warn other citizens of their suspect moral and public health status.[19] The capaciousness of the word *sodomy* also reflects the conjugation of sodomites and prostitutes in the popular imagination: in some parts of early modern Europe, the term defined a variety of sexual activities between men, while in others it included all non-procreative sexual acts between men, women, and, more rarely, animals.[20] Sodomy itself was viewed as contagious by such medieval authorities as Albertus Magnus; spread from person to person, it was very difficult to treat and particularly afflicted the rich.[21] Northern Italian religious authorities—in Venice, Lucca, and Florence, among other locations—viewed the visitation of the Black Death in the fourteenth century as a consequence of unpunished sodomy.[22] They were thus prepared to blame the arrival of a new disease at the end of the fifteenth century in a similar way. The great pox, erupting in that region during the lead-up to the Battle of Fornovo in 1495, would famously be blamed on many diverse groups—chiefly the French, but also Italians from Naples and Spanish Jews, with fingers pointed as far away as the Indies and Ethiopia.[23] As the disease spread over the next century, some, such as the Lucchese, linked it specifically to sodomitical practices.[24] Such linkages were solidified by a pa-

---

Cambridge University Press, 1986), 99; Jon Arrizabalaga, John Henderson, and Roger French, *The Great Pox: The French Disease in Renaissance Europe* (London: Yale University Press, 1997), 35–36.

19. Carmichael, *Plague and Poor*, 124.

20. N. S. Davidson, "Sodomy in Early Modern Venice," in *Sodomy in Early Modern Europe*, ed. Thomas Betteridge (Manchester, UK: Manchester University Press, 2002), 66. See also Jens Rydström, *Sinners and Citizens: Bestiality and Homosexuality in Sweden, 1880–1950* (London: University of Chicago Press, 2003), 1–25.

21. John Boswell, *Christianity, Social Tolerance, and Homosexuality: Gay People in Western Europe from the Beginning of the Christian Era to the Fourteenth Century* (London: University of Chicago Press, 1980), 53, 316.

22. See Guido Ruggiero, *The Boundaries of Eros: Sex Crime and Sexuality in Renaissance Venice* (Oxford: Oxford University Press, 1985), 113–14; Mary Hewlett, "The French Connection: Syphilis and Sodomy in Late-Renaissance Lucca," in *Sins of the Flesh: Responding to Sexual Disease in Early Modern Europe*, ed. Kevin Patrick Siena (Toronto: Centre for Reformation and Renaissance Studies, 2005), 240; Michael Rocke, *Forbidden Friendships: Homosexuality and Male Culture in Renaissance Florence* (New York: Oxford University Press, 1996), 28, 36–44.

23. Arrizabalaga, Henderson, and French, *Great Pox*, 24.

24. Hewlett, "French Connection," 244.

pal bull issued in 1566 that singled out sodomy as a chief cause of God's wrath.[25]

Christian responses to plague in late medieval and early modern England demonstrated similar attempts to understand the reasons for God's displeasure. While some Christians stressed the role of providence, others sought to intuit the offensive provocations and then act decisively, aiming to root out the sinners or social disorders to eliminate the risk of pestilence and other divine scourges.[26] Thus, during the infamous 1631 trial of the Earl of Castlehaven, who was found guilty of sodomitical practices and executed, the prosecuting attorney referred to the biblical plagues that were brought by "so abominable a Sin."[27] Several decades later the preacher David Jones warned London parishioners of the "abominable and execrable Sin" of male sodomy, which, he noted, "is now grown so common, *that several Persons have been lately executed for it.*" Reminding those listening of the devastation wrought by the city's great fire several decades before, he emphasized that "if you are guilty *but of this one Sin alone*, you do enough to provoke God to destroy this whole City, as he destroyed *Sodom* and *Gomorrah*, with *Fire from Heaven.*"[28]

25. Davidson, "Sodomy," 67.

26. Paul Slack, *The Impact of Plague in Tudor and Stuart England* (London: Routledge and Kegan Paul, 1985), 49.

27. "The Trial of Mervin Lord Audley, Earl of Castlehaven, for a Rape and Sodomy, on the 25th of April 1631," in *A Complete Collection of State-Trials, and Proceedings for High-Treason, and Other Crimes and Misdemeanours*, 4th ed., vol. 1 (London, 1776), 391, facsimile, Eighteenth Century Collections Online digital library, http://find.galegroup .com/ecco/infomark.do?&source=gale&prodId=ECCO&userGroupName=cambuni& tabID=T001&docId=CW3325058195&type=multipage&contentSet=ECCOArticles &version=1.0&docLevel=FASCIMILE. See also Cynthia B. Herrup, *A House in Great Disorder: Sex, Law, and the 2nd Earl of Castlehaven* (Oxford: Oxford University Press, 1999). Herrup also describes English views of sodomy being an unwanted import brought by European immigrants; *House*, 33–34.

28. D. Jones, *A Sermon Upon the Dreadful Fire of London, Preach'd in the Parish-church of St. Dunstan in the West in London, on Thursday, September 2. 1703* (London, 1703), 26, emphasis in original, facsimile, Eighteenth Century Collections Online digital library, http://find.galegroup.com/ecco/infomark.do?&source=gale&prodId=ECCO &userGroupName=cambuni&tabID=T001&docId=CW3321184722&type=multipage& contentSet=ECCOArticles&version=1.0&docLevel=FASCIMILE. Despite Jones's fiery language, it appears that seventeenth-century English courts took a negligible interest in prosecuting sodomy cases, let alone sentencing guilty parties to death; David F. Greenberg, *The Construction of Homosexuality* (Chicago: University of Chicago Press, 1988), 326.

Former British colonies including the United States and Canada traced much of their legislation to English statutes, and religious members of these societies would similarly link infectious disease with God's judgment on the practice of sodomy.[29] Gradually, over the course of the nineteenth century, same-sex offenses began to be seen more as acts of medical deviancy than crimes against God, a view which, in its turn, was challenged over the course of the twentieth century.[30] Nonetheless, there was a rich and well-established tradition upon which religious leaders like Jerry Falwell could draw when AIDS made its appearance in the 1980s and was heralded as the "gay plague."

Geographies and Genealogies of Blame: Tracing the Origins and Spread of Disease

The first cases in both New York City and Los Angeles could be linked to Gaetan, who himself was one of the first half-dozen or so patients on the continent . . . [31]

Attempts to understand plague and the great pox offer useful examples of a widespread fascination with disease origins, providing parallels to the reception of AIDS. For some observers, determining a disease's origin and how it spread through society was a matter of intellectual curiosity; for others it was motivated by a need to maintain order; for others still it was rooted in a desire to be found blameless of the misfortune.[32] Given the desperate amount of death and suffering caused by both diseases, many people who lived through times of pestilence attempted to locate specific secular causes for them and to identify and punish perpetrators.

During outbreaks of plague from the late Middle Ages onward, many

29. James R. Spence, "The Law of Crime against Nature," *North Carolina Law Review* 32, no. 3 (1954): 312–24.

30. D'Emilio and Freedman, *Intimate Matters*, 122.

31. Shilts, *Band*, 439. Shilts based his misleading claim about Dugas's relative priority among North American patients with AIDS on a mistaken reading of the Los Angeles cluster study and a New York health official's discussion of known cases within the gay community. See Bob Sipchen, "The AIDS Chronicles: Randy Shilts Writes the Biography of an Epidemic and Finds More Bunglers Than Heroes," *Los Angeles Times*, October 9, 1987, V9.

32. Sander L. Gilman, "AIDS and Syphilis: The Iconography of Disease," in Crimp, *AIDS*, 100.

attempts to act decisively focused on preventing travelers from plague-afflicted regions to visit others. The quarantine provisions emerging at this time for ships in Mediterranean ports are well known.[33] Perhaps less so was the the occasional willingness of contemporary chroniclers to single out and name individuals for their perceived transgressions. Lucia Cadorino, for example, and her lover Matteo Farcinatore, were alleged to have brought plague to Venice from the Trento region in 1575. A Milanese soldier, Pietro Antonio Lovato, traded garments with the German army and stood accused of bringing plague to his home city in 1629.[34] There is the suggestion of moral condemnation in these examples too: the perhaps illicit relationship between the two lovers from Trento or the possibly reckless trading of the Milanese soldier. These efforts to lay blame add a layer of complexity to one historian's observation that plague, with its complex ecology, can have "no human carriers . . . like a 'Typhoid Mary,' continually shedding the bacterium."[35] While technically true, this now-known fact did not stop people in the past from trying to attribute the plague's spread to human actors.

In addition to the widely held view that miasmatic airs were the main source of epidemics, ideas of contagion and infection have existed through the ages from Galen to Fracastoro, expressed through various explanatory models over time.[36] At the turn of the sixteenth century, the growing belief that the great pox might be spread through sexual contact coincided with and contributed to a gradual shift in conceptualizing disease causation. The emerging model viewed disease as owing less to communal transgressions and more to those of individuals.[37] Certainly, the propensity to identify single persons for the arrival of disease to a community existed before individual behavior became the general focus of condemnation. However, this tendency became more pronounced as the shift toward individual culpability gathered momentum, a develop-

---

33. George Rosen, *A History of Public Health*, expanded ed. (Baltimore: Johns Hopkins University Press, 1993), 43–45.

34. Pullan, "Plague and Perceptions," 112.

35. Carmichael, *Plague and Poor*, 5.

36. Nutton, "Seeds of Disease."

37. Jon Arrizabalaga, "Medical Responses to the 'French Disease' in Europe at the Turn of the Sixteenth Century," in Siena, *Sins of the Flesh*, 52; Laura McGough, *Gender, Sexuality, and Syphilis in Early Modern Venice: The Disease that Came to Stay* (Basingstoke, UK: Palgrave Macmillan, 2011), 67.

ment which the rise of bacteriological science would further consolidate in the late nineteenth century.

Immediately upon the appearance of the great pox at the end of the fifteenth century and in the centuries following its rapid spread across Europe, medical experts posited their explanations for the origins of this seemingly new disease. In 1736 Jean Astruc, the French royal physician, published *De morbis venereis*, his own scholarly contribution to the discussion, which went through several subsequent editions and translations during his lifetime. In his treatise, Astruc provided a catalog of the proposed causes ventured by generations of his predecessors. The physician recited and then refuted each claim before expounding the explanation he thought most reliable: "that the Venereal Disease was brought from Hispaniola into Spain before the Year 1495, by the Spanish Soldie[r]s who served under Gonsalvo Fernandez in Italy, and communicated to the French and Neapolitans by promiscuous Venery."[38] In his cataloging efforts, the physician listed several writers who emphasized the distant influence of the stars, or the miasmatic "Indisposition of the Air," before outlining diverse "particular causes."[39] These causes included a theory dating from 1525 of "an Harlot of Valencia who had lain with a Leper," which appeared in several variations, including one discussed in this chapter's next section.[40] Others held that Spanish soldiers poisoned the wells and bribed Italian bakers within the enemy's army to mix lime with their bread.[41] Astruc dismissed the suggestion of Francis Bacon that "certain dishonest Merchants, who sold human Flesh, new killed in Mauritania, pickled and put up in Vessels, instead of Tunney; and that to this abominable and heavy Food, the Origin of the Venereal Disease ought to be ascribed."[42] He also scorned two origin theories that may ap-

---

38. John Astruc, *A Treatise of Venereal Diseases, in Nine Books; Containing an Account of the Origin, Propagation, and Contagion of This Distemper*, vol. 1 (London, 1754), 67–84, quotation at 84, facsimile, Eighteenth Century Collections Online digital library, http://find.galegroup.com/ecco/infomark.do?&source=gale&prodId=ECCO&userGroupName=cambuni&tabID=T001&docId=CW108536016&type=multipage&contentSet=ECCOArticles&version=1.0&docLevel=FASCIMILE. Cynics might note that this conclusion would remove the blame for the "French pox" from Astruc's own country.

39. Ibid., 69–70.

40. Ibid., 70.

41. Ibid., 71.

42. Ibid., 74.

pear familiar to modern-day AIDS researchers. One was put forward in 1640 by the "credulous" Flemish physician Jan Baptist van Helmont, in which he proposed that the great pox had arisen as a variant of a disease that primarily affected horses. In this manner, at the siege of Naples, "some wicked Person had defiled himself with a Horse of that kind, and thus (by divine Permission) transplanted it into the human Race." Astruc was equally dismissive of the theory of the Swedish physician Johan Linder, who had asserted in an early eighteenth-century dissertation that "the Venereal Disease had its Origin in the Americas 'from Sodomy sometime committed between Men and "large Monkies or the Satyrs of the Antients [sic]."'" Of this theory, Astruc wrote that "nothing can possibly be more foolish or absurd, so nothing can be invented more affected or far fetched."[43]

More recently, questions about the origins of HIV have summoned concerns about bodily transgression and contamination that strongly resemble their seventeenth- and eighteenth-century forebears. Popular tendencies toward creating explanatory legends combined epidemiologic ideas of disease transmission with stories of primordial landscapes, exotic cultural practices, and political conflict to make sense of the disease's origins.[44] Three main scientific theories of origin were repeatedly posited for HIV: a disease previously existing in another animal species that had recently managed to transfer to humans; a mutation or wider transmission of a much older and previously unrecognized human disease; and a disease caused by a synthetic virus that was created either deliberately or accidentally in a laboratory. The overlap between and intermingling of the three basic theories served as a foundation for various popular explanations for the origins of HIV.[45]

Given the widespread consensus among researchers that now locates

43. Ibid., 74.

44. Diane E. Goldstein, *Once Upon a Virus: AIDS Legends and Vernacular Risk Perception* (Logan: Utah State University Press, 2004), 79; Wald, *Contagious*, 1–28. For more on the persistence of origin myths for venereal disease, see Marie E. McAllister, "Stories of the Origin of Syphilis in Eighteenth-Century England: Science, Myth, and Prejudice," *Eighteenth-Century Life* 24, no. 1 (2000): 22–44.

45. D. Goldstein, *Once Upon a Virus*, 80–81. A crude remixing of these theories appears in a short cartoon segment wherein a male flight attendant has sex with a chimpanzee and potentially infects the latter with a deadly virus; "AIDS Patient Zero," *Seth McFarlane's Cavalcade of Cartoon Comedy*, directed by Greg Colton (Beverly Hills, CA: Twentieth Century Fox, 2009), DVD.

the origins of HIV in Africa, it is important to remember that in the early 1980s, with the bulk of AIDS cases reported in the United States, the general assumption of non-Americans was that the United States was the source of the disease.[46] In June 1983, for instance, a journal in France referred to AIDS as "the curse which came from America." Similarly, it was common in the United Kingdom to attribute the arrival of the disease on gay men who had returned from "sex holidays" in the States.[47] Some Soviet observers, too, proposed the United States as the source, circulating a false story that the disease was the result of biological warfare experiments gone wrong at Fort Detrick, a US Army installation in Maryland.[48] This international response was in marked contrast to the assumptions of many American researchers who believed that a previously unnoticed disease in the United States, a country with comparatively strong disease surveillance abilities, was likely to have been introduced from abroad. Some observers, particularly members of other suspected origin countries, interpreted this view as an act of unjustified racial scapegoating, not to mention an unwillingness on the part of Americans to deal with what appeared to be domestic problems.

Much like the reaction of African physicians to Western suggestions that they had not recognized a disease in their midst for generations, Haitians and their supporters would assert that AIDS was in fact an epidemic brought by Americans to their country.[49] They could point to an American history which combined fears of infectious disease with a wariness and mistrust of foreigners, particularly immigrants.[50] Often underscored by racist attitudes, popular views of immigrants found ex-

46. See, for example, David M. Morens, Gregory K. Folkers, and Anthony S. Fauci, "The Challenge of Emerging and Re-Emerging Infectious Diseases," *Nature* 430 (July 8, 2004): 242–49. For a concise review of the literature discussing African origins, see John Iliffe, *The African AIDS Epidemic: A History* (Oxford: James Currey, 2006), 58–64.

47. Altman, *AIDS in the Mind of America*, 15–16.

48. Gilman, "AIDS and Syphilis," 101; Nattrass, *AIDS Conspiracy*, 27–28.

49. Treichler, *Theory in an Epidemic*, 205–34; Piot, *No Time to Lose*, 146–47; Sabatier, *Blaming Others*, 46–47, 59–61.

50. Sander L. Gilman and Dorothy Nelkin, "Placing Blame for Devastating Disease," *Social Research* 55, no. 3 (1988): 361–78; Alan M. Kraut, *Silent Travelers: Germs, Genes, and The "Immigrant Menace"* (New York: Johns Hopkins University Press, 1995); Howard Markel and Alexandra Minna Stern, "The Foreignness of Germs: The Persistent Association of Immigrants and Disease in American Society," *Milbank Quarterly* 80, no. 4 (2002): 757–88; Howard Markel, *Quarantine! East European Jewish Immigrants and the New York City Epidemics of 1892* (London: Johns Hopkins University Press, 1997).

pression in medical terms. The existence—or suspicion—of certain communicable diseases within an ethnocultural group led at times to the widespread view that all of the group's members were likely carriers of the disease.[51] Several authors, most notably Paul Farmer, argued that the "risk-grouping" of the Haitian immigrant community in 1982 and 1983 with regard to the threat of AIDS infection represented a reworking of this familiar response to epidemic disease. Such risk groups were soon used to posit potential origins for AIDS and resulted in what Farmer memorably labeled a "geography of blame."[52]

Beyond the geographic finger-pointing that memorably accompanied the emergence of both the great pox and AIDS, it is worth drawing attention to the ways in which tracing the person-to-person spread of both diseases within a country, region, or community enabled observers to construct a web of transmission or, to modify Farmer's phrase, a genealogy of blame. The next chapter will show how AIDS investigators, in their initial attempts to locate cases and establish the transmissibility of an infectious agent, made use of contact tracing techniques originally developed to deal with syphilis. This modern public health history is underpinned by a long-standing popular fascination with tracing the spread of venereal infections through society. A well-known example of this "strange genealogy" can be found in Voltaire's satire *Candide* (1759), published during a century in which venereal disease became more widely discussed in France.[53] When, after some misadventures, the story's naive and eponymous hero is reunited with his former tutor Pangloss, he scarcely recognizes him: the man has been reduced to a syphilitic wreck, "all covered with sores, his eyes dull as death, [and] the end of his nose eaten away." To Candide's worried question about the cause of his malady, Pangloss replies that a dalliance with a pretty chambermaid had produced his "torments of hell." This maid, he continues, "received this present from a very learned Franciscan, who had gone back to the source; for he had got it from an old countess, who had received it from a cavalry captain, who owed it to a marquise, who had it from a page, who had received it from a Jesuit, who as a novice had got it in a direct line

---

51. Kraut, *Silent Travelers*, 3.

52. Farmer, *AIDS and Accusation*, 2; Sabatier, *Blaming Others*, 42–47.

53. Susan P. Conner, "The Pox in Eighteenth-Century France," in *The Secret Malady: Venereal Disease in Eighteenth-Century Britain and France*, ed. Linda E. Merians (Lexington: University Press of Kentucky, 1996), 15–33.

from one of the companions of Christopher Columbus. For my part I shall give it to no one, for I am dying."[54] In this passage, Voltaire demonstrated his familiarity with authors like Astruc and the most up-to-date medical explanations for the great pox's "source." In addition, his ironic delineation of the spread of a disease—through opposite- and same-sex unions, across time and social class—accentuated the sexual and social taboos that venereal disease could render so painfully visible. By having Pangloss characterize the disease as a "present" being given, received, and—in the last sentence—withheld, Voltaire also hinted strongly that in some cases there was an element of volition involved in its transmission. In its most extreme form, this view would give expression to fears that some members of society might maliciously spread their sickness.

Deliberate Disease Spreading

It was around this time that rumors began on Castro Street about a strange guy at the Eighth and Howard bathhouse, a blond with a French accent. He would have sex with you, turn up the lights in the cubicle, and point out his Kaposi's sarcoma lesions. "I've got gay cancer," he'd say. "I'm going to die and so are you."[55]

Accusations of groups and individuals deliberately spreading contagion have gone hand in hand with epidemics of deadly and painful diseases like plague and the poxes, great and small. The widespread social disruptions caused by these outbreaks and a generalized fear of falling ill gave rise not only to allegations of people behaving carelessly, but also spreading disease maliciously. These allegations traveled widely in rumors, printed books, and plays, though in many circumstances they appear to have been culturally expressed fears rather than evidence of actual misconduct.

From the aforementioned linen washers in Geneva to others in Milan and England, accusations of individuals spreading plague-causing poisonous ointments have been documented across western Europe from the fourteenth to the seventeenth centuries. Brutal ends often befell those accused of such actions, as evidenced by one widely recirculated

54. Voltaire, *Candide, Zadig, and Selected Stories*, trans. Donald M. Frame (New York: New American Library, 1963), 21–23. See also McGough, *Gender, Sexuality, and Syphilis*, 17.

55. Shilts, *Band*, 165.

tale. Sebastian Münster's *Cosmographia*, first published in 1544, was an astronomical, historical, and geographic account of much of the known world. In a section that described the Alsatian town of Strasbourg, Münster recounted the violent punishment that befell the Jews during the devastation brought by the Black Death. Blamed for contaminating a water source and bringing plague to the town, hundreds of Jewish residents were burned to death in 1349. Much in demand, Münster's book went through more than thirty editions in five languages over the next eight decades.[56] While the story of this massacre remained relatively constant during this time, the accompanying woodcut illustrations, beginning with a simple depiction of a town well in 1544, underwent several metamorphoses, becoming increasingly dramatic and personified in later editions. By 1550, the German edition's recounting of the story featured a woodcut of a hooded individual standing at a well with both hands gripping the bucket's rope—an illustration which in many editions accompanied a description of a remarkable foot-operated well in the town of Breisach. The 1552 Latin text was complemented by a small and generic image of an elderly bearded Jewish man wearing robes and a prayer shawl half-covering his cap. In later German editions—including the final one published in Basel in 1628, as a massive epidemic of plague slowly and relentlessly advanced across Europe and eventually ensnared towns across Switzerland—the printers chose to accompany the anecdote with a depiction of two men being burned at the stake. In doing so, they reused woodcuts that had depicted the execution of the Bohemian dissidents Jan Hus and Jerome of Prague in earlier editions (see figure 1.1).[57] As well as exemplifying the pragmatic, budget-conscious approach to illustration adopted by many early modern printers, these examples of image repurposing demonstrate how different generations found new ways to interpret the same centuries-old story, making it relevant—perhaps even sounding a warning—for new audiences.[58] This reuse also foreshadows how images of Gaétan Dugas as "Patient Zero"—invoked as

56. Matthew McLean, *The Cosmographia of Sebastian Münster: Describing the World in the Reformation* (Aldershot, UK: Ashgate, 2007), 1.

57. For more on the 1628–1629 Swiss plague epidemic, see Edward A. Eckert, "Spatial and Temporal Distribution of Plague in a Region of Switzerland in the Years 1628 and 1629," *Bulletin of the History of Medicine* 56, no. 2 (1982): 175–94.

58. Sachiko Kusukawa, "Illustrating Nature," in *Books and the Sciences in History*, ed. Marina Frasca-Spada and Nicholas Jardine (Cambridge: Cambridge University Press, 2000), 97–100.

a "plague spreader" for the modern era—would be borrowed, adapted, and recycled in the late twentieth century.[59]

In 1898, a librarian at the Surgeon General's Office in Washington, DC, wrote a short treatise on an episode from the same early seventeenth-century plague epidemic. He described a column erected in 1630 to warn of the misdeeds and gruesome executions of two men found guilty of spreading plague in Milan during the previous year. While under torture, these men had admitted to spreading ointments—allegedly containing foam from the mouths of dead plague victims—to communicate the disease to unsuspecting passersby. The two, he wrote, had their flesh torn with hot pokers, their right hands cut off, their bones broken, and their bodies extended on a wheel for six hours before being put to death and burned. The librarian was writing at the height of the bacteriological age, a period which generated a newfound confidence in the power of science to trace diseases to specific causative germs. To him, the "column of infamy" in Milan served as a testament to the "ignorance and credulity" of the unfortunate men's inquisitors and the misplaced blame of an earlier time of fear and superstition.[60]

Fears aroused by plague and the newly recognized great pox commingled in the early sixteenth century, with both afflictions raising concerns that some of those afflicted had devilish motives. During one of the periodic outbreaks of plague affecting the German town of Wittenberg in 1527, the German theologian Martin Luther wrote a much reprinted open letter discussing whether Christians could, in good conscience, flee the pestilence. In it, he described reports of behavior by some individuals that was worse than careless:

> When they contract the pestilential disease they keep it secret, go out among other people, and think that if they can infect and defile others with the sickness they will themselves get rid of it and become well. With this notion they frequent streets and houses in the hope of saddling others or their children and servants with the pestilence and thus saving themselves. I can well

59. The ethicist Timothy F. Murphy notes the similarity between these historical figures and the role played by Dugas in Shilts's book; see Murphy, *Ethics in an Epidemic: AIDS, Morality, and Culture* (Berkeley: University of California Press, 1994), 11.

60. Robert Fletcher, *A Tragedy of the Great Plague of Milan in 1630* (Baltimore: Lord Baltimore Press, 1898), 5, Ebook and Texts Archive, https://ia800207.us.archive.org/9/items/atragedygreatpl00fletgoog/atragedygreatpl00fletgoog.pdf.

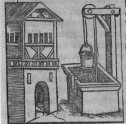

auch ein krieg wider den grauen võ pfirt/der des keysers hauptman was/vñ
lag vnder in einer schlacht bey dem dorff Blodeltzheim/dar von du hie fornen
folio 214. findest.   Anno Christi 1349.
erstünd im Elsaß ein grosser sterbet/vñ wüßt
doch niemand war von es were. Es was kein
pestiletz/aber man hett ein argwon vff die Ju
den/daß sie die brunnen hette vergifft. Es stur
bent allein zu Straßburg bey xvj. tausent/
iung vnd alt. Auß dissem argwon fieng man
zu Bern vnd Zofingen die Juden vnd streckt
sie/do veriahen sie das gifft/vnnd ward auch
also in den brünnen gefunden. So lieff das
volck zu Basel zusammen vnd zwüngen den
                    rhat/

A

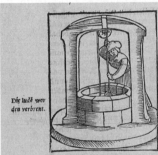

Die ludē wer
dē verbrent.

auff die Juden/das sie die brunnen hette vergifft.
Es sturben zu Straßburg bey 16000. iung vnd
alt. Auß disem argwon fieng man zu Bern vnd
Zofingen die Juden vnd streckt sie / do veriahen
sie das gifft/vñ ward auch also in brunnen gefun
den. So lieff das volck zu Basel zusammen vnd
zwungen den rhat/zu tödē die Juden. Des gleī
chen geschah zu Straßburg/ dañ do wurdē etwā
200. in einem hauffen auff dē Juden kirchoff ver
brent. Aber die sich wolten lassen tauffen/die ließ
man bey leben. Es wurden auch vil kinder wider
irer ältern willen auß dē hauffen gezuckt vnd zū
dē tauff behalten. Zu diser zeit wordē die bauren
auch auffrürig vnd wurffen ein künig auff/der
hieß künig Armleder/was auch ein bauwer/die
erschlugent mer dañ 5000. Juden anno 1338.

B

nobilis, inter quos fuerat comes unus de Tierstein, & Hermannus de Geroldseck fra-
ter episcopi, & populares multi. Fuerunt quoqჳ multi capti & in ciui
tatem ducti, multa etiã damna utrinqჳ illata. Postremo mortuo episco
po, pax est reformata. Circa annum Christi 148. tanta fuit pestis per
Europam graffans, qualem in historijs nemo legerat fuisse inter mor
tales. Fuerant autem de ea infamati Iudæi quod eam prouocauē-
rint fontibus infectis, & propterea cremati sunt ubiqჳ locorum. Ha-
bitus fuit etiam super hac re tractatus in Benfeld oppido Alsatiæ, &
ut scribitur, quidam ex Iudæis inuenti fuerunt ceu omnium malefi-
ciorum autores atque in Hispania de ueneficijs conuenisse. Item de
nece multorum puerorum, de falsificatione super debitis instrumen-
torum & monetæ, unde plebs furens omnes traxit ad supplicium,
                        S   Cremati

C

FIGURE 1.1 Woodcuts (*A–E*) accompanying various editions of Sebastian Münster's *Cosmographia*, 1544–1628. Presenting more personalized and violent visual commentar-
ies over time, bookmakers in Basel used and reused different woodcuts to illustrate the
story of Jews being punished for the arrival of plague in Strasbourg in 1349. The fourth
woodcut image (*D*)—originally employed in the book's 1545 edition to depict the burning of two religious dissidents, Jan Hus and Jerome of Prague—was later reappropriated in 1614, at a time of increasingly brutal punishment for those accused of spreading

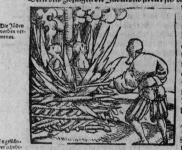

D

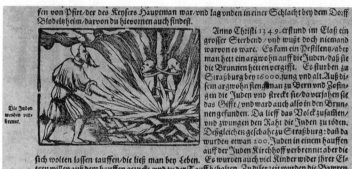

E

the plague. The same image was later reprinted, with the generic caption "Burning of the Plague Spreaders," in Johannes Nohl, *The Black Death: A Chronicle of the Plague*, translated by C. H. Clarke (London: George Allen and Unwin, 1926), 179. A, Woodcut, 5.7 × 5.8 cm. Sebastian Münster, *Cosmographia, beschreibung aller lender. . . .* (Basel: Henrichum Petri, 1544), cccxvii, http://gallica.bnf.fr/ark:/12148/btv1b55007851n/f402, Bibliothèque nationale de France. B, Woodcut, 5.6 × 7.0 cm. Sebastian Münster, *Cosmographei: oder beschreibung aller länder. . . .* (Basel, 1550), dlviii, Digital Collections Freiburg, University of Freiburg, http://dl.ub.uni-freiburg.de/diglit/muenster1550/0630. C, Woodcut, 3.7 × 4.7 cm. Sebastian Münster, *Cosmographiae universalis libri VI in quibus. . . .* (Basel: H. Petrus, 1552), 457, image no. L0077447 (cropped), Wellcome Library, London, https://wellcomeimages.org/indexplus/image/L0077447.html. D, Woodcut, 6.3 × 5.8 cm. Sebastian Münster, *Cosmographey: das ist Beschreibung aller Länder. . . .* (Basel: Sebastianum Henricpetri, 1614), 868, Central Library of Geography and Environmental Protection, Institute of Geography and Spatial Organization, Polish Academy of Sciences, http://rcin.org.pl/publication/18809. E, Woodcut, 8.2 × 5.8 cm. Sebastian Münster, *Cosmographia, das ist: Beschreibung der gantzen Welt. . . .* (Basel: Henricpetrinischen, 1628), 834.

believe that the devil obliges and helps to further this notion so that it actually comes to pass. I am also told that some individuals are so desperately wicked that they carry the pestilence among the people and into houses for no other reason than that they regret that the disease has not struck there, and so they spread the pestilence as if this were a great joke, like slyly putting lice in somebody's clothes or gnats in somebody's room.

Luther questioned, though, whether he should believe these rumors, and concluded, "If it is true, I do not know whether we Germans are human beings or devils. To be sure, there are immoderately coarse and wicked people, and the devil is not inactive."[61] The same decade, the humanist scholar Erasmus of Rotterdam voiced very similar views relating to venereal disease in his writings on marriage. In a colloquy he published in 1529 on an "Unequal Match"—between a beautiful young woman and a pox-infested old man—one speaker observes of the pox that "this disease is accompanied by a mortal hatred, so that whoever is in its clutches takes pleasure in infecting as many others as possible, even though doing so is no help to him. If deported, they may possibly escape; they can fool others at night or take advantage of persons who don't know them."[62] Nearly two centuries later, Daniel Defoe would reprise such concerns in his fictionalized *A Journal of the Plague Year*. The author included a self-consciously tentative account, set off with a parenthetical note—"(if the Story be true)"—of a woman attacked by a sick man in the streets of London, who kissed her and declared that "he had the Plague, and why should not she have it as well as he."[63]

Others envisioned harnessing disease to achieve political revenge and warfare. In *Timon of Athens*, a satirical play Shakespeare wrote for the London stage in the early seventeenth century, the titular charac-

61. Martin Luther, *Luther: Letters of Spiritual Counsel*, ed. and trans. Theodore G. Tappert (London: SCM Press, 1955), 243. Readers may wish to compare Luther's words with the widely reported belief held by some people that sex with a virgin might cure venereal disease and, later, HIV infection; see Rachel Jewkes, "Child Sexual Abuse and HIV Infection," *Sexual Abuse of Young Children in Southern Africa*, ed. Linda Richter, Andrew Dawes, and Craig Higson-Smith (Cape Town: HSRC Press, 2004), 130–36.

62. Desiderius Erasmus, "A Marriage in Name Only, or the Unequal Match," *Collected Works of Erasmus: Colloquies*, trans. and annot. Craig R. Thompson (Toronto: University of Toronto Press, 1997), 852.

63. Daniel Defoe, *A Journal of the Plague Year*, ed. Louis Landa (Oxford: Oxford University Press, 1990), 160.

ter urges two prostitutes, Phrynia and Timandra, to spread their infection across Athens and bring infectious revenge upon his former-friends-turned-enemies and social chaos to the city he has abandoned.[64] Such a desire to use disease to sow terror later became realized in a North American colonial context more than a century later. Correspondence between two senior British army officers in 1763 outlines plans for an incident of biological warfare. Dismayed at the threat posed by Native American uprisings, Sir Jeffery Amherst asked: "Could it not be contrived to send the small-pox among these disaffected tribes of Indians?" Colonel Henry Bouquet replied that he would "try to inoculate the —— with some blankets that may fall in their hands, and take care not to get the disease myself."[65]

Focussing on syphilis permits us to further trace the theme of revenge through the nineteenth and twentieth centuries, with examples that blur divisions between fiction and reality. In "Bed No. 29" (1884), a short story by Guy de Maupassant, the mistress of a French army captain becomes infected by the Prussian soldiers who invade her town while he is away at the front. When the captain later visits his sick lover in hospital, she explains her desire to avenge herself, by foreaking treatment and sleeping with as many enemy soldiers as possible. "'And I poisoned them too, all, all that I could.'"[66] Even more resonant for our purposes, however, is a letter Maupassant wrote in 1877 to a friend, in which he shared news of his recent diagnosis with syphilis. The writer also provided, with a shockingly boastful misogyny, a rare instance of an individual claiming to pass on his disease intentionally. With words that eerily anticipate those attributed to the French Canadian Dugas in Shilts's book a century later, Maupassant wrote, "Allelujah, I've got the pox, so I don't have to worry about catching it any more, and I screw the street whores and trollops, and afterwards I say to them 'I've got the pox.' They are afraid and I just laugh."[67]

---

64. Louis F. Qualtiere and William W. E. Slights, "Contagion and Blame in Early Modern England: The Case of the French Pox," *Literature and Medicine* 22, no. 1 (2003): 1–24.

65. John Joseph Heagerty, *Four Centuries of Medical History in Canada and a Sketch of the Medical History of Newfoundland* (Toronto: Macmillan Canada, 1928), 43.

66. "Bed No. 29," *The Complete Short Stories of Guy de Maupassant* (New York: P. F. Collier and Son, 1903), 390; Claude Quétel, *History of Syphilis*, trans. Judith Braddock and Brian Pike (Cambridge: Polity Press, 1992), 124.

67. Maupassant quoted in Quétel, *History of Syphilis*, 130. Beyond coincidence, it is difficult to explain the unusual similarity between Maupassant's words and their context

More typical than his personal exploits may be the way that Maupassant infused contemporary worries surrounding venereal disease into his
fictional writing. It is worth noting that similar concerns about syphilis
and other sexually transmitted infections were on the increase in American urban gay communities in the 1970s and early 1980s. This period
also witnessed an efflorescence of American gay literature, with novels
from such New York authors as Larry Kramer and Andrew Holleran
exploring the haunts and pastimes of urban gay men.[68] Holleran's 1978
novel, *Dancer from the Dance,* featured a brief reference to a "vengeful
queen" whose alleged actions are reminiscent of the mistress in Maupassant's short story. Sutherland, one of the book's main characters, scorn-
fully describes one blond man as the bearer of a very small penis, declaring that "the boy became so bitter about his fate that when he developed
a case of syphilis he went to the Baths and infected everyone he could
who sported an enormous organ."[69]

Given the ease with which many stories of deliberate disease transmission have been fictionalized, there is a cautionary tale to be told
about how some of them have recirculated. For instance, in 2003 a political analyst produced a study of a young man in New York state who
stood accused of infecting thirteen young women with HIV. In one section of his book, the author surveyed past epidemics and, citing a history of the plague written in 1926, found that "some did intentionally infect others . . . [and in several] cases, those who were infected preferred
not to suffer alone." The doubtful stories in the book he cited included
a jealous tale of a classics scholar who deliberately infected his archri-
val with a contaminated manuscript—originally published as a fictional
short story by Bettina von Arnim, a German literary scholar closely connected with Goethe and the Grimm brothers—and Luther's fearful pass-

---

with the rumors associated with Dugas more than a century later. Scholars knew of the
existence of Maupassant's letter to Robert Pinchon before it appeared for auction in late
1984, but it seems that only fragments of this document were published—and crucially not
the passage referring to "street whores and trollops"—while it remained in private hands.
See Quétel, *History of Syphilis,* 128, 295n52; and Guy de Maupassant, *Correspondance /
Guy de Maupassant,* vol. 1, ed. Jacques Suffel (Geneva: Edito-service, 1973), 117.

68. Jennifer Brier, *Infectious Ideas: U.S. Political Responses to the AIDS Crisis*
(Chapel Hill, NC: University of North Carolina Press, 2009), 15–19.

69. Andrew Holleran, *Dancer from the Dance* (1978; repr., New York: Perennial Press,
2001), 53.

ing on of tales he had heard.[70] It is relatively easy to uncover tales of deliberate disease spreading when surveying the history of disease.[71] It is
far more difficult, however, to infer human motivation and intentional-
ity, or to demonstrate that the stories represent anything more than the
cultural fears of a historically specific period.[72] Unless there there is substantial evidence to the contrary, one might do well, therefore, to exercise strong skepticism of any story alleging that a sick person was deliberately attempting to infect others.

Beauty, Sexual Activity, and the Threat of Disease

"I am the prettiest one."[73]

The readers of *And the Band Played On* would receive their main introduction to Gaétan Dugas with these words, a few pages after catching an initial glimpse of the character in a mirror—a fitting first appearance given the narcissistic role Shilts had him play.[74] The setting Shilts
chose to present Dugas's backstory is a San Francisco dance venue during the city's Gay Freedom Day celebrations in 1980. The scene is filled
with drugs, loud music, and sexual competition, aspects of the commer-

70. Thomas Shevory, *Notorious H.I.V.: The Media Spectacle of Nushawn Williams*
(Minneapolis: University of Minnesota Press, 2004), 113–14; Johannes Nohl, *The Black
Death: A Chronicle of the Plague*, trans. C. H. Clarke (London: George Allen and Unwin,
1926), 136–38, 161–80; [Bettina von] Arnim, "Les aventures d'un manuscrit," *Revue germanique* 9, no. 26 (1837): 149–85.

71. Compare Baldwin, *Disease and Democracy*, 90, 127.

72. See, for example, Paul Slack's assessment of such accusations during plague outbreaks in sixteenth- and seventeenth-century England. He concludes that they reside in
the realm of hearsay and rumor and are more clearly indicative of the divisive impact of
the plague on social relationships; Slack, *Impact of Plague*, 292–93. For a discussion of the
urban legends surrounding AIDS, see Gary Alan Fine, "Welcome to the World of AIDS:
Fantasies of Female Revenge," *Western Folklore* 46, no. 3 (1987): 192–97; Jan Harold
Brunvand, *Curses! Broiled Again!* (London: W. W. Norton, 1989), 195–205.

73. Shilts, *Band*, 21. Dugas is seen closely examining his reflection in a mirror on p. 11.

74. See Robin Metcalfe, "Light in the Loafers: The Gaynor Photographs of Gaëtan
[*sic*] Dugas and the Invention of Patient Zero," in *Image and Inscription: An Anthology of
Contemporary Canadian Photography*, ed. Robert Bean (Toronto, 2005), 72–73. Metcalfe
suggests that the depiction of Dugas could represent a modern version of Oscar Wilde's
Dorian Gray.

cialized gay male life in urban San Francisco of which Shilts was known to be critical. "Gaetan," Shilts wrote, "was the man everyone wanted, the ideal for this community, at this time and in this place. His sandy hair fell boyishly over his forehead. His mouth easily curled into an inviting smile, and his laugh could flood color into a room of black and white. He bought his clothes in the trendiest shops of Paris and London. He vacationed in Mexico and on the Caribbean beaches. Americans tumbled for his soft Quebeçois [sic] accent and his sensual magnetism."[75] Shilts allowed little room for irony in the flight attendant's remark about his own attractiveness, which suggests his opinion that Dugas believed his own joke completely and belies a narrow reading of Shilts's source material, the notes from his interviews with Dugas's friends. Soon after in the book, like a vampire closing in on his prey—on Halloween, no less— Dugas lures a victim at an upscale nightclub by smiling "in a particularly winning way." His target cannot resist; "and before long Jack and Gaetan Dugas slipped away from the crowd and into the night."[76]

Beauty that masked an underlying danger of infection is another theme that can claim a long history. Medieval literature drew on mythological and biblical references for the construction of beautiful women as dangerous temptresses. As one early modern writer noted, Helen of Troy, the quintessential beautiful woman, was unable to remain faithful to her husband and generated an unparalleled war in the ancient world. Eve, Delilah, and Judith were similarly seen to have tempted men and led them to their downfall. Under the Renaissance ideas of balance, women granted greater than normal attributes of beauty would also have received greater than normal capacities for vice. Not only was this a tale that built on medical and ecclesiastical images of women as ready vessels

75. Shilts, Band, 21. Metcalfe remarks on the book's insistence on "misspelling the word 'Québécois,' as if to emphasize the otherness of a language whose strange rules of orthography normal people really cannot be expected to master" ("Light in the Loafers," 74).

76. Shilts, Band, 41. Some have noted the similarity between Dugas's depiction as "the very Dracula of AIDS," particularly his employment as a flight attendant, and the cosmopolitan, mobile vampires of the nineteenth century and in gothic literature. See Judith Williamson, "Aids and Perceptions of the Grim Reaper," Metro 80 (1989): 2–6; Ellis Hanson, "Undead," in Inside/Out: Lesbian Theories, Gay Theories, ed. Diana Fuss (London: Routledge, 1991), 332; Teresa A. Goddu, "Vampire Gothic," American Literary History 11, no. 1 (1999): 126.

of contagion, but it was also deemed a warning against the dangers of extreme beauty, which men found difficult to resist.[77]

In her examination of early modern Venetian attempts to isolate prostitutes, as well as women so beautiful they were seen to risk drawing sin to themselves, the historian Laura McGough outlines a tale of syphilis origins in which the disease could be traced to "the most beautiful prostitute."[78] According to Pietro Rostinio, a sixteenth-century Italian medical writer, the prostitute had a putrefying sore at the opening of her womb and was blamed not only for spreading the disease but also for creating it within her own body. The friction and warmth of intercourse combined with the humidity of her vagina led to the contamination of the penetrating male member. As Rostinio explained, "And this illness began to stain one man, then two, and three, & one hundred, because this woman was a prostitute and most beautiful, and since human nature is desirous of coitus, many women had sexual relations with these men (and became) infected with this illness."[79] McGough defines this figure as a sixteenth-century "Patient Zero"—fulfilling the criteria of attractiveness and point of origin—and noted that Renaissance writers viewed extreme beauty as rarely occurring in nature. If it did, it was almost a deformity, which defied the importance of balance, moderation, and harmony advocated by Renaissance aesthetics. Any overallocation of beauty would, it was thought, be accompanied by an equivalent endowment of vice.[80] Later works would also hold both beauty and vice in the same frame. The embodiment of the pox shifted from the image of the lone male sufferer to that of the female "source" between the sixteenth and eighteenth centuries; by the nineteenth century, the illustration for a French translation of Fracastoro's *Syphilis* was the image of a skull-faced female, suggestive of syphilitic decay, luring a man behind the guise of a beautiful mask.[81]

The idea of beauty out of balance was also suggested by some members of New York's urban gay community in the early 1980s. In an article in *Christopher Street* magazine, one critic referred to his own gay

77. Laura J. McGough, "Quarantining Beauty: The French Disease in Early Modern Venice," in Siena, *Sins of the Flesh*, 221.

78. Ibid., 211–37.

79. Quoted in ibid., 211.

80. Ibid., 222.

81. Gilman, "AIDS and Syphilis," 97.

subculture as "Gaycult" and pondered its concern with "the question of beauty": "One might further acknowledge that there is a certain continuity between the classical sense of beauty and exercise in Gaycult's gymnasium addiction. Whereas in classical terms there was a necessary relationship between the well-proportioned body and the well-trained mind and, in turn, the compassionate soul, there appears to be a more one-dimensional obsession nowadays." The writer linked this imbalance, rendered visible by gay men's attempts to construct well-muscled bodies, to their fears of demonstrating any feminine attributes.[82] Being more sexually attractive meant one could find partners more easily when cruising in bars, discotheques, and bathhouses, though this attractiveness also brought risks of its own. One man later recalled New York City nightlife during the late 1970s, which for some gay men offered the possibility of having sex at the Saint, a popular nightclub. He noted the precautions taken beforehand: "At these parties there was a bowl of penicillin outside, right before you left the house, and everybody would just reach in and take some penicillin and put the penicillin in their mouths as a preventative for the diseases."[83] Early AIDS reports suggested that it was gay men with a very active sexual lifestyle who were most represented in the ranks of the sick. Among them, the good-looking men who typified those attending nights at the Saint featured so prominently that early discussions in Manhattan made reference to the "Saint's Disease."[84] Indeed, the author Edmund White suggested that an ulterior motive shaped by physical insecurities might underlie some of the publicity AIDS drew in late 1982 and early 1983. "It's cruel to say," he told a reporter, "but a lot of the people who are the loudest on this issue are men in their forties who, perhaps by the harsh standards set by our community, no longer have the sort of attractiveness that's required in settings where one is likely to have multiple, anonymous encounters."[85] Debates about sexual activity—often provocatively

82. Neil Alan Marks, "New York Gaycult, the Jewish Question . . . and Me," *Christopher Street*, November 1981, 20.

83. Zvi Howard Rosenman, interview with author, Los Angeles, July 6, 2007, recording C1491/01, tape 1, side A, BLSA.

84. Charles Kaiser, *The Gay Metropolis* (London: Weidenfeld and Nicholson, 1998), 283. Compare this reference with "the saints among us" in Bill Russell's poem at the beginning of the present book, preceding the table of contents.

85. Quoted in Lindsy Van Gelder, "Death in the Family," *Rolling Stone*, February 3, 1983, 18.

labeled *promiscuity*—consumed gay communities.[86] Mainstream amazement, meanwhile, at the number of partners reported by some early gay cases with AIDS was not uncommon, as was demonstrated by the reactions of those present at the NCAB meeting discussed in this book's introduction.[87]

The "Healthy Carrier"

Gaetan, the Quebeçois [*sic*] version of Typhoid Mary[88]

Direct comparisons between "Typhoid Mary" Mallon and Gaétan Dugas —from Alvin Friedman-Kien's recollection that begins this chapter to the widely circulated line from Shilts's book that opens this section— have been frequent. Mallon was an Irish-born woman who arrived in the United States in 1883, early in a period of mass immigration between 1880 and 1924 that attracted more than twenty-three million people.[89] She settled in New York City and, seeking domestic employment as did many other Irish American single women of the period, found work as a cook for a series of wealthy families.[90] In the summers, she traveled with her employers to their summer estates on the Jersey shore or on

86. Brier, *Infectious Ideas*, 11–44.

87. Douglas Elliott, the only openly gay counsel in regular attendance at the Commission of Inquiry on the Blood System in Canada, and whose work there is discussed in detail in chapter 5 of this book, later remembered similar astonishment at one stage of the inquiry's hearings. When one expert giving testimony explained that some of the persons diagnosed with AIDS in 1982 and 1983 had reported more than one thousand lifetime sexual partners, Elliott recalled that "there was this audible *gasp* in the room . . . and then, not the witness, but everyone else in the room, including Justice [Horace] Krever, they all looked over at *me* [*laughing*]." Elliott, C1491/39, tape 2 side B, August 27, 2008; emphasis on recording. A review of the inquiry's verbatim transcripts suggests that Elliott was thinking of Dr. Brian Willoughby's testimony at the regional hearings held in Vancouver on April 8, 1994; *Verbatim Transcripts of Commission of Inquiry on the Blood System in Canada*, 247 vols. (Gloucester, ON: International Rose Reporting, 1997), 30:5897–98, CD-ROM.

88. Shilts, *Band*, 158.

89. Kraut, *Silent Travelers*, 52. During that period, there was also a corresponding rise in nativist prejudice from an anti-immigrant movement that, Kraut demonstrates, employed biomedical arguments to gain acceptance for its views.

90. Leavitt, *Typhoid Mary*, 164.

Long Island.[91] To her knowledge, as she protested repeatedly in her later years, she had never been sick with typhoid fever.[92]

By the time that Mallon's story first captured the public's attention in 1907 through articles published in New York newspapers, the concept of healthy human beings who were able to pass on infectious "germs" without themselves being sick was not widely held. For a period of almost thirty years, bacteriologists in North America and Europe had drawn on the scientific work of Louis Pasteur and Robert Koch, championing the primacy of microorganisms in the etiology of disease and arguing that specific germs were at the root of specific diseases. The adoption of a bacteriological theory of disease causation was gradual and was resisted by many observers who contended that its reductionistic focus on the transmission of microbes from person to person ignored the apparent success of sanitationists in reducing mortality from epidemic diseases, particularly cholera and typhoid, with improvements in water delivery and urban cleanliness.[93] With regard to tuberculosis, the new theory divided experts on the relative importance of "seed"(the infectious germ) and "soil" (the constitutional and social conditions affecting an individual's general health and his or her likelihood of falling ill).[94] One particular failing of the "germ theory," as seen by one of its ardent later supporters, was its inability to account for epidemic outbreaks that did not appear to stem from a sick individual.[95]

With the cultivation of diphtheria bacilli from the throat of a healthy patient in 1884, the German bacteriologist Friedrich Loeffler theorized the existence of a "healthy carrier" state.[96] Koch confirmed this possibility with comparable findings for cholera in 1893; studies of typhoid infection over the next thirteen years, particularly in Germany, confirmed

91. Ibid., xvii.

92. Ibid., 185–89, 194.

93. Margaret Pelling, *Cholera, Fever and English Medicine, 1825–1865* (Oxford: Oxford University Press, 1978); Charles E. Rosenberg, *The Cholera Years: the United States in 1832, 1849, and 1866, with a New Afterword* (London: University of Chicago Press, 1987).

94. David S. Barnes, *The Making of a Social Disease: Tuberculosis in Nineteenth-Century France* (Berkeley: University of California Press, 1995), 74–111.

95. Charles-Edward Amory Winslow, *The Conquest of Epidemic Disease: A Chapter in the History of Ideas* (1943; repr., London: University of Wisconsin Press, 1980), vii.

96. Ibid., 339.

that this disease could also have its human carriers.[97] Contemporary medical publications in England and the United States indicate a familiarity on the part of doctors in both countries with such studies. Doctors and medical officers of health of the time referred liberally to disease carriers on both sides of the Atlantic to develop their ideas on disease etiology.[98] The case of Mallon, described by George Soper in 1907, drew wide comment.

In the first published account of the case, Soper, a sanitary engineer, articulated a narrative structured similarly to Friedman-Kien's recollection at the opening of this chapter—in the format of a detective story.[99] Soper had been hired by a wealthy Long Islander to investigate an outbreak of typhoid that had taken place in his holiday home during the summer of 1906. Using a standardized sequence of inquiries that built on fieldwork techniques dating from before the bacteriological period and relying considerably on recently developed laboratory tests, Soper was able to eliminate common environmental sources of typhoid infection such as contaminated well water and soft clams.[100] Learning that the household had switched cooks just before the outbreak of typhoid, Soper first attempted to contact Mallon, the replacement cook in question. With no luck, he did some research into her work history, using information provided by her employment agency. Ultimately he was

97. Ibid. See also William H. Park, "Typhoid Bacilli Carriers," *Journal of the American Medical Association* 51, no. 12 (1908): 981–82.

98. See, for example, Park, "Typhoid Bacilli Carriers," 981–82; D. S. Davies and I. Walker Hall, "A Discussion on the Etiology and Epidemiology of Typhoid (Enteric) Fever: Typhoid Carriers, with an Account of Two Institution Outbreaks Traced to the Same 'Carrier,'" *Proceedings of the Royal Society of Medicine* 1 (1907–8): 191.

99. George A. Soper, "The Work of a Chronic Typhoid Germ Distributor," *Journal of the American Medical Association* 48 (1907): 2019–22. Several commentators have remarked on the detective-like narrative style of medical investigations: see Leavitt, *Typhoid Mary*, 16; Wald, *Contagious*, 23–25; and chapter 2 of this book for further discussion. Soper himself refers to the discovery that the household in question had changed cooks shortly before the outbreak of typhoid as a "clue" ("Typhoid Germ Distributor," 2021).

100. For the prebacteriological origins of epidemiologic investigations, and particularly his discussion of the importance attributed to the first case, or cases, in an attempt to discover, in the words of hygienist Edmund A. Parkes, "the influence of essential antecedents," see W. Coleman, *Yellow Fever in the North*, 183. See also William Coleman, "Epidemiological Method in the 1860s: Yellow Fever at Saint-Nazaire," *Bulletin of the History of Medicine* 58, no. 2 (1984): 145–63.

able to posit Mallon as the cause of seven separate typhoid outbreaks occurring in the families for which she had worked, despite her appearing, as Soper put it, to be "in perfect health."[101] Deciding that Mallon was a "chronic typhoid germ distributor," Soper shared his information with the medical officer of the New York City Department of Health.[102] Mallon was forcibly removed and detained on North Brother Island in the East River, where she remained for three years before being released in 1911 on the condition that she not work as a cook. She achieved notoriety in the media in 1915 when she was discovered cooking again under an assumed name at a maternity hospital. A typhoid outbreak that occurred after she started work there resulted in illness in twenty-five people and death for two others. Subsequently, Mallon was apprehended and spent her remaining twenty-three years living in isolation on North Brother Island.[103] The stories that were told about her experience over the following decades varied. In some, she was the hapless victim of an overaggressive public health department. Others overlooked her limited financial means and viewed her as a careless transmitter. More forceful versions of the story declared that she had willfully infected and killed the unlucky consumers of the food she prepared.[104]

Mallon's case was brought up in similar debates about the role of healthy carriers in England, particularly when the first recorded example of a carrier-induced typhoid outbreak in that country drew, in the words of medical journal the *Lancet,* "the deepest interest in Parliamentary circles."[105] In the Brentry Home for Inebriates, near Bristol, a "continuing outbreak of enteric fever," occurring between September 1906 and November 1907, led to twenty-eight cases of typhoid and two deaths.[106] Dr. D. S. Davies, the medical officer of health for Bristol, who was described as "fresh from a perusal of German literature relative to 'carrier' cases," was able to trace the Brentry cases to a healthy carrier cook, whom he subsequently determined to be the outbreak's solitary

101. Leavitt, *Typhoid Mary*, 16; Soper, "Typhoid Germ Distributor," 2022.

102. Soper, "Typhoid Germ Distributor," 2022.

103. Leavitt, *Typhoid Mary*, xviii.

104. Ibid., 202–30.

105. "An Outbreak of Enteric Fever and Human 'Carriers,'" *Lancet* 171, no. 4409 (1908): 685.

106. "Dissemination of Enteric Fever Due to a 'Typhoid Carrier,'" *Lancet* 171, no. 4404 (1908): 246.

cause.[107] At a meeting of the Epidemiological Section of the Royal Society of Medicine, Dr. Davies and Dr. I. Walker Hall, a pathologist, presented their findings to colleagues[108] and surprised them with the announcement that the female inmate at the Brentry home in question had also been linked to an earlier outbreak of typhoid at a girls' home near Bristol in 1904, where she had also worked as a cook.[109]

While Davies and Hall's report presented compelling evidence for the case of an infective chronic carrier of typhoid, it is also worth noting the element of threat, pollution, and social irresponsibility suggested by their use of language throughout. Chronic carriers are noted to be "obviously the most dangerous class" of contagious individual; "when these chronic carriers are engaged in the preparation of food, or in dairy work, they are apt to give rise to intermittent local outbreaks of typhoid fever, probably by contamination of the food with the hand after daefecation or micturition."[110] Mrs. H., the cook in question, had been "entrusted" with dairy work and to prepare milk for children to drink.[111] There was little doubt, according to Davies and Hall, that such an offensive and "'gross'" transfer of infection, "through carelessness and neglect to wash the hands after attending to the calls of Nature," amounted to an abuse of such trust. They associated cooks with waitresses and schoolboys as a group whose dirty fingernails were teeming with microorganisms, suggesting "uncomfortable thoughts anent 'our daily bread'"—a potent phrase which succinctly linked class anxieties, germ phobia through meal preparation, and Christian prayer.[112] Davies and Hall closed their paper by looking dually to bacteriology and the law for answers, wondering whether there was a solution to be found in "bacterial methods" or whether a carrier "capable of distributing disease and death" could be placed under any statutory restrictions.[113]

107. "The 'Bacillus Carriers' of Enteric Fever," *Lancet* 171, no. 4410 (1908): 733; "Outbreak of Enteric Fever," 685.

108. Ibid., 733.

109. Davies and Hall, "On Typhoid Fever," 187.

110. Ibid., 177.

111. Ibid., 180.

112. Ibid., 187.

113. Ibid., 189. Such fears would be captured in discussions about AIDS "carriers" a century later. For a critical overview of the manner in which "the need to find the vector of infection demonstrates our human obsession with origins and causation," see the entire special issue of *Sexuality Research and Social Policy* entitled "Reckless Vectors," 2,

The pair's carrier hypothesis was not met with universal support. In his own paper at the same session and in the ensuing discussion, Dr. W. H. Hamer voiced a strong opposition to the importance of the carrier and criticized Soper's investigation of the New York case for not paying sufficient attention to other likely causes, such as infected seafood.[114] He also challenged the authority of the laboratory, noting that "the conditions of scientific experiment were not rigorously fulfilled in these laboratory experiments."[115] Moreover, in an argument which strikingly anticipated one put forward more than eighty years later regarding HIV/AIDS, Hamer contended that the typhoid bacillus was not necessarily the cause of typhoid and that it might be one of "a number of organisms, believed at one time to be 'causal,' [which] are now classed as 'secondary invaders.'"[116]

While Hamer's objections can be taken to represent the resistance from some members of the scientific community to the concept of the healthy carrier, a balanced history must also consider those raised by members of the lay public, and particularly by affected carriers.[117] Despite a varied reception to ideas of contagion in educated circles during the mid-nineteenth century, many historians have noted how regular citizens adhered to the ancient and strongly held belief that many diseases were spread from person to person, from the sick to the healthy.[118] With cholera, the conviction that the disease was noncontagious was limited to the

no. 2 (2005). This quote is drawn from Heather Worth, Cindy Patton, and Diane Goldstein, "Introduction to Special Issue: Reckless Vectors: The Infecting 'Other' In HIV/AIDS Law," 4.

114. W. H. Hamer, "A Discussion on the Etiology and Epidemiology of Typhoid (Enteric) Fever: The Relation of the Bacillus typhosus to Typhoid Fever," *Proceedings of the Royal Society of Medicine* 1 (1907–8): 205.

115. "A Discussion on the Etiology and Epidemiology of Typhoid (Enteric) Fever: Discussion," *Proceedings of the Royal Society of Medicine* 1 (1907–08): 227–28.

116. Hamer, "Bacillus typhosis," 217. Hamer's argument would be echoed many years later by Peter Duesberg, as noted in the introduction to this book.

117. In "Methods of Outbreak Investigation in the 'Era of Bacteriology' 1880–1920," *Sozial-und Präventivmedizin/Social and Preventive Medicine* 46, no. 6 (2001): 355–60, Anne Hardy argues that, although perhaps extreme, Hamer's critical approach to the idea of the carrier was representative of a widely held English reluctance to adopt an overly authoritative public health approach.

118. Indeed, such popular belief was often associated with "primitive" societies and no doubt a contributing reason for many elite members to distance themselves from such views. See Pelling, "Meaning of Contagion," 17.

medical profession and educated members of the public during the nine-teenth century; most laypeople believed in some sort of contagion, mak-ing it difficult for authorities to set up hospitals to treat patients or to staff these buildings with nurses.[119] Yellow fever, another epidemic disease whose manner of spread was contested by medical experts, was thought by most of the population to be communicable.[120] Typhoid was held to be similarly transmitted, either through exposure to sick individuals or to contaminated water and milk products. Within this understanding of transmission, it would have seemed particularly nonsensical to suggest that healthy people could harbor disease-causing agents for a sickness they had experienced long ago or with which they had never thought themselves to have been afflicted.[121] Thus, just as Mary Mallon found it incomprehensible that she might bear responsibility for infecting others with typhoid when she did not feel sick, one can understand how, years later, Gaétan Dugas rejected as unlikely the idea that his "cancer"—or the hypothesized infection underlying it—could be transmissible.

* * *

As we have seen, the popular impulse to allocate blame for disease has often gravitated toward nominating cultural outsiders for the role of dis-ease "carriers." This distancing process has resulted in a history of ac-cused disease carriers sharing the discriminated role and finding them-selves in that position in part due to their different sex, sexuality, gender, race, ethnicity, or religion. Also, as the germ theory of disease gained ac-ceptance, an increased emphasis on cleanliness and individual respon-sibility reinforced earlier notions of moral failure and contamination which epidemics brought to light.

These historical themes lay the groundwork for understanding why Randy Shilts recognized that the investigations of a sexual network link-ing early AIDS cases would serve as a compelling thread for his book and, in particular, why his characterization of Dugas as "Patient Zero" would capture the public imagination. By emphasizing the flight atten-

119. Rosenberg, *Cholera Years*, 81.

120. See Margaret Humphreys, "No Safe Place: Disease and Panic in American History," *American Literary History* 14, no. 4 (2002): 851; as well as her monograph *Yellow Fever and the South* (New Brunswick, NJ: Rutgers University Press, 1992), 18.

121. Leavitt, *Typhoid Mary*, 170.

dant's sexuality, his early diagnosis with an AIDS-related illness and sexual liaisons with other cases, his alleged bathhouse encounters facilitated through an unnatural beauty, and his initial subclinical and mostly hidden infection, Shilts's portrayal resonated with and reproduced sometimes centuries-old ideas of irresponsible behavior associated with epidemic disease. Similarly, accusations of deliberate disease spreading have long played a role in times of epidemic, often representing a sense of social helplessness and paranoia at what other members of society *might* do rather than, necessarily, a sense of what they *actually* do. Given this history, it is utterly unsurprising that accusations of disease spreading should have occurred during the AIDS epidemic, with ill intentions ascribed to the socially vulnerable and marginalized "deviant," without a rigid adherence to evidence. It also helps to understand the interpretive frames many people used to make sense of the CDC's early AIDS investigations, a subject to which this book now turns.

CHAPTER TWO

The Cluster Study

The CDC cluster study . . . is pivotal to the research that will be done in the next 2–5 years, for it strongly suggests that the recent outbreak of Kaposi's sarcoma and pneumocystis pneumonia is caused by an infectious agent which is being sexually transmitted. — *Marcus A. Conant*, dermatologist, San Francisco, 1982[1]

The cluster is in fact a textbook example of constructing your empirical evidence to fit your theory. — *Andrew R. Moss*, epidemiologist, San Francisco, 1988[2]

In the autumn of 1988, a San Francisco–based epidemiologist wrote to a New York literary journal to critique an AIDS study conducted by one of his professional colleagues several years earlier. In many ways, the *New York Review of Books* was an unusual forum for a disagreement about epidemiology. One might normally expect a challenge of this sort to take place within the discussion pages of an academic publication or at a conference session. This, however, was not a typical case.

In his letter, published in early December, Andrew Moss addressed a review that had appeared in a previous issue of the periodical. This article had contrasted two accounts of the impact of AIDS in the United States: one a report from a presidential commission on the HIV epidemic

---

1. Marcus Conant, letter to Sheldon Andelson (a Los Angeles–based gay political fund-raiser who had expressed concerns about the study's accuracy), 17 September 1982, folder 16, box 1, Marcus A. Conant Papers, Archives and Special Collections, Library and Center for Knowledge Management, University of California–San Francisco (hereafter cited as Conant Papers).

2. Andrew R. Moss, "AIDS without End," letter to the editor, *New York Review of Books* 35, no. 19 (1988): 60.

and the other Randy Shilts's popular history, *And the Band Played On*.[3] Moss took issue with one section of the review in which the authors discussed a theory that suggested the North American epidemic could be traced to one individual. The epidemiologist complained that the authors had misattributed the "'patient zero' story" to him and had also indicated that most scientists, particularly his colleague William Darrow, were of the opinion that the story was no longer true. "This is not correct," Moss insisted, "the study on which the story is based was Darrow's; the opinion is mine." To drive the point home, he added: "I do however feel that it should be his as well."[4]

In his letter, Moss went on to deconstruct the cluster study, which had been conducted by Darrow and his colleagues at the US Centers for Disease Control (CDC) in 1982, during the early phase of that institution's response to AIDS.[5] The study had been published twice, first as a brief report in June 1982 and later as a more detailed peer-reviewed article in March 1984.[6] Moss noted that the study had reported "a 'cluster'"

3. Ibid. See also the original review: Diane Johnson and John F. Murray, "AIDS without End," *New York Review of Books* 35, no. 13 (1988): 57–63.

4. Moss, "AIDS without End," 60.

5. For a detailed investigation of the phases of this organization's growth and its many name changes, see William H. Foege, "Centers for Disease Control," *Journal of Public Health Policy* 2, no. 1 (1981): 8–18; Elizabeth W. Etheridge, *Sentinel for Health: A History of the Centers for Disease Control* (Berkeley: University of California Press, 1992). The institution was first a unit of the Public Health Service, or PHS (Malaria Control in War Areas, 1942), then an expanded field station of the Bureau of State Services (Communicable Disease Center, 1946). In 1967 its name changed to the National Communicable Disease Center, and in 1968 it became a bureau of the PHS. In 1970, the organization regained its old initials with a name change to the Center for Disease Control, and in 1973 it became a PHS agency. In October 1980, CDC's name changed to the Centers for Disease Control; finally, in October 1992, it became the Centers for Disease Control and Prevention. For simplicity, I will use the acronym CDC throughout.

6. Task Force on Kaposi's Sarcoma and Opportunistic Infections, CDC, "A Cluster of Kaposi's Sarcoma and *Pneumocystis carinii* Pneumonia among Homosexual Male Residents of Los Angeles and Range Counties, California," *MMWR* 31, no. 23 (1982): 305–7; David M. Auerbach et al., "Cluster of Cases of the Acquired Immune Deficiency Syndrome: Patients Linked by Sexual Contact," *American Journal of Medicine* 76, no. 3 (1984): 487–92. Further information was also contained in Roger C. Grimson and William W. Darrow, "Association between Acquired Immune Deficiency Syndrome and Sexual Contact: An Analysis of the Incidence Pattern," in *Infectious Complications of Neoplastic Disease: Controversies in Management*, ed. Arthur E. Brown and Donald Armstrong (New York: York Medical Books, 1985), 221–27; William W. Darrow, E. Michael Gorman, and Brad P. Glick, "The Social Origins of AIDS: Social Change, Sexual Behav-

of 40 cases of AIDS—taken from among the first 248 reported cases of AIDS in homosexual men in the United States—who had been shown to be linked through sexual contact up to five years prior to their displaying symptoms suggestive of AIDS (see fig. 2.1). One man—labeled "Patient 0"—was "placed at the center of the cluster: the inference is that he infected the persons who reported having sex with him, they infected the persons who reported having sex with them, and so on." Yet, as Moss would go on to argue, "when the evidence given is examined in detail the cluster dissolves." In condemnatory prose, the epidemiologist reduced the cluster to "a myth" and argued that the study represented "a textbook example of constructing your empirical evidence to fit your theory."[7]

The cluster study carried out by Darrow and his colleagues drew on techniques and approaches that were developed during an earlier era of public health efforts to control sexually transmitted infections with short incubation periods. Andrew Moss's criticisms in his letter to the *New York Review of Books* say as much about changes in the training, research focus, and professional self-image of epidemiologists in the late twentieth century as they do about his disagreement over the significance of a "Patient 0." These shifts and conflicts are more easily understood in historical perspective. Thus, instead of placing the cluster study near the beginning of research into the North American AIDS epidemic, this chapter situates that investigation at the end of a longer history of venereal disease (VD) control. Doing so makes it easier to understand how historical precedent shaped the ways in which the study was carried out, communicated, and resisted, and how some of the results worked against the investigators' stated intentions.

The chapter explores the circumstances that gave rise to the cluster study and the epidemiological phrase "Patient 0," and how, over time, this notion became embellished with new meanings and was rechristened as "Patient Zero." It suggests that the modes of professional thought and practice underpinning contact epidemiology—work that traces infection from contact to contact through a population—may have worked against

---

ior, and Disease Trends," in *The Social Dimensions of AIDS: Method and Theory*, ed. Douglas A. Feldman and Thomas M. Johnson (New York: Praeger, 1986), 95–107; William W. Darrow, "AIDS: Socioepidemiologic Responses to an Epidemic," in *AIDS and the Social Sciences: Common Threads*, ed. Richard Ulack and William F. Skinner (Lexington: University Press of Kentucky, 1991), 82–99.

7. Moss, "AIDS without End," 60.

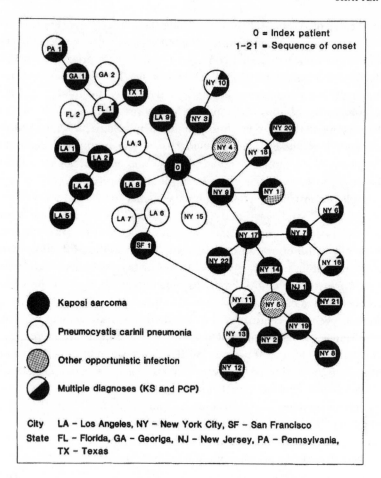

FIGURE 2.1 The extended Los Angeles cluster diagram, as it appeared in the *American Journal of Medicine* 76, no. 3 (1984): 488; 11 × 13.5 cm.

the aims of the cluster study's authors. Although William Darrow and his colleagues at the CDC may not have intended the study to position "Patient 0" as a source case for the North American epidemic, there exists, at the root of the cluster approach they used, the desire to trace an outbreak back to "the source." Decades of work in VD control had built faith in certain truths: that sexually active gay men were at high risk of acquiring and transmitting VD and that the contact tracing method typified by the "cluster" approach could eventually lead investigators to the root of an outbreak. In other words, structural forces—in terms of the objectives, methods, hypotheses, language, and other aspects of the working culture of a public health agency such as the CDC—placed constraints on the agency of historical actors, restricted their ability to break from tradition, and contributed to popular misreadings of their work.

The chapter begins with a consideration of general shifts in the field of epidemiology following the Second World War, and the trends in VD investigation at the CDC in particular. We will see how the changing understanding of disease patterns and at-risk populations, as well as the training of VD investigators, served to build faith in the power of the contact tracing method, on the one hand, and to pathologize men who had sex with other men, on the other. In 1981 and 1982, the initial activities of the CDC's Kaposi's Sarcoma and Opportunistic Infections (KS/OI) Task Force—made up of many individuals from the organization's VD division—were shaped by these historical legacies. In response to the appearance of a deadly and unknown condition, previous practice came together with the CDC's disease detective tradition to create a study whose terminology and findings were ripe for reinterpretation in subsequent years. The final sections of the chapter demonstrate how certain choices—word selections and decisions about how to visually represent the study's data—frequently steered audiences' interpretations in a direction contrary to the investigators' intentions.

I would like to stress an additional point. This chapter offers a critical analysis of the ways in which the cluster study has been communicated and interpreted since 1982 and, following Moss's 1988 letter to the *New York Review of Books,* emphasizes the implausibility of some of its underlying hypotheses based on what would subsequently become known about AIDS and HIV in the years after the study's completion. In doing so, there is no wish to diminish the work undertaken by the CDC investigators. Indeed, their efforts at this early stage, on a limited budget and under high pressure, are a testament to public health workers who undertake challenging assignments with fragmentary information in high-stake situations.

Mid-Twentieth-Century Shifts in Epidemiology

From its early work in malaria control, and its later acquisition of the US Public Health Service's Venereal Disease Division, the CDC had for decades been associated with control of infectious disease. While it did stretch its efforts into the realms of prevention and chronic illnesses in the 1970s, the organization's history and its efforts to eradicate first syphilis, then smallpox, kept it firmly associated with infectious disease outbreaks in the public mind.[8] Alexander Langmuir, the CDC's chief of epidemiology from 1949 to 1971, had done much during his tenure to secure this link by promoting the activities of the agency's best-known representatives: the Epidemic Intelligence Service (EIS) officers. After completing the CDC's six-week training course, these medical doctors were posted around the country, ready to assist state health officials with any challenging local outbreaks, often at a moment's notice.[9] Due to the combination of their good work and Langmuir's talent for publicity, the EIS officers became known as infectious "disease detectives" in popular accounts from the 1950s onward, most notably in the short stories of the *New Yorker* writer Berton Roueché. The detective image was not imprinted solely in the popular mind-set. The EIS self-consciously embraced this characterization too, adopting as its symbol a tie emblazoned with a well-worn shoe—indicative of detectives, or "gum-shoes," chasing down leads in the field.[10] Harold Jaffe, an infectious disease specialist who was one of the lead members of the KS/OI Task Force that conducted the initial investigations into AIDS, would later reflect, "I have often been asked what it was like to be one of the early AIDS investigators. To me, it all began as a medical mystery. I was caught up in being a 'medical detective' without much thought of the broader implications of what we were investigating. As time went on, however, I gradually began to see that what we were studying was much bigger than I had first imagined."[11]

The detective image also influenced, in an oppositional manner, the professional identity of a separate group of epidemiologists. From the midcentury onward, these researchers saw the techniques of their field shift away from those employed by the CDC disease investigators. This

---

8. For a discussion of the CDC's expansion into broader areas of health prevention, see Etheridge, *Sentinel for Health*, 276–320.

9. For a historical view of the CDC's less widely celebrated yet indispensable public health advisors, see Beth E. Meyerson, Frederick A. Martich, and Gerald P. Naehr, *Ready to Go: The History and Contributions of U.S. Public Health Advisors* (Research Triangle Park, NC: American Social Health Association, 2008).

10. Ibid., 36–48; Wald, *Contagious*, 23–25.

11. Harold W. Jaffe, "The Early Days of the HIV-AIDS Epidemic in the USA," *Nature Immunology* 9, no. 11 (2008): 1203.

group of epidemiologists began to deal with the increasingly prevalent cancers and chronic conditions which formed the bulk of American morbidity and mortality in the post–World War II period.[12] As historian Allan Brandt has argued persuasively with regard to researchers assessing the harms of smoking, a "new epidemiology" emerged in the middle of the twentieth century. Investigators at this time revisited the use of statistical inference and population studies, methods that had been popular in the nineteenth century before the powerful ascendancy of ideas related to germ theory. From the 1880s onward, scientists who followed the bacteriologist Robert Koch's postulates of causation—searching for specific mechanisms as the causes of specific diseases—had achieved great successes in the laboratory. However, the chronic diseases emerging as a concern in the mid-twentieth century required a different set of analytical tools. Researchers returned to the use of statistics—an approach displaced for decades by germ theory's emphasis on laboratory evidence of a disease's cause—to develop ever more sophisticated means of investigating disease causation.[13] Andrew Moss's training, first in statistics and then for a PhD in cancer epidemiology, might be seen as indicative of the field's developing professional divide.[14]

While this shift toward population-based epidemiology was under way, it is important to recognize that at the CDC's Venereal Disease Branch, and at other city, county, and state public health departments around the country, the traditional approach of laboratory-supported person-to-person disease investigation—"contact epidemiology"—was still going strong, particularly in the control of venereal disease. In 1957, the Washington-based VD Division of the Public Health Service was relocated to Atlanta, absorbed by a growing CDC. In the large-scale national campaign to eradicate syphilis that followed a special task force

12. Mervyn Susser, "Epidemiology in the United States after World War II: The Evolution of Technique," *Epidemiologic Reviews* 7, no. 1 (1985): 147–77; Mervyn Susser and Ezra Susser, "Choosing a Future for Epidemiology: I. Eras and Paradigms," *American Journal of Public Health* 86, no. 5 (1996): 668–73.

13. Allan M. Brandt, *The Cigarette Century: The Rise, Fall, and Deadly Persistence of the Product that Defined America* (New York: Basic Books, 2007), 118–23, 148–52.

14. Andrew R. Moss, "AIDS Epidemiology: Investigating and Getting the Word Out," oral history interview conducted in 1992 by Sally Smith Hughes, in *The AIDS Epidemic in San Francisco: The Medical Response, 1981–1984, Volume II*, Regional Oral History Office, Bancroft Library, University of California–Berkeley, 1996, Online Archive of California, 2009, http://ark.cdlib.org/ark:/13030/kt7b69n8jn.

report to the surgeon general in 1961, more than half of the CDC's personnel were working on VD control.[15] The report called for increased funding to support expanded syphilis case-finding and public-education efforts. The resulting case-finding program, Operation Pursuit, viewed every index case—the first sick individual brought to investigators' attention—as a potential cause of an epidemic, requiring more health workers to interview and reinterview individuals with syphilis for the names and contact information of their sex contacts.[16]

VD Control and the Cluster Method

It was in this climate that Bill Darrow joined the CDC in 1963 as a public health advisor, shortly after his graduation from university and following a yearlong contract of work as a venereal disease investigator for the New York City Department of Health. His early work with the CDC was representative of the optimistic aims of Operation Pursuit: to eradicate the scourge of syphilis by tracking down every index case, interviewing each of them for the names of potential contacts, and treating with penicillin those suspected of being infected. Young, educated, male, and white (Darrow would later recall playing a role in challenging this stereotype as a CDC recruiter), the public health advisor was viewed as an essential player in the investigation of potential syphilis cases and

15. Etheridge, *Sentinel for Health*, 87–92, 119.
16. Ibid., 121; John Parascandola, *Sex, Sin, and Science: A History of Syphilis* (Westport, CT: Praeger, 2008), 140–42; Amy L. Fairchild, "The Democratization of Privacy: Public-Health Surveillance and Changing Perceptions of Privacy in Twentieth-Century America," in *History and Health Policy in the United States: Putting the Past Back In*, ed. Rosemary A. Stevens, Charles E. Rosenberg, and Lawton R. Burns (London: Rutgers University Press, 2006), 121–22. A 1936 report on tuberculosis offers a useful working definition of *index case*: "that person through whom attention was drawn to the household, and may not be the only case in the household, or the initial case in the household in point of time"; H. C. Stewart, R. S. Gass, and Ruth R. Puffer, "Tuberculosis Studies in Tennessee: A Clinic Study with Reference to Epidemiology within the Family," *American Journal of Public Health and the Nation's Health* 26, no. 7 (1936): 689–90. Note also the following definition of the word *case*: "In epidemiology, a person in the population or study group identified as having the particular disease, health disorder, or condition under investigation"; *A Dictionary of Epidemiology*. ed. John Last (New York: Oxford University Press, 1983), s.v. "case."

bringing them to treatment.[17] Such investigators were "carefully selected for their tact, integrity, intelligence, interviewing ability, personality, and their understanding of the confidential nature of their work."[18] Idealistic in outlook, the young Darrow had felt as though President John F. Kennedy "was talking to me when he said, 'Ask not what your country can do for you, but rather ask what you can do for your country.'"[19]

Darrow and other public health advisors like him had at their disposal a newly developed technique of syphilis control: the cluster method. Whereas venereal disease case finding had traditionally relied on interviewing solely the sexual contacts named by the patient with syphilis, "cluster testing" extended this traditional practice by having investigators interview and test the patient's friends and acquaintances as well.[20] Incorporating a language that was strongly suggestive of detective fiction, a syphilis cluster was expanded beyond the usual contacts to include "suspects," those acquaintances whom the person with syphilis suspected might also have the disease, and "associates," who "may be a friend or social acquaintance who is named by or found in the company of sex contacts or 'suspects.'"[21] The cluster method emerged at a time when certain populations in the United States were being increasingly viewed as mobile disease threats requiring screening, identification, and control. Sex workers and African Americans, for example, had long and problematically been associated in the medical and popular imagination with higher levels of syphilis.[22] To these traditional "res-

17. Despite the fact that women had performed contact tracing duties for decades, it was thought that only men were able to undertake this risky occupation: see William W. Darrow, "A Few Minutes with Venus, A Lifetime with Mercury," in *The Sex Scientists*, ed. Gary G. Brannigan, Elizabeth R. Allgeier, and A. Richard Allgeier (New York: Addison, Wesley, Longman, 1998), 162–63.

18. William J. Brown, Thomas F. Sellers, and Evan W. Thomas, "Challenge to the Private Physician in the Epidemiology of Syphilis," *Journal of the American Medical Association* 171, no. 4 (1959): 392.

19. Darrow, "Few Minutes," 157.

20. William J. Brown, "Cluster Testing—A New Development in Syphilis Case Finding," *American Journal of Public Health* 51, no. 7 (1961): 1043–48; Etheridge, *Sentinel for Health*, 91–92.

21. W. Brown, "Cluster Testing," 1045.

22. See, for example, Elizabeth Fee, "Sin versus Science: Venereal Disease in Twentieth-Century Baltimore," in Fee and Fox, *AIDS: The Burdens of History*, 125; Brandt, *No Magic Bullet*, 31–32; James H. Jones, *Bad Blood: The Tuskegee Syphilis Experiment*, rev. and expanded ed. (New York: Free Press, 1993), 16–29.

ervoirs" of VD—the terminology employed by public health workers at the time, evoking connections with polluted wells and a residual social pool of infection—were added two other marginal and frequently mobile groups: migrant laborers from Mexico and homosexual men.

In 1959, as part of a series that profiled the CDC's work, a *Washington Post* reporter outlined how officials were "Meeting the Health Threat of Mexican Migrants."[23] He described how each year roughly four hundred thousand Mexican "braceros," or hand laborers, legally entered the United States to work on farms "from the Rio Grande border as far north as Michigan." These workers, he wrote, had until recently "posed an annual threat to this Nation's efforts to control venereal diseases." Without elaborating on why authorities thought there might be a higher prevalence of venereal disease in this population, the reporter warned that an unfettered US need for laborers had resulted in these Mexican workers being hired without attention to their health. In his view, the result of such an indiscriminate search for labor was clear: "the ready reception was perpetuating self-imported contagions of syphilis, gonorrhea and other venereal diseases." The reporter quoted William J. Brown, the director of Venereal Disease Control at the CDC, who praised the "newly developed technique" of cluster testing, which he assured the nation could halt the rising incidence of syphilis. According to Brown, by interviewing and testing those in the "living and travel environments" of the individuals with syphilis, investigators could raise the ratio of uncovered cases from 34 for every 100 checked using conventional methods to 54 for every 100 checked. One might wonder whether the approach simply allowed medical authorities to test based on race, class, and later sexual behavior, providing a scientific scaffold onto which cultural stereotypes could be erected. Perhaps seeking to neutralize such criticism, the reporter pointed out that Mexico benefited from the inspections too, "since the names and addresses of the VD-infected and their home community sex contacts are supplied to the appropriate Mexican local health departments."[24]

23. Nate Haseltine, "Meeting the Health Threat of Mexican Migrants," *Washington Post*, February 25, 1959, B7.

24. All quotations in the paragraph in ibid. Brown headed the Venereal Disease Division of the CDC from 1957 to 1971, working for years to promote the need to seek out and treat venereal disease in most of the American population. He would subsequently receive less favorable attention for his role in the continuation of the Tuskegee syphilis experiment: see Jones, *Bad Blood*, 180–209.

Brown published a separate article dealing with the difficulties that mobile populations presented for VD control efforts, in which he outlined the modern solutions that disease control workers had at their disposal. While the article's text acknowledged the effects of mobile Americans in spreading disease—particularly those taking part in the massive postwar increase in leisure travel by automobile—the accompanying photographs suggested a racialized understanding of disease spread, one which viewed national health security as under threat. White male health officials out "in the field," resplendent in white shirts and dark ties, extended the virtues of science by performing rapid syphilis tests, in one photo on a darker-skinned seaman and in another on a group of Mexican workers. A map positioned above the photograph of these workers suggests a slow, northward spread of VD, unchecked but for the unrelenting efforts of the CDC's scientific testing and treatment (see fig. 2.2).[25]

"Reservoirs of Infectious Venereal Disease"

To this group was added another population that had begun to attract heightened concern among public health workers: homosexuals. While homosexual men had for decades wrestled with a medical discourse that constructed them as pathological, during the first half of the twentieth century they had generally not been associated in the medical and scientific literature with higher levels of venereal diseases. Instead, medical science had interpreted their difference largely in terms of psychological and psychiatric deviance.[26] Gradually this focus began to broaden at midcentury, with public health officials and physicians increasingly discussing men having sex with other men as a group at higher risk of acquiring VD.[27]

25. William J. Brown, "Migration as a Factor in Venereal Disease Programmes in the United States," *British Journal of Venereal Diseases* 36, no. 1 (1960): 49–58. This reading coexists uncomfortably alongside other photographs from this period showing PHS employees drawing blood from black participants in the Tuskegee syphilis study; see images following p. 108 in Susan M. Reverby, *Examining Tuskegee: The Infamous Syphilis Study and Its Legacy* (Chapel Hill: University of North Carolina Press, 2009).

26. See Jennifer Terry, "The Seductive Power of Science in the Making of Deviant Subjectivity," in *Science and Homosexualities*, ed. Vernon A. Rosario (New York: Routledge, 1997), 271–96.

27. Herman Goodman, "An Epidemic of Genital Chancres from Perversion," *Ameri-

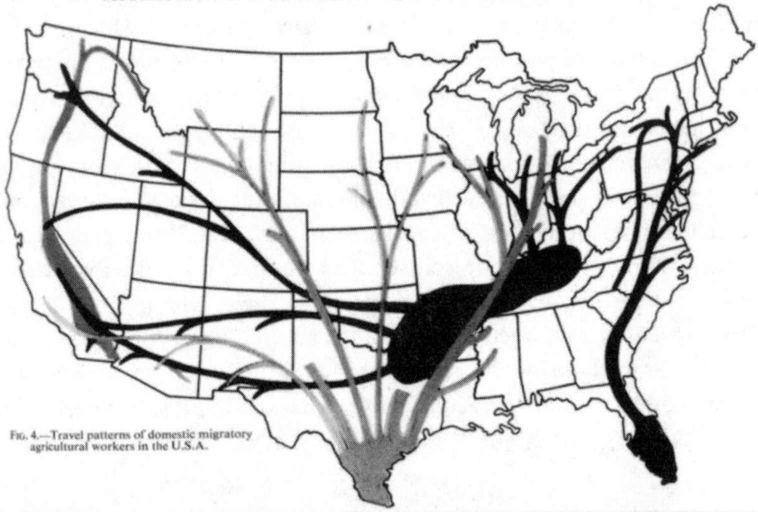

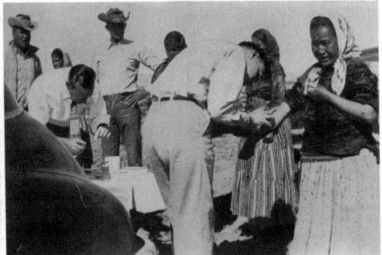

FIG. 4.—Travel patterns of domestic migratory agricultural workers in the U.S.A.

FIG. 5.—Field testing station for migratory agricultural workers.

FIGURE 2.2 Map depicting travel patterns of domestic migratory agricultural workers and photograph of rapid syphilis testing in the United States, 1960, both in William J. Brown, "Migration as a Factor in Venereal Disease Programmes in the United States," *British Journal of Venereal Diseases* 36, no. 1 (1960): 53, map and photograph each 14.5 × 9.5 cm. The original captions accompanying the images have been retained to provide context. Readers are invited to compare this map of the United States, which suggests the external threat of syphilis—pumped slowly throughout the country via the arterial-like migration of agricultural workers—with the very different image in chapter 4, figure 4.1.

"Homosexuality as a Source of Venereal Disease," the title of an article published in 1951 by two concerned venereal specialists in Vancouver, Canada, succinctly captured the emerging view of "a hitherto unsuspected source" of VD transmission.[28] The physicians' language here echoed centuries-old views that perceived certain individuals—particularly female prostitutes and wet nurses—to be not simply conduits but sources of venereal disease.[29] While these physicians were by no means to first to report that sexual contact between men could transmit infections, a long-practiced cultural silence surrounding same-sex sexual practices would mean that a number of physicians over hundreds of years would "discover" this particular mode of transmission anew.[30]

---

can Journal of Syphilis, Gonorrhea, and Venereal Diseases 28 (1944): 310–14; this article is also cited in William W. Darrow et al., "The Gay Report on Sexually Transmitted Diseases," American Journal of Public Health 71, no. 9 (1981): 1004, 1010; Parascandola, Sex, Sin, and Science, 146–47. For an examination of the mid-twentieth-century associations linking sex between men with venereal disease, which expands upon the material in this section, see Richard A. McKay, "Before HIV: Venereal Disease among Homosexually Active Men in England and North America," in The Routledge History of Disease, ed. Mark Jackson, 441–59 (London: Routledge, 2017), http://www.tandfebooks.com/userimages/ContentEditor/1489134497468/9780415720014_oachapter24.pdf.

28. B. Kanee and C. L. Hunt, "Homosexuality as a Source of Venereal Disease," Canadian Medical Association Journal 65, no. 2 (1951): 138–40.

29. William Naphy, Sex Crimes: From Renaissance to Enlightenment (Stroud: Tempus, 2002), 57–58. Roger Davidson relates how in 1973 a Scottish committee tasked with controlling sexually transmitted diseases described "passive homosexuals" as "reservoirs of infection": see "'The Price of the Permissive Society': The Epidemiology and Control of VD and STDs in Late-Twentieth-Century Scotland," in Sex, Sin and Suffering: Venereal Disease and European Society since 1870, ed. Roger Davidson and Lesley A. Hall (London: Routledge, 2001), 220–36.

30. For a possible mid-nineteenth-century suggestion that male prisoners could transmit diseases through "libidinous indiscretions," see Jonathan Ned Katz, Gay American History: Lesbians and Gay Men in the U.S.A. (New York: Thomas Y. Crowell, 1976), 572. By 1892, Katz reports that a professor of nervous diseases in Washington, DC, presented a paper to his colleagues about the spread of venereal disease through same-sex acts (40–42). Work on the early modern period in Spain, France, and England suggests that physicians and patients may have been aware of this mode of venereal disease transmission but practiced a well-kept silence. See Cristian Berco, "Syphilis and the Silencing of Sodomy in Juan Calvo's Tratado Del Morbo Gálico," in The Sciences of Homosexuality in Early Modern Europe, ed. Kenneth Borris and George Rousseau (New York: Routledge, 2008, 92–113; Kevin Siena, "The Strange Medical Silence on Same-Sex Transmission of the Pox, c. 1660–1760," in Borris and Rousseau, Sciences of Homosexuality in Early Modern Europe, 115–33.

The Vancouver physicians' comments were amplified a decade later at the World Forum on Syphilis and other Treponematoses, held in Washington, DC, in 1962. Twelve hundred participants attended the conference, organized as part of an American-led drive to eradicate syphilis—among them, the newly appointed VD investigator Bill Darrow.[31] To assembled delegates, one speaker, a medical representative of the Los Angeles City Health Department, declared that the "social clustering" of homosexual men in urban environments "creates a huge reservoir when syphilis is introduced." This trend, he noted, had been witnessed in Los Angeles—where early case rates had tripled over the last decade—as well as other urban centers. Of the 506 male syphilis patients his department's staff had interviewed for contact information, one half had revealed exclusively homosexual contacts, and less than a third named only female contacts. "Unquestionably," the speaker concluded, "the white male homosexual has replaced the female prostitute as a major focus of syphilis infection."[32]

Researchers in New York further cemented the connection between homosexual men and VD in a 1963 article, noting the "mounting concern that this is one of the important reservoirs of infectious venereal disease."[33] The authors emphasized that homosexual men made up 15 percent of all new VD cases treated by physicians in solo practice in Manhattan during a study conducted in 1960 and 1961, and that epi-

31. Nate Haseltine, "Complacency Slowed Anti-Syphilis Drive in U.S., Health Chief Admits," *Washington Post*, September 5, 1962, A3.

32. Ralph R. Sachs, "Effect of Urbanization on the Spread of Syphilis," in *Proceedings of World Forum*, by U.S. Department of Health, Education and Welfare (Washington, DC: US Government Printing Office, 1964), 154–55. The racial specificity of this remark is striking, particularly when compared to other contemporary links being made between VD and certain racial/ethnic groups. It raises questions about the use of public clinics by different groups, racial segregation in sexual networks in Los Angeles during this period, and the possibility of differing levels of comfort among men of different racial and ethnic groups in acknowledging partners of the same sex to public health officials. The last point resonates with more recent discussions of "secretive sex," between non-gay-identified men who have sex with men, in the context of HIV prevention; see Lena D. Saleh and Don Operario, "Moving Beyond 'the Down Low': A Critical Analysis of Terminology Guiding HIV Prevention Efforts for African American Men Who Have Secretive Sex with Men," *Social Science and Medicine* 68 (2009): 390–95.

33. Anna C. Gelman, Jules E. Vandow, and Nathan Sobel, "Current Status of Venereal Disease in New York City: A Survey of 6,649 Physicians in Solo Practice," *American Journal of Public Health* 53, no. 12 (1963): 1912.

demiologic investigations of this population were of "vital importance," given their potential to uncover chains of sexual contacts numbering in the hundreds.[34] From the late 1950s onward, investigators responded to this growing sense of urgency with vigor. Author and later AIDS activist Larry Kramer recalled in an interview the tenacious qualities of a VD investigator attempting such an inquiry: "In 1958 when I came to New York, after the army, I got syphilis from somebody. And in those days syphilis was a reportable thing to the public health people and they'd contact you. And this health care worker came to interview me, and he wanted to know everybody I'd been to bed with. And I had no idea and we would get in his car and we would drive around, and I'd say, 'Oh, up there on the third floor.' Literally."[35]

From a public health perspective that viewed male homosexuals as an undrained "reservoir" of infection, the cluster interviewing technique appeared to be effective. The author of a report of a "Homosexual Syphilis Epidemic" in Fort Worth, Texas, explained that repeatedly interviewing infected patients, as well as their sexual partners and associates, allowed investigators to detect more infected individuals and to break through what they perceived to be a protective wall of silence. This approach was likely to succeed, in the author's view, due to "the fact that the homosexual group is an exclusive fraternity and that friends of homosexuals are, in most instances, sex partners as well. In a large homosexual group it is impossible to show by epidemiologic charting the widespread inter-relation of the group. During an interview of one of the last patients diagnosed as infectious, the request for names of contacts incurred the remark, 'I'll be glad to tell you who I've been with, but you have already checked all the people like me in town.'"[36]

This quotation invites several observations. First, it suggests the investigator's faith in the effectiveness of the cluster technique in identifying suspected infections by casting wide the net of suspicion. Second, it points crudely to one of the challenges faced by contact epidemiologists. With

34. Ibid., 1915.

35. Larry Kramer, interview with author, New York City, April 14, 2008, recording C1491/23, tape 1, side B, BLSA.

36. W. V. Bradshaw Jr., "Homosexual Syphilis Epidemic," *Texas State Journal of Medicine* 57 (1961): 909. The author urged readers to look beneath appearances, as one married man—who was "an alert, intelligent person with none of the characteristics normally attributed to the homosexual"—nevertheless yielded the names of twenty-eight homosexual contacts under the duress of a 2½-hour interview.

the widespread interrelatedness of sexual partners in some homosexual networks, it was extremely difficult to represent all of the connections between members, a point that would again be recognized in the AIDS era. Third, it highlights the extent to which some investigators believed that they were dealing with a secretive, and potentially hostile, band of deviants. The curiously ambivalent final remark from the patient appears to have been received as a confirmation of the cluster technique's effectiveness, though it may also read as a studied refusal to supply names.

Certainly, venereal disease investigators were taught to expect that many homosexual men would attempt to conceal their sexual identity and the names of their sexual partners, and that it was the investigator's responsibility to deftly wrest the information from them. Darrow later wrote, self-deprecatingly, of his youthful enthusiasm and skill in applying the taught interview technique "to discover the patients' most intimate secrets and to elicit information from them about other people who might be infected with syphilis."[37] The 1962 *Field Manual* of the Venereal Disease Division of the CDC, which was prescribed training material for all new investigators, emphasized the benefits of such diligent and persistent interviewing: "Although laws and circumstances differ in various states, and elaborate safeguards are invariably thrown around the right of the physician to protect his patient's reputation, it is often possible by persuasion to ferret out the chain of contacts, frequently with rewarding—though astonishing—results."[38]

The manual's description of the investigator invokes the familiar persona of a detective, further demonstrating the Venereal Disease Division's self-identification with the popular image of CDC workers being presented in the press. The good investigator, it explained, "must know the places where people gather to spend leisure and socialization time. It is advisable to become friends of the owners, managers, waitresses, bartenders, etc. of certain establishments. These people can give him the three-monkey act, 'hear nothing, see nothing, speak nothing' or, on the other hand, supply him with much helpful information if proper relationships have been made."[39] Though much of the contact-tracing work

37. Darrow, "Few Minutes," 158.

38. US Department of Health, Education, and Welfare, *Venereal Disease Branch Field Manual* (Atlanta: Communicable Disease Center, 1962), H18. When I met with Darrow in March 2008, he suggested that the manual was "where I learned it all."

39. Ibid., E27.

would focus on urban areas, the manual helpfully noted that "in rural areas the cross-road storekeeper and the rural route mailman are good sources of information."[40] The book's euphemistic reference to "certain establishments" suggests known trouble spots or hideaways and hints at the background role of alcohol, which facilitated the sexual interactions enabling the spread of VD. The manual also emphasized that the investigator, in fulfilling his "enigmatic" function, needed to recognize that his work could have him interact with anyone. "He may use his facts in a somewhat evasive manner, if necessary," the text explained, "to effect the examination of a husband, a wife, a teenager from a prominent family, a child, a prostitute, or a homosexual executive, so as not to disturb the status of any of them." To protect the people he investigated from social sanction, the investigator would "learn through experience to become a master at evasion and a professional purveyor of silence."[41]

Investigators were to be attentive to clues suggested by comments made by the subject, paying early attention to the subject's field of employment: "Here the interviewer may receive his first indication as to the sexual behavior of the patient. Certain known occupations may suggest deviant sexual activity to the interviewer."[42] Similarly, the manual highlighted the qualities investigators could expect to find and were explicitly seeking to confirm: "With this and subsequent sexual behavior questions, the interviewer attempts to establish the fact that the patient is a sexually promiscuous person and that this promiscuity has developed into a continuous pattern from early in life."[43] Given the mid-twentieth-century concerns linking homosexuality with venereal disease, the manual gave detailed instructions to investigators on how to elicit such information and assess whether someone was being untruthful when asked whether he had any same-sex sexual partners. "Based on past experiences, the observant interviewer may obtain some indication about the patient's sexual adjustment from the manner in which a negative

40. Ibid.
41. Ibid., E29.
42. Ibid., E15. A sociological study of the Montreal gay community had claimed that "overt homosexuals" tended to work in occupations either with "traditionally accepted homosexual linkages," such as the artist, the interior decorator, and the hairdresser, or ones "of such low rank" to allow them to be open, such as the counterman or the bellhop. See Maurice Leznoff and William A. Westley, "The Homosexual Community," *Social Problems* 3, no. 4 (1956): 257–63.
43. US Department of Health, Education, and Welfare, *Field Manual*, E16.

response is delivered. A hostile "no" or a labored, thoughtful "no" can be indicative of a deviant sexual adjustment. A completely heterosexually oriented person will usually respond with an amused and/or humorous 'no.'"[44] Investigators were encouraged to rephrase the question in a number of ways if they were answered in the negative, in a manner that implied to the interviewee:

> That the patient needs help with his problem and the interviewer can provide this help.
> That the interviewer has received and handled this confidence before.
> 3. That this behavior is quite "normal" for many people."[45]

Certainly, an ambivalent tension exists throughout the manual, one which is perhaps representative of VD control efforts in the penicillin era. On the one hand, the authors construct the syphilitic patient in general, and the homosexual patient in particular, as deviant and pathological. On the other hand, they recognize that the investigator will achieve more success if he appears sympathetic to the patient to gain the information he needs. As the CDC-trained head of New York City's VD investigators told a reporter in 1961, "We're not involved in questions of morality. We don't judge people. We don't care who they are or what they are. No court in the land could get us to give them a name from our files. We have only one job: Find the people who may be exposed, get them to treatment."[46]

Gay and Lesbian Health Activism in the 1970s

While these efforts to control VD were under way, dramatic legal, social, and cultural shifts in the 1960s and early 1970s continued to thrust homosexuality into the public eye. These changes mounted a challenge to the previously dominant views of homosexuality as criminal behavior and psychiatric disturbance, while simultaneously strengthening the link between venereal disease and gay men. The Canadian government, follow-

44. Ibid., E17.
45. Ibid.
46. Joseph Giordano, quoted in Bernard Gavner, "U.S. Wages War on Rise in VD: Medical Sleuths Have Job of Tracking Down Disease," *Niagara Falls Gazette*, April 23, 1961, 9A.

ing the lead of the United Kingdom, which in 1967 had partially decriminalized sex between men, implemented law reforms that amended the Criminal Code in 1969 by removing penalties for sexual contact between two adult males in private.[47] Meanwhile, across North America, a culture of youth-driven protest surrounding the Vietnam War, women's rights, and the civil rights movement contributed to an escalated and more radicalized form of confrontation regarding homosexuality. These newly energized efforts built on the work of the homophile groups that had been slowly organizing since the 1950s.[48] Two of the most powerful symbols of this trend were the 1969 Stonewall riots in New York City and the 1973 decision by the American Psychiatry Association to delist homosexuality as a mental illness in the organization's *Diagnostic and Statistical Manual of Mental Disorders*. The first served as a rallying point for an increasingly vocal gay liberation movement, while the second called into question the authority of medicine to label homosexuality as deviant.[49]

The CDC's VD control efforts met with mixed results during this period. Sexual mores had undergone a profound transformation since the Second World War, a series of changes catalyzed by the more general rise of antiauthoritarian protest and the introduction of the birth control pill.[50] The organization's work to eradicate syphilis fell victim to funding cuts at the moments when they demonstrated signs of success; despite some initial progress, it became evident that the 1972 eradication goal would not be met. The CDC also weathered controversy when leaked information revealed that it was overseeing the Tuskegee study, which for forty years had charted the effects of untreated syphilis in black male patients.[51] Despite these setbacks, the organization expanded its VD control efforts to include an assault on the growing epidemic of gonor-

47. Gary Kinsman, "Wolfenden in Canada: Within and beyond Official Discourse in Law Reform Struggles," in *Human Rights, Sexual Orientation and Gender Identity in the Commonwealth: Struggles for Decriminalisation and Change*, ed. Corinne Lennox and Matthew Waites (London: School of Advanced Study, University of London, 2013), 183–205.

48. D'Emilio, *Sexual Politics, Sexual Communities*.

49. Martin B. Duberman, *Stonewall* (New York: Plume, 1994), 169–212, 224; Ronald Bayer, *Homosexuality and American Psychiatry: The Politics of Diagnosis* (New York: Basic Books, 1981); Minton, *Departing from Deviance*, 219–64.

50. Cokie Roberts and Steven V. Roberts, "The Venereal Disease Pandemic," *New York Times*, November 7, 1971, SM62–81.

51. Jean Heller, "Syphilis Victims in U.S. Study Went Untreated for 40 Years," *New York Times*, July 26, 1972, 1, 8; Reverby, *Examining Tuskegee*.

rhea, as well as preventive work with the development of a vaccine for hepatitis B that involved increasingly close collaboration with the gay community.[52]

Bill Darrow continued to work on venereal disease, studying behavioral aspects of sexuality that thwarted prevention efforts. His doctoral thesis in sociology, completed in 1973, examined the low condom usage of heterosexual patients attending public health clinics in Sacramento, California, and the associated impact on VD control efforts. He was part of a team "investigating the source and spread" of a penicillin-resistant strain of gonorrhea in the United States in 1976, and in 1977 he joined another group studying hepatitis B incidence, prevalence, and prevention in gay men.[53] Darrow's work on hepatitis B allowed him to develop collaborative relationships with gay physicians in five US cities. These medical professionals were part of a wave of lesbian and gay health activism that emerged in the 1970s and which saw the creation of health services as an intrinsic part of gay liberation and community building.[54] One of the gay doctors, David Ostrow, who worked at Chicago's Howard Brown Clinic, provided Darrow with the tip that two gay liberation activist-journalists, Karla Jay and Allen Young, were in the process of compiling a study entitled *The Gay Report*. This study sought to compile the responses of more than five thousand gays and lesbians to surveys sent out in a number of American and Canadian gay periodicals, undertaking, in the authors' words, not "a 'scientific' approach to homosexuality, but rather a personal one."[55] Darrow wrote to Jay to inquire whether he could undertake secondary analyses of the data related to sexually transmitted infections and gay men. This self-reported information would offer a useful comparative with the existing data, which had predominantly been gathered from men reporting to public clinics.[56]

Darrow's letter to Jay politely and conscientiously indicated that the sociologist was well aware of the ongoing development and multifaceted nature of the increasingly public gay world, suggesting that "these data

52. Etheridge, *Sentinel for Health*, 235–44.

53. Darrow, "Few Minutes," 166–67; William Darrow, interview with author, Miami, March 28, 2008, recording C1491/21, tape 1, side A, BLSA.

54. Catherine P. Batza, "Before AIDS: Gay and Lesbian Community Health Activism in the 1970s" (DPhil diss., University of Illinois at Chicago, 2012).

55. Karla Jay and Allen Young, *The Gay Report: Lesbians and Gay Men Speak Out about Sexual Experiences and Lifestyles* (New York: Summit Books, 1979), 16.

56. Darrow et al., "Gay Report on STDs," 1004.

may help us develop more effective venereal disease control programs for the Gay Community (or is it communities?)."[57] His "hope that we will meet and be able to share our observations" was granted: Jay replied with an ebullient enthusiasm, commenting that "the original prospectus probably greatly underestimated how many gay people we could reach with our efforts, and the number will probably be over 500,000. Thus, this will be the largest study done of gay people—or probably of any people!"[58] Jay noted that she and Young had already depleted their publisher's advance by mailing out the questionnaires and could benefit from financial support to assist with computer analysis of the survey results: "Let us know whether your center will be willing to help us. I don't have to convince you that this information will be absolutely invaluable in understanding the relations between sex acts and incidence of venereal disease, and in spotting any possible patterns of venereal disease and hepatitis occurrence across the United States and Canada (perhaps the Canadian health agency you work with would be interested in co-funding?)."[59]

Ultimately Jay wrote to Paul Wiesner, the director of the Venereal Disease Control Division, and offered the CDC access to coded computer results of the survey at a cost of $7,000. Jay articulated the potential for venereal diseases to spread beyond gay men—anticipating a rationale that would be voiced with regard to AIDS a few years later—and argued that the data would be "of great service to the homosexual and heterosexual communities alike (since some gay men are not exclusively homosexual)."[60] The agency eventually agreed in 1978, paying $7,202.00 for data from approximately four thousand respondents. This exchange resulted, ironically, in a US government agency cofunding a project devoted to the explicit exploration of diverse gay and lesbian sexual practices during one of the more virulently antihomosexual periods of the twentieth century.[61]

57. William Darrow to Karla Jay, 26 May 1977, folder: *Gay Report*: responses to surveys, box 22, Karla Jay Papers, Manuscripts and Archives Division, New York Public Library (hereafter cited as Jay Papers).

58. Karla Jay to William Darrow, 17 June 1977, p. 2, *Gay Report*, Jay Papers.

59. Ibid., 3; "venereal disease and hepatitis occurrence" corrected from "veneral disease and hepetitis occurence" in original.

60. Karla Jay to Paul Wiesner, 16 November 1977, *Gay Report*, Jay Papers.

61. CDC, Contract Order Form #35854, June 1, 1978, *Gay Report*, Jay Papers. The contract order form took care to stipulate that no personal identifiers be provided. The CDC's

Darrow conducted secondary analyses on these data and was at work preparing them for publication in February 1981 when, at a regular meeting, he heard his colleague Mary Guinan report on an unusual case involving a gay man in New York City.[62] The patient had been diagnosed with disseminated herpes, had very few T cells, and was dying from a disease of unknown origin. In the years to come, Darrow would make use of all his previous training and experience to search for a cause and understand this condition.

"A Jigsaw Puzzle"

When Darrow flew out to Los Angeles in March 1982 in response to a call from his EIS officer colleague David Auerbach, he had been considering the geographic distribution of the early reported cases of Kaposi's sarcoma and opportunistic infections in the United States for some nine months. Since June 1981, reports of young homosexual men afflicted with unusual illnesses were reaching the CDC with increasing frequency, predominantly from New York, Los Angeles, and San Francisco. Darrow had been co-opted onto the CDC's KS/OI Task Force soon after its formation that month, chosen for his many years of work and interviewing experience within the CDC's Venereal Disease Control Division (VDCD) and his links with gay researchers across the country. The task force brought together members from various CDC divisions, including immunology, parasitic diseases, and virology, in addition to a core group from VDCD. The group's activities took place under financial strain: the recent 1981 Omnibus Budget Reconciliation Act had led to staff reductions at the CDC. Thus, the KS/OI Task Force had been set up on a tem-

---

forging of ties with gay groups during the 1970s is discussed in Batza, "Before AIDS," 233–65; Etheridge, *Sentinel for Health*, 326–27. For more on opposition to the gay rights movement in the 1970s—namely, the much-publicized work of Anita Bryant and John V. Briggs—see Randy Shilts, *The Mayor of Castro Street: The Life and Times of Harvey Milk* (New York: St. Martin's Press, 1982), 153–68, 211–45; Dudley Clendinen and Adam Nagourney, *Out for Good: The Struggle to Build a Gay Rights Movement in America* (New York: Simon & Schuster, 1999), 291–390.

62. The article would be published in September of that year, in collaboration with Jay and Young: Darrow et al., "Gay Report on STDs," 1004–11; Darrow, recording C1491/21, tape 1, side A.

porary basis within the Sexually Transmitted Disease Division and had to operate within the division's existing budget.[63]

Minutes from an early meeting held on June 10, 1981, suggested the directions that would steer the group's later inquiries. Representatives from the CDC's Center for Infectious Diseases (CID), Center for Prevention Services (CPS), Center for Environmental Health (CEH), and the Epidemiology Program Office (EPO) had gathered to discuss the cases of KS in male homosexuals, prompted by a telephone call on June 5, 1981, from Alvin Friedman-Kien, which coincided with the first report in the *Morbidity and Mortality Weekly Report* (*MMWR*) about pneumonia cases among five gay men in Los Angeles.[64] This cancer specialist at New York University had phoned to report thirty cases of KS diagnosed in New York City over the previous two years. In the meeting, James Curran, chief of the Operational Research Branch for VD Control in CPS, shared reports of additional cases of *Pneumocystis carinii* pneumonia (PCP), cytomegalovirus (CMV), *Campylobacter*, and severe herpes infection among homosexual men in San Francisco, Palo Alto, and New York City. David Gordon, an immunology specialist, ventured that immune suppression seemed to be the common factor underlying the cases of PCP, CMV, and KS which had been reported, and that "one or more co-factors would explain the occurrence of these diseases in homosexuals better than a single specific infectious organism such as CMV." Harold Jaffe of VDCD responded that "a new, more virulent strain of CMV might explain the recent clustering," since CMV in itself was thought to be immunosuppressive, and that the "high mobility in this population would lead to rapid dissemination."[65] Other hypotheses were discussed, including the effects of drugs on immunity, "unusually high doses" of a virus like CMV, and, more speculatively, "unusual routes of inoculation of infectious agents, e.g., direct inoculation of virus into the blood through microfissures in the rectum."[66] Thus, from the be-

63. Etheridge, *Sentinel for Health*, 323–25.

64. Michael S. Gottlieb et al., "*Pneumocystis* Pneumonia—Los Angeles." *MMWR* 30 (1981): 250–52, https://www.cdc.gov/mmwr/preview/mmwrhtml/june_5.htm.

65. A recent study had found that 93.5 percent of randomly selected male homosexuals at a venereal disease clinic in San Francisco showed antibodies to CMV; see W. Lawrence Drew et al., "Prevalence of Cytomegalovirus Infection in Homosexual Men," *Journal of Infectious Diseases* 143, no. 2 (1981): 188–92.

66. Dennis Juranek, "Kaposi's Sarcoma in Male Homosexuals," memo for the record, June 11, 1981, pp. 2–3, folder: AIDS Task Force: 1981, William Darrow's Professional

ginning, the CDC hypothesized that they were dealing with "unusual" practices and exposures in relation to these ill homosexual men.

Dennis Juranek of Parasitic Division, CID, and Curran were dispatched to New York City the next day to gather more information. They interviewed a number of private and hospital physicians, including Friedman-Kien, and were able to establish, based on cancer registry and hospital records, that a real increase in the number of KS patients seemed to be occurring in New York City. Their report also indicated an early estimate of illness duration: "The median duration of illness from time of presentation for those who died was 15 months (mean 13 months); for patients living the median duration was 10 months (mean 12 months)."[67] This information would prove important in influencing investigators' ongoing conceptions of the syndrome, as it would shape subsequent estimates of disease duration and later suggest a shorter incubation period (as opposed to one lasting several years).[68]

The task force decided that its first major effort was to be a case control study, to gather more information on what was different about the cases of the apparently new syndrome. In meetings and correspondence in July and August 1981, members debated how best to set a case definition, select cases, and undertake the more challenging aspect of choosing appropriately matched controls. They also attempted to make sense of the preliminary data they had gathered in early case interviews un-

---

Papers, Miami (hereafter cited as Darrow Papers). There was some evidentiary basis for such speculation, given the knowledge that some infectious agents (for instance, anthrax) produced different host responses depending on the inoculation route; see Wilhelm S. Albrink et al., "Human Inhalation Anthrax: A Report of Three Fatal Cases," *American Journal of Pathology* 36, no. 4 (1960): 457–71. At the same time, the researchers' guesswork was suggestive of the lack of knowledge about and antipathy toward homosexual practices that characterized many parts of the medical and scientific establishment in the early 1980s and before.

67. James W. Curran and Dennis D. Juranek, "Trip Report—Kaposi's Sarcoma in New York City," memo, June 17, 1981, pp. 1–3, folder: AIDS Task Force: 1981, Darrow Papers.

68. Since KS presents after a lengthy subclinical period of HIV infection and the presence of a separate herpes virus, the "faster" course of the illness is thought to have been due to the fact that the immune deficiency was recognized at a relatively late stage. Some clinicians, though, were of the opinion that the patients falling ill in the late 1970s and early 1980s had a more virulent form of HIV infection, which killed patients more swiftly. See, for example, Reminiscences of Dan William, 1996, pp. 77–79, Physicians and AIDS Oral History Project, Columbia Center for Oral History Archives (CCOHA), Columbia University in the City of New York.

dertaken since June. They decided that the "likely strong association of these disorders with active homosexual men" was most suggestive of "environmental and/or behavioral factors as the primary cause(s)." They acknowledged that genetic factors might play a role in *"determining susceptibility among* homosexual men," but those factors were unlikely to provide an explanation for the noted increase in cases or for the concentration of the disorders in this population group.[69]

The clues guiding the construction of the case control study, gathered in the early interviews, noted the concentration of cases in New York City and California ("Undoubtedly there is a bias in reporting, but what hypotheses would this geographic concentration suggest if it is real?"). Also of note was a larger number of sexual partners than expected from comparison with other data such as the Jay–Young set (which Darrow had provided), a frequent use of nitrite inhalants, the overt nature of their homosexuality ("These men are not 'new' to the homosexual lifestyle, nor do they seem to *currently* lead 'dual' lives"), and a high level of education ("They do *not* seem to be lower SES [socioeconomic status]"). The group members were puzzled by reports of related cases ("What about the report of 3 cases of PCP in a family?") and what such relationships might suggest about an incubation period. They also discussed cases occurring in women and heterosexual men ("Why no KS? (or only one case)"), and PCP occurring in "drug addicts."[70] Based on these clues and the questions they raised, the task force settled on the following working hypotheses:

1. An environmental agent (microbial or chemical) is causing lasting immunosuppression among homosexual men. As an intermediate variable, immunosuppression is rendering some of these men susceptible to OI's and allowing the expression of KS.

---

69. James W. Curran, "Case Control Study Issues and Hypotheses," memo and attachment, August 11, 1981, p. 1 of attachment, folder: AIDS Task Force: 1981, Darrow Papers; emphasis in original.

70. Ibid., pp. 1–2 of attachment; emphases in original. The scientific and medical research communities would later face criticism for their delay in incorporating the first female and injecting drug user cases into their initial response to AIDS, which focused primarily on homosexual men; see, for example, Treichler, "AIDS, Gender, and Biomedical Discourse," 190–266; Gerald M. Oppenheimer, "Causes, Cases, and Cohorts: The Role of Epidemiology in the Historical Construction of AIDS," in *AIDS: The Making of a Chronic Disease*, edited by Elizabeth Fee and Daniel M. Fox, 49–76 (Berkeley: University of California Press, 1992).

2. Repeated CMV infection or reactivation is occurring resulting in immunosuppression, etc. This "continuous antigenic stimulation" may lead to
   an increased synthesis of defective viruses. These defective viruses may
   be oncogenic in certain individuals.
3. A heavy total body infection burden is exhausting the individual's ability
   to respond, resulting in immunosuppression, etc.[71]

While initially task force members explored a number of hypotheses
of causation—in particular, the recreational drug use of nitrite inhalants,
commonly known as "poppers," by gay men—they became more convinced that an infectious disease was causing the immune suppression
that underlay the Karposi's sarcoma and opportunistic infections. This
view was underscored by an early analysis of the case control study data
in late December 1981, which indicated that "the number of lifetime
[male] sex partners appears to be an important risk factor."[72] Nevertheless, they needed strong evidence to demonstrate this infectious disease
hypothesis, particularly since research published by scientists at the National Institutes of Health in mid-February 1982 suggested that other researchers were moving away from a sexually transmitted disease (STD)
etiology and back toward the use of nitrites.[73] As Darrow recalled in an
interview:

> And so when we suggested to them and other scientists that we think it's sexu-
> ally transmitted, they said, "That's because [*in mocking tone*] *you guys are all
> in the Venereal Disease Program*, you think that *everything* is sexually trans-
> mitted including *sunburn*." You know, so they thought that we were speaking
> from a certain point of view or bias, and that we didn't have any credible evi-
> dence along those lines, so we had to be very cautious and careful about mak-
> ing recommendations about sexual behaviour.[74]

71. Curran, "Study Issues and Hypotheses," p. 3 of attachment.
72. James W. Curran, "Briefing, Task Force on Kaposi's Sarcoma and Opportunistic
Infections," memo, December 30, 1981, folder: AIDS Task Force: 1981, Darrow Papers.
On the archival copy of the document, *male* is inserted in handwriting, likely as a correction by Darrow. This same briefing makes note of an initial report of a dermatologist in
Port-au-Prince, Haiti, treating eleven young men with KS, foreshadowing the later appearance of Haitians as one of the "risk groups" for AIDS.
73. James J. Goedert et al., "Amyl Nitrite May Alter T Lymphocytes in Homosexual
Men," *Lancet* 319, no. 8269 (1982): 412–16.
74. Darrow, recording C1491/21, tape 1, side B.

Although the bulk of the attention on sexual transmission focused on gay men, heterosexual cases accounted for more than 10 percent of the cases by January 1982.[75] While investigators primarily focused on the injection drug use that was widespread among these cases, several individuals had traveled substantially and reported a large number of sexual partners. For example, one early case reported to the CDC was a heterosexual Haitian man under the age of fifty who had come down with PCP in early 1981. Beginning in the late 1960s, he had lived for nearly a decade on the East Coast of the United States, returning occasionally for visits to Haiti, and reported more than forty lifetime female sexual partners. He had also traveled to Europe in the mid-1970s, and he disclosed intravenous (IV) heroin use during 1980 and 1981.[76] Cases like this individual, as well as others which doubtlessly escaped the CDC's retrospective surveillance efforts, suggest the implausibility of later attempts to pin the emergence of AIDS in North America to a single, identifiable "Patient Zero." They also illustrate the point made by the sociologist Steven Epstein, who suggested the possibility that the infectious agent spread simultaneously among IV drug users and among men who had sex with men but was first recognized in the latter group because it spread more quickly and widely within it and because the first such case subjects were middle-class men with better access to health care.[77]

In February 1982, EIS officer and task force member Harry Haverkos wrote a memo emphasizing the need to interview surviving case subjects from outside New York City, San Francisco, and Los Angeles, to access further "epidemiologic clues":

75. "Kaposi's Sarcoma and Opportunistic Infections in Heterosexuals," memo, Harold Jaffe to James Curran, 22 January 1982, folder: AIDS Task Force: 1982, Darrow Papers.

76. "Summary of Interview Data from Heterosexual Cases of Kaposi's Sarcoma and Pneumocystis Pneumonia," attachment to memo from Mary Guinan to James Curran, 4 January 1982, folder: AIDS Task Force: 1982, Darrow Papers.

77. Epstein, *Impure Science*, 49–50; Don C. Des Jarlais et al., "HIV-1 Infection among Intravenous Drug Users in Manhattan, New York City, from 1977 through 1987," *Journal of the American Medical Association* 261, no. 7 (1989): 1008–12. James Curran's comments at the NCAB meeting in December 1982 reinforce the likelihood of this point: "They're not difficult to recognize syndromes, they're 35 years old, prosperous, previously healthy men who come in looking like they're going to die, spend the next six or seven months in hospital, run up a hospital bill of $100,000 to $150,000 and then die. So it's not something that's missed, each case is a grand rounds case in its individual hospital"; "NCAB Meeting," 17.

A theory of a point source in New York City could be strengthened by show-ing that all cases have some connection with the "Big Apple." Could it be one place, i.e., one specific bathhouse, in New York City? Contact with New York City may help us to define the incubation period of these diseases. Leads into the distinction between drugs and transmissible agents as the cause of the epidemic could be unearthed.[78]

In an attachment to Haverkos's memo, the individual identified as Case 57 —one of twenty-three living male case subjects with a residence outside of metropolitan New York, Los Angeles, and San Francisco—is listed as a Canadian from Toronto with an early onset of KS in July 1978. Dar-row, who had until this time been closely involved with the case control study in the design of the questionnaire and the training of interviewers, circled this case for follow-up, as well as Case 154, a gay man in his early fifties from a European country, whose onset of KS was listed as Janu-ary 1975.[79]

On February 25, 1982, Darrow wrote to Polly Thomas, an EIS offi-cer at the New York Department of Public Health who was responsible for the city's investigations into the new illness, requesting further infor-mation about some of the earliest cases in that city. "I am trying to put together the pieces of a jigsaw puzzle I found locked away in a cabinet at CDC," he wrote, "and I find many of the important pieces missing." Darrow believed there to be "a geographic focus to the current outbreak of Kaposi's sarcoma before 1980," a hypothesis he attempted to disprove by revisiting the data about the earliest recorded cases.[80] Shortly there-after he wrote a memo in which he examined the possibility of "the Hor-

78. Harry W. Haverkos, "Cases Outside New York City, San Francisco, and Los Ange-les," memo and attachment, February 8, 1982, p. 1, folder: AIDS Task Force: 1982, Darrow Papers; *transmissible* typed as "trsnsmissible" in original.

79. Ibid., p. 1 of attachment. Case 154 was lost to subsequent follow-up when he re-turned to Europe shortly after his diagnosis with KS in July 1981. Due to this individual's early symptom onset, Darrow wrote that "one could assume that this international travel-ler was a source of all subsequent infections seen in the U.S."; Darrow, "Time-Space Clus-tering of KS Cases in the City of New York: Evidence for Horizontal Transmission of Some Mysterious Microbe," memo, March 3, 1982, p. 2. The onset date for the individual identi-fied as Case 57 was later determined to be December 1979. In the task force documenta-tion, investigators often used the terms *patient* and *case* interchangeably, and they referred to individuals by both two-digit and three-digit identifiers (for example, 57 and 057).

80. William Darrow to Pauline A. Thomas, 25 February 1982, pp. 1–2, folder: KSOI: Cases and Contacts in New York City: July 12–16, August 4–6, 1982, Darrow et al., Dar-

izontal Transmission of Some Mysterious Microbe" in New York City, Darrow found that "of those experiencing symptoms before 1980, all but one lived in the metropolitan New York City area and could be linked to Manhattan in one way or another." While the possibility could not be dismissed, "no evidence for direct transmission is available. . . . We need more data."[81] Darrow suggested that some of the individuals in these cases needed to be interviewed or, as in the instance of Case 57, reinterviewed.[82]

AIDS Project Number 6: The Los Angeles Cluster Study

An unexpected opportunity to gather more data was presented in March 1982 when David Auerbach, an EIS officer stationed in Los Angeles, contacted Atlanta to let the KS/OI Task Force team know that four men with KS/OI were in the same Los Angeles hospital and had apparently been one another's sexual partners. To investigate the possibility that AIDS patients could be linked sexually, Darrow was dispatched to Los Angeles, and together he and Auerbach attempted to interview as many surviving KS/OI case subjects as possible. The Los Angeles cluster[83] was one of two possible clusters that appeared at this time; the other—three cases of PCP among male prisoners in New York's Taconic Prison—was also investigated, though CDC physicians were unable to establish any direct links in the latter case.[84]

It was here that Darrow's training was vitally useful. "I felt confident," he recalled, "that I could talk to the people who were infected, make them feel comfortable, not embarrass them, assure them that I would

row Papers. Thomas's work on AIDS is featured in James Colgrove, *Epidemic City: The Politics of Public Health in New York* (New York: Russell Sage Foundation, 2011), 107–41.

81. William Darrow, "Time-Space Clustering of KS Cases in the City of New York: Evidence for Horizontal Transmission of Some Mysterious Microbe," memo, March 3, 1982, pp. 1, 3, folder: KSOI: Cases and Contacts in New York City, Darrow Papers.

82. Shilts explained in his history that task force member Mary Guinan had conducted the first interview with the man known as Case 57. See Shilts, *Band*, 83–84.

83. The Los Angeles cluster study was also known within CDC as AIDS Project Number 6: Harold Jaffe, "AIDS Project Codes," memo, April 9, 1985, p. 2, folder: AIDS Task Force 1983–85, Darrow Papers.

84. James W. Curran, "Briefing, Task Force on Kaposi's Sarcoma and Opportunistic Infections," April 2, 1982, folder: AIDS Task Force: 1982, Darrow Papers.

not violate their trust, and assure them that although I was not a medical doctor and couldn't help them at all, that whatever I learned I would try to see to it [that] it would be beneficial for them and other people that they were concerned about."[85] Darrow also had years of experience in terms of prompting VD patients to name their sexual partners, obtaining important information by inference, and maintaining the commitment to the legwork required in VD control. Still, there was a key difference in this instance: "I had worked on problems related to syphilis, gonorrhea, herpes, and lots of other sexually transmitted diseases that were very annoying and disturbing but rarely killed people. And suddenly we were finding a disease that was fatal, and for the first time I was going to come face-to-face with some people who . . . were dying from this disease."[86] At a time when declarations of homosexual activity could lead to felony charges in several states, the CDC investigators were well aware of many possible reasons for noncooperation. Darrow and Auerbach were struck by the men's concern, their desire to help researchers learn more about the syndrome, and the willingness of most to speak freely. They later gave special thanks to these men for their openness and trust.[87] Through their interviewing efforts in March and April 1982, Auerbach and Darrow were able to establish sexual links between nine out of thirteen of the twenty-six earliest reported KS/OI cases in southern California. To their excitement, four men named the same out-of-town patient—the CDC's Case 57, whose details Darrow already knew since he was an individual with an early date of symptom onset—as a sexual contact. These four men reported that they or their acquaintances had had sexual exposures with this man between nine and eighteen months before the onset of their symptoms.[88] Locating and reinterviewing this individual became a top priority.

Given subsequent misunderstandings, it might be useful at this point to emphasize how unlikely it would be that the cases reported to the CDC by the spring of 1982 would represent all existent cases of the disease in California at that time. It is worth drawing on our current knowl-

85. Darrow, recording C1491/21, tape 1, side A.

86. Ibid.

87. Auerbach et al., "Cluster of Cases," 491.

88. "Documentation for MMWR Article: 'A Cluster of Cases of Kaposi's Sarcoma and *Pneumocystis Carinii* Pneumonia among Homosexual Male Residents of Los Angeles and Orange Counties, California,'" May 12, 1982, p. 8, folder: AIDS Task Force: 1982, Darrow Papers.

edge of HIV infection to consider the hurdles a prospective case subject would need to clear to be included in the cluster study. Such an individual would have had to be infected with HIV some time before, likely for several years. Subsequently he (and it was almost entirely men being investigated during this period) would have had to feel sufficiently unwell to seek medical attention. If he received a medical examination, the health care staff would have needed to be aware of the CDC's case definition, recognize that his presenting signs and symptoms conformed to it, and then report this individual to the CDC. Failing such a report, the CDC's task force members would have had to uncover the case in their retrospective surveillance activities. Finally, the task force members would have needed to be able to gather sufficient information about the patient's sexual history to link him to the cluster. In short, it would be a mistake to interpret, as some observers subsequently did, the twenty-six earliest cases reported in California by April 1982 as the twenty-six first cases of infection, in absolute terms, caused by the transmissible agent that would subsequently be identified as HIV.

Letters and Numbers

The Los Angeles cluster study, as this work became known, was first published on June 20, 1982, in the CDC's *Morbidity and Mortality Weekly Report* and would soon be cited as evidence supporting the theory that a sexually transmissible agent caused the immune suppression leading to AIDS.[89] While there was no suggestion in the initial report that the epidemic had begun in California, subsequent communications between KS/OI Task Force members suggested that they believed the cluster might lead them to the root of the problem. "In order to discover *the source* of the current outbreak of acquired cellular immunodeficiency," Darrow and a colleague wrote in an internal proposal to extend the cluster, "the interconnected series of cases uncovered in southern California should be followed as far as it may go."[90] This distance proved to be

89. Task Force on Kaposi's Sarcoma and Opportunistic Infections, CDC, "A Cluster," 305–7.

90. "Relationships among Cases of and Contacts to Kaposi's Sarcoma and Opportunistic Infections in New York City: A Proposal," final draft of report, July 8, 1982, p. 1, folder: KSOI: Cases and Contacts in New York City, Darrow Papers; emphasis added.

to New York and beyond, as the follow-up article published in 1984 demonstrated. In it, Auerbach and Darrow were able to link forty cases of AIDS in ten cities in an implied web of transmission, though ultimately they did not speculate as to the geographic point of entry for the transmissible agent.

Key to their success was the assistance of Case 57, an individual who received the designation "Patient 0" in the 1984 article and whose personal sexual network extended to a large number of men in many cities. This non-Californian resident was able to provide them with a list of 72 contacts from his personal address book, nearly 10 percent of the 750 partners he estimated he had had sex with in the previous three years, through whom they were able to continue their cluster research. His ability to provide names stood out sharply in contrast to the other men linked to the cluster. More than 65 percent of these men had reported more than 1,000 lifetime sexual partners, and more than 75 percent had reported more than 50 partners in the year before they experienced symptoms. Yet most of these men were able to provide only a handful of names. For example, in the year before the onset of his KS in February 1978, the man known as Case 335 (LA 1 in the cluster) reported 240 sexual partners and named 6. Case 32 (the cluster's LA 6) reported an estimated 500 sexual partners in the twelve months prior to his becoming sick in November 1980; he was able to name 5 of them.[91] Thus, by comparison, the trove of information possessed by Case 57 was quite remarkable. By 1982, the man was spending more time in San Francisco and had recently updated his book, discarding, to the disappointment of some task force members, many older names from other cities.[92]

Both the desire to locate the source of the epidemic, implicit in contact epidemiological practice and long part of its history, and the transformative coding assigned to cluster cases appear to have worked against the originally stated intentions of the study.[93] Auerbach and Darrow

91. "Table 1: Cases of KS/OI Reported among Homosexual Men in LA or Linked to LA Cluster," in Auerbach and Darrow, "Los Angeles Cluster: Background," May 12, 1982, p. 6, folder: AIDS Task Force: 1982, Darrow Papers.

92. Some task force investigators, including Harold Jaffe, would subsequently wonder whether discarding these names may have been an excuse to protect some of his contacts, though there is no additional evidence to suggest that this was the case.

93. William Coleman describes the work of mid-nineteenth-century French and British epidemiologists who emphasized the importance of attempting to locate the "initial victims" of epidemics of yellow fever and cholera to determine whether they shared exposures

needed to integrate numerical identifiers from several sources into their study and to simplify the complex webs of sexual contact that they had uncovered. Each patient had been assigned a unique case number when reported to the CDC but also likely had another unique coding in the local public health district. For example, "Patient 0" had been CDC's "Case 57," while at the same time in San Francisco, he was labelled "D (K+) (Montreal, NY, SF)" by Selma Dritz, the city's public health department epidemiologist who was investigating the outbreak there (see fig. 2.3).[94] By May 1982, in an unpublished report leading up the June *MMWR* article about the Los Angeles cluster, he became "Patient O"— short for "Out[side]-of-California" or "non-Californian KS"—before acquiring his final, numerical designation. In early September 1982, Darrow wrote an internal report to his colleagues, summarizing his New York investigations during July and August, in which he used the CDC's case numbers to designate individual cases and employed the prefix *Patient* for each one. One month later, he annotated a separate copy of the report by hand to be typed up for distribution beyond the CDC to partner organizations in New York and elsewhere. On this report, he replaced each cluster-linked case number with a sequential city-based number in order of symptom onset date within each city's cluster cases— the style of designation which would eventually feature in the 1984 article—and wrote the letter *O* in substitution for Patient 57's number to abbreviate "Out-of-California." What happened next may have been the result of a secretarial error, or indeed due to the fact that the CDC's typewriters produced a capital letter *O* and a numeral 0 that were virtually indistinguishable. In any event, while Darrow and Auerbach would continue to refer to "Patient O" using a letter in conversation (sounding like "Patient Oh") and in print, others discussing the investigation began to use the numeral 0 (resulting in speech sounding like "Patient Zero"), interpreting the ambiguous oval as a digit, alongside the other city case numbers.[95] Thus the term "Patient 0" was born, and it was this code that

---

to hazardous local conditions or to other sick individuals; see W. Coleman, *Yellow Fever in the North*, 20–21, 182–87.

94. In the portrait of Dritz shown in figure 2.3, the positioning of the subject in front of her work apparatus, representing the "proof" of her authority, links this photograph to other works of scientific portraiture; see Ludmilla Jordanova, *Defining Features: Scientific and Medical Portraits 1660–2000* (London: Reaktion Books with National Portrait Gallery, London, 2000).

95. Copies of the original, the annotated, and the retyped versions of this memo are

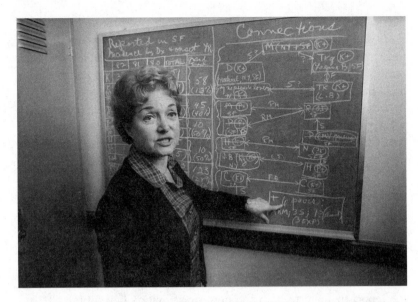

FIGURE 2.3 Selma Dritz in her office, November 15, 1982. Photograph by Jerry Telfer for the *San Francisco Chronicle*. © Jerry Telfer / San Francisco Chronicle / Corbis. This portrait shows the public health official standing in her small office, next to a locker, pointing to a blackboard that depicts known connections between early cases of AIDS in gay men. On the right half of the blackboard behind her, Gaétan Dugas's information is listed in a rectangle at top left—"D Ⓚ (Montreal, NY, SF)"—the first, and perhaps most important, example on her list, and the man whom she would confront that month about his continuing sexual activity. Arrows linking cases were labeled as "RM" for "roommate" and "S?" to query whether there had been sexual contact between them. These notations can be compared with similar images in Dritz's presentation slides, which are now held in the special collections of the University of California–San Francisco. A cropped version of this photograph, covering roughly one-quarter of the width of the newspaper's page, accompanied an article by the *Chronicle*'s science editor: David Perlman, "A War against 'Gay Plague,'" *San Francisco Chronicle*, November 17, 1982, 5.

designated the CDC's Case 57 in the most well-known publication of the cluster study in 1984.

The consequences of this change cannot be overemphasized, given the multitude of meanings for the word *zero*. Particularly noteworthy definitions include: "a worthless thing or person," "an absence or lack

in Darrow's files: "Trip Report to New York City: July 12–16 and August 3–6, 1982," September 3, 1982, folder: KSOI: Cases and Contacts in New York City. A copy of one page from the retyped version, in the archived files of the New York City Department of Public Health, is reproduced in Colgrove, *Epidemic City*, 112.

of anything," "the initial point of a process or reckoning . . . the starting-point, [and] the absolute beginning."[96] Such a shift was further compli-cated by the rather nonspecific identification of "Patient 0," in the 1984 publication, as the "index case," which in contemporary usage usually meant the first case to come to the investigators' attention, as opposed to the *primary case*—which was the earliest to occur in time—although neither was true for "Patient 0" in this scenario.[97] Judging from previ-ous CDC-reported outbreaks, such as one of smallpox in Sweden in 1963, it appears to have been the agency's practice to use the term *index case* to refer to the "source" case—a case to which other, more specific terms such as *primary* or *initial* might be applied. A report of the Swed-ish smallpox outbreak in *MMWR* noted that "the first case to be iden-tified occurred in an unvaccinated 19-year-old bricklayer (Case 7) who had onset of fever, vomiting, and backache on May 5." He later died, as did three of the other twenty-four confirmed case subjects. Epidemio-logic research determined that the "original source of the outbreak was a 24-year-old seaman who after two weeks residence in Australia left Darwin on March 22 on BOAC Flight #709," stopping briefly at Dja-karta, Singapore, Rangoon, Calcutta, Karachi, Teheran, and Damascus on the way to Zurich, where he boarded another plane and flew to Swe-den. A figure accompanying reports of the smallpox investigation indi-cated three generations of confirmed and suspected "indigenous" cases that stemmed from the twenty-four-year-old. The seaman was labeled as the "index case" in the figure, even though he was not the first pa-tient to come to investigators' attention in the outbreak. A tabular rep-resentation of the investigation numbered the cases in order of the indi-viduals' symptom onset and listed the "presumed source of infection" for each. While the indigenous cases were each linked to an earlier case number (Cases 2 to 5 linked to Case 1, Cases 6 and 7 to Case 2, etc.), the presumed source of Case 1's infection was listed far more vaguely—and problematically—as "Southeast Asia." This historical example not only demonstrates the ambiguities of the CDC's use of the term *index case*

---

96. *Oxford English Dictionary Online*, s.v. "zero," accessed February 22, 2017, http://www.oed.com/view/Entry/232803?rskey=SMeMCR&result=1.

97. *Index case* was defined as "the first case in a family or other defined group to come to the attention of the investigator" in Last, *Dictionary of Epidemiology*, s.v. "index case." It may not be not surprising, therefore, that *patient zero* is even now used interchangeably as a term denoting *index case* and *primary case*.

but also indicates the ease with which reports of well-resourced epidemiologic investigations in one country can, in a few words, construct whole regions of the world as the source of an infectious outbreak.[98]

Returning to the cluster study, in mid-1983 Darrow and Auerbach were revising their work for publication and seeking peer review. One experienced epidemiologist, who had seen Auerbach present the study at a CDC conference that spring, entered into correspondence with the physician about the study. In addition to commenting on the role of age as a variable and the high numbers of cluster cases who practiced fisting (manual-rectal intercourse), he remarked that "Patient 'O'" was "interesting" and drew what would become a common inference. He pointed out that "Patient 'O'" had a date of symptom onset of November–December 1979, while one of his contacts had an onset date of August 1979, and another contracted PCP in November 1979. The public health professional queried, "Is this inconsistent with an hypothesis of 'O' as source case?"[99]

Here, an experienced epidemiologist appears to have interpreted the reference to "Patient 'O'" and this individual's prominence in the study to imply the cluster's source. It is not surprising, then, that members of the media and the public also took away that impression in the news coverage that accompanied the study's publication in March 1984, and which emphasized the "mysterious" central figure. For example, in an interview given to the *Los Angeles Herald Examiner*, coauthor David Auerbach tried to emphasize that "Patient O" was "not the source." (Auerbach's use of the letter *O*, which was reproduced in this article and the accompanying illustration, suggests that he and Darrow continued to refer to this patient by letter when discussing the cluster study in person, preserving the connection to their original adjectival phrase "Out-of-California.") Auerbach's efforts were undermined, however, by the

98. The reports, which appeared in the May 24, May 31, June 7, June 14, and July 3, 1963, issues of *MMWR*, were assembled and reprinted in a special edition of the periodical in honor of the CDC's fiftieth anniversary; see "*International Notes—Quarantine Measures*: Smallpox—Stockholm, Sweden, 1963," *MMWR* 45, no. 25 (1996): 538–45.

99. Andrew C. Fleck Jr. to David M. Auerbach, 17 May 1983, pp. 3–4, folder L.A. Cluster FF! Personal and Professional Papers of Joseph Sonnabend, London (hereafter cited as Sonnabend Papers). In this typed letter, it is impossible to distinguish whether Fleck was using a number or a letter to designate the non-Californian KS case. However, since he had seen Auerbach present the material in person, it seems likely that Fleck, following Auerbach's oral delivery, would have been using the letter.

article's disease-detective focus and his evident enthusiasm to be, in the reporter's words, "one of the sleuths who tracked down the mysterious 'Patient O,' . . . [who was] the missing piece in a puzzle." Auerbach remarked, "It was real exciting. . . . In two interviews both men spontaneously mentioned to us the name of one man, Patient O . . . I can tell you we were both startled." The former EIS officer emphasized the man's perceived importance: "Patient O is at the center of our study. . . . He was the link between the West Coast cases and New York. He was the key." The result was decidedly mixed. The article's text claimed, somewhat vaguely, that the man "was a link between all 40 cases" and carried Auerbach's assertion that he was not the source. The accompanying graphic led readers in the opposite direction. While a small disclaimer admitted that "Patient O" was "not necessarily the source of the disease," the largest print, apart from the title, was the word at the top of the image labeling the central figure as "Originator" (see fig. 2.4).[100]

For his part, Darrow took pains to explain to reporters in an inter-

---

100. Auerbach quotations in Richard Nordwind, "Doctor Helped Track Down Sexual Link between Cluster of 40 AIDS Victims," *Los Angeles Herald Examiner*, March 28, 1984, A6. The representation of the cluster shown in figure 2.4 has constituted it as a family tree, with visual similarities to the "trees of life" used to represent evolutionary relationships in biology; Theodore W. Pietsch, *Trees of Life: A Visual History of Evolution* (Baltimore: Johns Hopkins University Press, 2012). The perceived importance of "Patient O" has resulted in this individual being defined as "Originator," despite text on the very same graphic stating that "Patient O . . . was not necessarily the source of the disease." This example vividly demonstrates the recurrent desire to find a way of tracing a disease to its origins. And even when designated by the letter *O* and not the number 0, the figure seen to be centrally important to the cluster collapses back to zero in the context of a family tree because the originating line is known as "generation zero" in genetics. Michael Keegan, the *Herald Examiner*'s design director from 1979 to 1985, suggested in an e-mail to the author in October 2014 that the image was most likely created by one of the newspaper's two staff artists on short notice and for a quick turnaround, probably in one day or less. The artist would have set the image's type on a photocomposition machine before cutting it out and pasting it into position on the drawn diagram. The artwork would then have been engraved and placed on a page to undergo letterpress printing. One gay reader who clipped this article for his personal files cut out a similar one in the *Los Angeles Times*. The second article designated the central individual as "Patient 0." The reader stated with excitement, much as Randy Shilts would later do, that this was a "fascinating story!" He underlined the article's text where it explained: "It appears that Patient 0 transmitted the disease to at least two others before he had any signs of it himself, the CDC investigators found." The reader then wrote, on the margins of the paper to which he affixed the clipping, "So he infected 38 others when he had signs and symptoms? The guy's a monster"; "Homosexual Linked to 40 AIDS Cases May Have Carried Infection," *Los Angeles Times,* March 27, 1984, 10 [an-

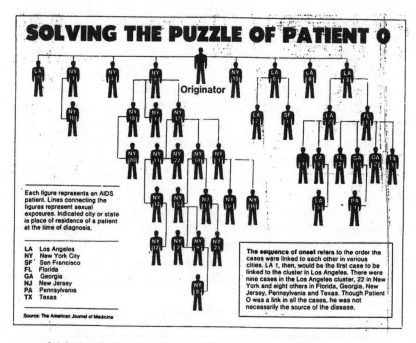

FIGURE 2.4 Patient O labeled as "Originator" in illustration accompanying newspaper article. Scan from microfilmed paper. Richard Nordwind, "Doctor Helped Track Down Sexual Link Between Cluster of 40 AIDS Victims." *Los Angeles Herald Examiner*, March 28, 1984, A6. The image's original printed size would have been roughly 17.5 ×13.5 cm, covering approximately half the width of one newspaper page.

view that "Patient 0" was probably not the first patient to get AIDS, suggesting that the man was an "unwitting carrier" who "may have unknowingly spread the disease across the country." An Associated Press reporter explained, "Darrow thinks Patient 0 picked it up from a contact in Los Angeles or New York and then carried it across the country to the others." The reporter quoted Darrow as stating, "One of the problems we had, of course, was determining the source of the infection and the spread."[101] The terms *source* and *spread* had been used by VD investiga-

notated clipping]; in untitled folder, box 5, Frank Robinson Papers, GLBT Historical Society, San Francisco.

101. Paul Raeburn, "40 AIDS Cases in 10 Cities Linked to One Carrier," Associated Press newswire, March 27, 1984, LexisNexis News. In this instance the reporter followed the published study's use of the number zero in numeral form.

tors at least as early as the 1940s to denote the order of infection among cases. A handbook produced in 1945 wisely cautioned these health workers not to ask the patients being interviewed "Who gave you VD?" (the "*source contact*") or "To whom did you give VD?"(the "*spread contact*") since the two were often difficult to distinguish in practice. The handbook also noted that such an approach "diverts the patient from the important objective of naming *all* contacts."[102]

In retrospect, Darrow also believed that the designation "O" is where a number of people were led astray:

> I didn't start using the term "Patient 0" until other people had used it, and I don't—it probably came from CDC, but I don't know who did it, you know, who the first one was. But probably when they wrote it down "Patient O," they went around talking to one another about "Patient 0" and so that's how he got his name. . . . Because everybody said that this is "ground zero," you know, this is how the epidemic started, and I want you to know that I never said that he was the first case in the United States, that he brought . . . this condition to America. He *may have* brought it to Los Angeles, there's a possibility that could have happened—that these other men would have never become infected if they hadn't had sex with him—but certainly they had other sex partners who may have been the source of their infection.[103]

CDC investigators would later express surprise at the resilience of the phrase "Patient Zero" and the generalized assumption that the man denoted by the term represented the origin of AIDS in North America. Darrow would note that "there's a conventional wisdom that he started the whole epidemic, but that's not true. . . . Nobody said he was the first case."[104] Though strictly true, such statements downplay the contributions to this misunderstanding made by the CDC's eventual—and largely accidental—use of the phrase "Patient 0," and, as we shall see, the visual depiction of the cluster. Indeed, KS/OI Task Force members may have inadvertently shaped the welcoming public reception of "Patient 0" by

102. S. W. Evans, *VD Case-Finding Manual: For Use in Training Programs*, trial ed. (Raleigh, NC: VD Education Institute, 1945), V-5; emphasis in original.

103. Darrow, recording C1491/21, tape 1, side B; emphasis on recording.

104. Wyatt Olson, "The Protection Racket: And the Band Plays On," *Broward-Palm Beach New Times*, February 2, 2006, http://www.browardpalmbeach.com/2006–02–02/news/the-protection-racket/.

furnishing him with an "infectious" name.[105] Randy Shilts later recalled being alerted in 1982 to the likelihood of a sexually transmissible causative agent through the first publication of the cluster study. Later, in the course of researching his book on the history of the American AIDS epidemic, he was also struck by the term's sensational potential after consulting with CDC researchers. As Shilts related in an interview, "In the middle of that study was a circle with an *O* [letter] next to it, and I always thought it was Patient O. When I went to the CDC, they started talking about Patient Zero. I thought, *Ooh, that's catchy.*"[106] At the very least, Shilts's response ought to serve as a cautionary tale of the risks of using "catchy" promotional metaphors in scientific publications.[107]

Reception and Reproduction

As soon as the initial reports of the ongoing cluster investigation were published in June 1982, gay community groups, physicians, and public health officials relayed the information. The New York–based Gay Men's Health Crisis included a stop-the-presses announcement regarding its implications in the organization's first newsletter about "Acquired Immune Deficiency"—which it abbreviated as AID—printed in July 1982: "The upshot of this information is that one or more infectious agents—germs, microbes, viruses, bacteria—were likely passed through sexual contact from one gay man to another in [Los Angeles and Orange Counties] and from there on to men in possibly 16 more cases in eight other cities."[108]

The study reached national prominence again in February 1983 when a *New York Times* feature on AIDS highlighted the Los Angeles cluster

---

105. The process by which "Patient O" became "Patient 0" brings to mind the "microprocessing" described by Bruno Latour and Steve Woolgar in *Laboratory Life: The Social Construction of Scientific Facts* (London: Sage, 1979), 151–86. Playing on one synonym for the word *computer*, Latour and Woolgar define *microprocessing* as the manner in which the day-to-day interactions of the laboratory lead to the production of a scientific "fact."

106. Jeff Yarbrough, "The Life and Times of Randy Shilts," *Advocate*, June 15, 1993, 37; emphasis in original.

107. Dorothy Nelkin, "Promotional Metaphors and Their Popular Appeal," *Public Understanding of Science* 3, no. 1 (1994): 25–31.

108. Gay Men's Health Crisis, "Late Evidence on Contagious Causes," *G.M.H.C. Newsletter* 1 (July 1982): 2.

and explained that, "later, a missing link was found between Los Angeles and New York."[109] The next month, in San Francisco, a reporter interpreted the use by local physicians of the cluster and this "missing link" as two separate examples demonstrating the infectious nature of the disease. At a meeting held to alert gay men to the threat of AIDS, Marcus Conant, a dermatologist who played an active role in mounting the city's response, explained that the incubation period for the syndrome now appeared to stretch to eighteen months. As far as evidence for a sexually transmissible causative agent, Paul Volberding, his oncologist colleague at the Kaposi's Sarcoma Clinic at the University of California–San Francisco—a group in close contact with the CDC—explained that nine of nineteen AIDS cases in Los Angeles had had sex with one another. The reporter noted that Volberding also cited the example of "a Canadian man who traveled frequently between the coasts of the United States . . . [who] came down with AIDS," as did some of his sexual partners.[110]

In mid-1984, Michael Callen, the New York AIDS activist, wrote to Mervyn Silverman, chief of the San Francisco Department of Health, to ask about that city's ongoing bathhouse deliberations. Silverman replied that "three important published epidemiological papers" had guided the decision making of the city attorney's office and the health department to focus on "decreasing multiple anonymous sexual partners." A case control study in New York led by Michael Marmor and another by the CDC had both "showed that the greater the number of sexual partners the higher risk for the onset of the disease." He added that the LA cluster study was also "considered important," since it established sexual links between a number of cases. "This," Silverman explained, "was consistent with the infectious etiology of AIDS."[111]

Some members of the gay community were also convinced by the study. As Randy Shilts recollected, "The L.A. Cluster Study made it very clear that we were dealing with a sexually transmitted disease. Being a gay man, I could see what that meant, and in 1983 I started get-

109. Robin Marantz Henig, "AIDS: A New Disease's Deadly Odyssey," *New York Times*, February 6, 1983, SM30.

110. Wayne April, "Doctors Brief 'Gay Leaders' On AIDS," *Bay Area Reporter* [San Francisco], April 7, 1983, 3, 18.

111. Mervyn Silverman to Michael Callen, 25 July 1984, p. 1, folder: Merv Silverman, Correspondence Out, 1984, Carton 1, San Francisco Department of Public Health AIDS Office Records (SFH 4), San Francisco History Center, San Francisco Public Library.

ting very heavy into AIDS coverage at the *Chronicle*."[112] Neil Schram, a
gay physician based in Los Angeles, later recalled the importance of the
study for him, particularly in the absence of an antibody test:

> My view was that people could change behavior without an antibody test. Be-
> cause I had. And I figured if I had, everybody could. . . . I had changed my
> behavior in '82, when what's-his-name, David Auerbach, from the CDC, had
> reported in Orange County that something like 16 of 21 gay men who devel-
> oped AIDS had had sex with each other. That was the day I knew, one, we
> were in trouble and, two, this was a sexually transmitted disease. No mat-
> ter what anybody said after that. And I changed my behavior . . . I figured if I
> could do it, then everybody could do it, and they didn't need an antibody test
> to do it.[113]

Not everyone, however, was satisfied by the study's conclusions or its
methods. Joseph Sonnabend—a New York-based physician who had begun to treat a number of KS/OI patients and who would later go on to
question the singular role of the virus in AIDS—was an early proponent
of a multifactorial model of AIDS causation. He was concerned by the
prospect—unfounded, in his view—that gay men might be singled out
as carriers of a virus. Sonnabend wrote angry letters to David Sencer,
the commissioner of the New York City Department of Health and former chief of CDC; to the Democratic congressman Henry Waxman; and
to Michael D. Gregg, the editor of *MMWR*. To Sencer, he declared that
"CDC has shown in this matter an unfortunate lapse in their abilities
to undertake research of this kind, and what is perhaps more serious, a
lapse in appreciation of their responsibilities. It is indeed a very serious
matter to suggest that members of any minority group may be carriers of
what in effect is a cancer virus."[114] To Waxman, he complained, with reference to the *Gay Report*, that "the fact that material from a survey conducted in part through pornographic magazines (reference no. 2) is cited
in support of the contention is a further indication of an oversight on

---

112. Ron Bluestein, "Cries and Whispers of an Epidemic," *Advocate*, November 24,
1987, 64.
113. Reminiscences of Neil Schram, 1996, p. 47, Physicians and AIDS Oral History
Project, CCOHA.
114. Joseph Sonnabend to David J. Sencer, 19 July 1982, folder: L.A. Cluster FF! Sonnabend Papers.

the part of the editors with respect to the responsibilities associated with their position."[115] Sonnabend was particularly concerned with the cluster study's reliance on "generalizations contained in the Kinsey report of 1948," used to estimate the size of the gay populations in California and thus the likelihood that the individuals in the AIDS cases included in the cluster might know each other by chance. He suggested to Gregg that the *Gay Report*, upon which some of the study's evidence relied, "can hardly be regarded as a valid scientific reference," since it could "support any point of view." Sonnabend angrily wrote that "these are the flimsiest of referral sources to support a contention with such far-reaching implications. These derive from the perception of gay men as carriers of a cancer virus."[116]

Andrew Moss, the San Francisco epidemiologist, was also critical of the CDC's epidemiologic abilities, as well as the cluster study's approach. "I met the CDC people that came out here," he later recalled in an oral history interview, "Curran and Jaffe, and I drove them around in my hideous beat-up Volkswagen. Both of them said, 'Well, I'm not really an epidemiologist,' meaning, 'I don't know what I'm doing.' Which is true; they had no idea what they were doing." He continued, dismissively:

They had the CDC kind of three-week course, or whatever it is they get. They were not formal epidemiologists. They were insecure about their ability as formal epidemiologists. . . .

The CDC didn't in those days give them a lot of training before pitching them in. Infectious disease epidemiology is sort of like, "Get in there and see what's going on!" Outbreak investigation—stamp it out. AIDS is a bit different.

See, the interesting thing about AIDS from a professional point of view is it's an infectious disease that looks like a chronic disease. It takes a long time [to develop]. You don't go and stamp it out. It's not like salmonella or something. You don't stamp out an outbreak by finding the infected chicken. Although that's what Darrow tried to do. That's what all that Patient Zero stuff was about.

It's like trying to visualize AIDS in the model of an infectious disease out-

115. Joseph Sonnabend to Representative [Henry] Waxman, 15 July 1982, folder: L.A. Cluster FF! Sonnabend Papers.
116. Joseph Sonnabend to Michael D. Gregg, 14 July 1982, folder: L.A. Cluster FF! Sonnabend Papers.

break. It's quick; it spreads from person to person; you go in there and you find the prime cause, and you remove it. This is not the way AIDS works.[117]

Moss acknowledged that, while more confident in his training, he felt less connected to the CDC than his rival San Francisco epidemiologist, Selma Dritz of the city's health department.[118] This insecurity in a possible turf war in San Francisco over access to information about cases may have colored his frank recollections. Still, by making clear his belief that the type of work done by the CDC was distinct from that done by "formal epidemiologists," Moss exhibits views that are suggestive of the divisions rendered by shifts in epidemiological practice in the mid-twentieth century.

Lengthening Incubation Periods

Following the isolation and identification of a virus in 1983 and 1984 and the increasingly widespread ability to test for viral antibodies in 1985, the practical importance of the cluster study waned. Additional research clarified the virus's transmission routes, and the key questions shifted from whether sexual contact spread the virus to the types of activities that presented the highest risk and, more problematically, to what extent the disease posed a threat to the "general public."[119] The cluster study receded from the spotlight, having served its role in helping to redirect the attention of researchers and concerned members of the public to the likelihood of a sexually transmissible agent as a cause for AIDS. The hypotheses on which the study had been based and which provided significance to its central visual representation did not receive explicit challenge—despite evolving knowledge about the time between HIV infection and the appearance of an AIDS-related illness. Early estimates of an incubation period were hampered by difficulties in testing for subclinical infections and by a lack of historical data, as well as by an ini-

117. Moss, "AIDS Epidemiology," 246–47.

118. Andrew Moss, interview with author, San Francisco, July 24, 2007, recording C1491/09, tape 1, side A, BLSA.

119. For criticism of the discourse that posited the threat of infection shifting from "risk groups" to the "general population" or "general public," see, for example, Grover, "AIDS: Keywords," 23–30; Patton, *Inventing AIDS*, 25.

tial hypothesis that AIDS patients were likely to develop complications at the same speed as patients taking immunosuppressant drugs after organ transplants.

Scientists would soon note that the incubation period seemed to be lengthening. In 1986, for example, three public health researchers suggested that it was "becoming apparent from several lines of evidence that the period of latency from exposure to illness may be five years or longer."[120] And the authors of a paper published in 1988 noted drily, "In past studies the estimated average incubation period has been disconcertingly close to the time span over which data are available, suggesting that the average could lengthen as more information accumulates." The paper also noted that the most up-to-date analysis then available suggested that the average incubation period between HIV infection and the onset of AIDS was seven to eight years—an estimate which would grow to a median of just over ten years for adult men in the absence of treatment.[121]

In his 1988 letter to the *New York Review of Books*, Andrew Moss pointed out that this evolving understanding of HIV's incubation period made it highly unlikely that the neatly arranged cluster continued to indicate what it had once appeared to do.[122] Before, when researchers relied on the comparison to renal transplant recipients, who developed KS an average 14.9 months after taking immunosuppressive drugs, the cases making up the cluster could be assumed to link together in a manner which suggested that the patient who first demonstrated symptoms likely passed the infection to one displaying symptoms afterward.[123] While James Curran had qualified his statement at the NCAB meeting in December 1982 with the caution that this was "certainly a very loose figure," he maintained that the "out of California case" showed that the incubation period between sexual contact and onset of illness was ap-

120. Victor De Gruttola, Kenneth Mayer, and William Bennett, "AIDS: Has the Problem Been Adequately Assessed?" *Reviews of Infectious Diseases* 8, no. 2 (1986): 297.

121. Roy M. Anderson and Robert M. May, "Epidemiological Parameters of HIV Transmission," *Nature* 333, no. 6173 (1988): 514; Nancy A. Hessol et al., "Progression of Human Immunodeficiency Virus Type 1 (HIV-1) Infection among Homosexual Men in Hepatitis B Vaccine Trial Cohorts in Amsterdam, New York City, and San Francisco, 1978–1991," *American Journal of Epidemiology* 139, no. 11 (1994): 1077–87.

122. Moss, "AIDS without End," 60.

123. Auerbach, Darrow, Jaffe, and Curran, "A Cluster of AIDS: Patients Linked by Sexual Contact," second prepublication draft, May 10, 1983, p. 8, folder: L.A. Cluster FF! Sonnabend Papers.

proximately 14 months, since "he had contact with the people about 9 to 22 months prior to the onset of their symptoms."[124] By the late 1980s, however, when an average incubation period was understood to be at least six times that long, some of the supposed transmission events noted in the cluster and represented in its commonly cited diagram might better be interpreted as epidemiological red herrings. The actual exposures that had infected the cluster's patients had almost certainly occurred several months or years before the ones depicted, with different partners than those denoted by the diagram's links. These names and faces would have lain beyond the recall of some of the patients and likely beyond the historical period examined in the study too. In other words, the cluster most likely represents a network of gay men who had sex with each other *after* they had become HIV-positive, and not a web of transmission of a causative agent.[125]

Certainly, a patient's health and other conditions would affect the speed at which he or she would experience the onset of AIDS. It is possible that one or more of the men included in the cluster, many of whom had extensive histories of sexually transmitted infections, could have advanced along the HIV continuum to an AIDS diagnosis faster as a result of their previous or concurrent infections.[126] It is highly unlikely, though, that it would be enough to cause them to advance at a rate suggested by the cluster study's calculated incubation period.

124. "NCAB Meeting," 29–30.

125. Recent molecular evolutionary analysis of stored serum samples collected from gay and bisexual men has found that extensive genetic diversity of HIV already existed in these groups in New York City and San Francisco by 1978–1979. Furthermore, the research used serum and blood product drawn in 1983 from the CDC's "Patient 0" to generate an HIV genomic sequence for this individual and to compare its genetic diversity to sequences obtained from eight other samples, as well as sequences from genomes stored in a national database at Los Alamos. The research found that Patient 0's HIV sequence appeared "typical" of the strains of HIV circulating undetected in the United States in the mid-1970s; in other words, it was not foundational to the North American epidemic. See Michael Worobey et al., "1970s and 'Patient 0' genomes Illuminate Early HIV/AIDS History in North America," *Nature* 539, no. 7627 (2016): 98–101.

126. Deschamps et al., "HIV Infection in Haiti," 2515–21. This study determined that the median time from infection to AIDS was three to five years in a resource-deprived country in a population with high levels of respiratory, diarrheal, and skin infections. Such data offer a tentative point of comparison for the claim that the first homosexual men infected with HIV in the United States, having weathered many STDs already, had compromised immune systems and may have progressed more swiftly to AIDS.

"A Picture Is Worth a Thousand Words"

Given the centrality of the cluster diagram to later interpretations of the cluster study and the role of "Patient 0," it is worth examining the production and reception of this illustration in greater detail. This chapter's final section draws on insights furnished by historians and sociologists of science since the 1990s to chart the evolution of this scientific image. As a number of authors have pointed out, scientific visual representations are important, socially produced documents crucial to the development of ideas and theory. They assist scientists in arranging data, testing hypotheses, and convincing colleagues. Although they are often treated as subordinate to the text, images often play a powerful role in the overall process of knowledge production and communication. Recent work in the sociology of science encourages readers to consider the broad trajectory of an image's life span—its conception, the work it needs to accomplish, and the various ways in which it is interpreted, by particular audiences in varying contexts beyond the specific working environment in which it was produced—paying attention at each stage to factors influencing its development. Visual representations convey information, but they conceal it as well, and they can occasionally, and unwittingly, communicate the worldviews of the working environment in which they are produced.[127]

Translation or conversion is involved in every process of scientific representation, whether taking a photograph, recording an interview, tallying a survey, or drawing an image. A number of actors—including researchers, artists, and technicians—make a series of decisions that will affect the final appearance of the representation. These choices—some deliberately made, others outside of conscious thought—will determine which features of a referent (the object, phenomenon, or concept being represented) are included and emphasized, which are downplayed or obscured, and which are left out. Institutional context, disciplinary con-

127. Michael Lynch and Steve Woolgar, eds., *Representation in Scientific Practice* (Cambridge, MA: MIT Press, 1990); Luc Pauwels, ed., *Visual Cultures of Science: Rethinking Representational Practices in Knowledge Building and Science Communication* (Lebanon, NH: Dartmouth College Press / University Press of New England, 2006); Regula Valérie Burri and Joseph Dumit, "Social Studies of Scientific Imaging and Visualization," in *The Handbook of Science and Technology Studies*, 3rd ed., ed. Edward J. Hackett et al., 297–317 (Cambridge, MA: MIT Press, 2008).

ventions, cost, and individual aesthetic preferences may all play a role.[128] For the representation of conceptual phenomena not visible to the eye— relationships between individuals, for example—standardization is difficult, and the representation will depend a great deal on the individual producing the original work.

In our example, Darrow faced the challenging task of representing complex conceptual data—the sexual relationships within a network of early reported AIDS patients, first in Los Angeles and Orange Counties, later across the country—in a resource-constrained public health setting. Darrow used the rudimentary and low-cost tools at hand to make his first attempts to create visual order from the hundreds of names, places, and dates of sexual contact gleaned from his interviews and other CDC data sources. These tools included quarters and paper clips to represent patients and connections between them, and pencil, pen, and paper to create figures that would accompany the trip reports he produced for his California and New York research trips, first in May and later in the summer of 1982.[129] The first representations of the Los Angeles cluster clearly demonstrate this provenance (see fig. 2.5), as do the subsequent images that would result in the final cluster diagram in the 1984 article. Other efforts to organize the additional data Darrow gathered in New York involved a graph of early known cases (see fig. 2.6), which drew on earlier techniques used to chart syphilis cases, and an early pencil sketch arranging the contacts (see fig. 2.7), which is a prototypical version of a color-coded cluster diagram (see fig. 2.8).

Darrow's task was difficult. He was attempting to represent schematically a highly mobile population of gay men with a large number of sexual interconnections over several years. Even assigning a city or state classification was not straightforward, since some cases moved between cities. Patient 0 was not the only one to travel frequently and switch residences between 1978 and 1982. The man identified as SF 1, for example, had moved to San Francisco in 1979, where he would receive a diagnosis of KS in March 1982. He had also spent time in New York and Los

128. Luc Pauwels, "A Theoretical Framework for Assessing Visual Representational Practices in Knowledge Building and Science Communications," in Pauwels, *Visual Cultures of Science*, 4–5.

129. Darrow reenacted his research practice for the documentary film *The Zero Factor*, the first in the multipart televised documentary series *A Time of AIDS*, directed by Anne Moir (Princeton, NJ: Films for the Humanities, 1992), videocassette (VHS).

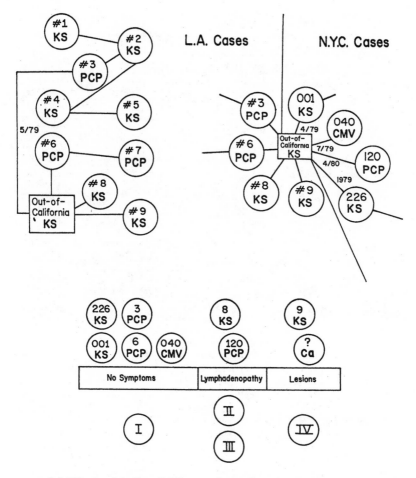

FIGURE 2.5 "Cluster—LA Cases," "Cluster—Connection of LA and NYC Cases," and "Cluster—Relationship of Symptom Onset to Sex Contact," AIDS Slides for Dr Foege, AIDS TRACER M 1983 Jan–June (1 of 2), AIDS correspondence (TRACER) archives, US Department of Health and Human Services, MS C 607, National Library of Medicine, Bethesda. Three slide reproductions on letter-size papers, 21.6 × 27.9 cm. Courtesy of the National Library of Medicine. Note the simple representational devices of circles and straight lines used by the CDC sociologist William Darrow, which bear the influence of the sociograms in figure 2.9 but also the fiscal constraints of working with the tools at hand—in this case, pencils, coins, and paper clips. "Out-of-California KS" appears here in its earliest form, prior to being abbreviated as "Patient O," and later "Patient 0." Photocopies of these slides, along with one depicting the extended cluster of forty cases, were shared through the Department of Health and Human Services in early 1983. It is highly likely that James Curran used these images in his presentation to the National Cancer Advisory Board at the National Cancer Institute in December 1982, as detailed in this book's introduction.

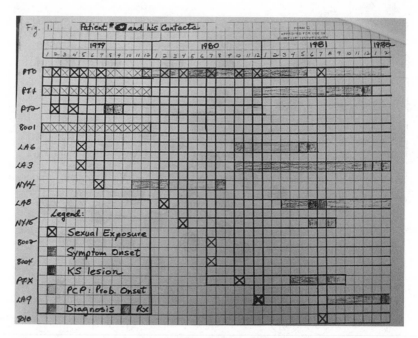

FIGURE 2.6 "Patient #O and his Contacts," pencil, ink, and colored crayon, 27.9 × 21.6 cm, 1982, Professional Papers of William Darrow, Miami. Courtesy of William Darrow. The original caption accompanying this image has been retained to provide context for the reader. This figure accompanied the original use of the cluster diagram (shown in figs. 2.1 and 2.8) in Darrow's report to his colleagues of his New York research during the summer of 1982. It offered additional information to contextualize the cluster representation and formed an important part of the cluster diagram's initial environment of use. Without it—as, for example, when the article was published in the *American Journal of Medicine* in 1984—the cluster diagram is unable to demonstrate the dates and frequency of "sexual exposures" nor the dates of symptom onset. In the title, one can see that the originally written "Patient #57" has been overwritten with the letter *O*, indicating that this particular version was destined for readers outside the CDC. Individuals denoted by the 8000 number series indicate sexual contacts of "Patient #O" who had not yet been diagnosed with an AIDS-related illness.

Angeles, and "was known by several cases" in those cities; indeed, two of these sexual connections would be captured in the cluster diagram.[130] Despite these challenges, location was one of the features Darrow emphasized in the cluster diagram, along with the type of illness each patient had, and the sequence, though not the date, of the onset of these illnesses. This set of choices made sense, given that the image was intended

130. Darrow, "Trip Report," pp. 4, 10, Darrow Papers.

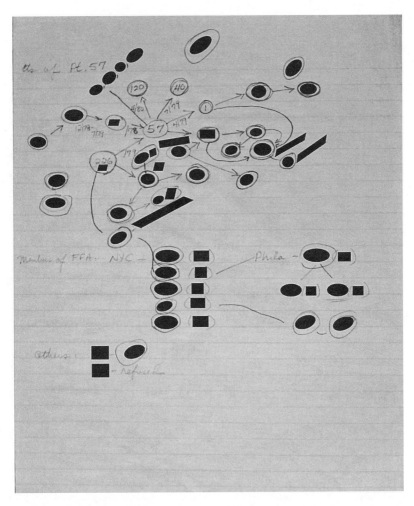

FIGURE 2.7 "Cts of Pt. 57; Members of FFA; Others," early draft of the cluster diagram in regular and colored pencil, 21.6 × 27.9 cm, 1982, Professional Papers of William Darrow. Courtesy of William Darrow. This draft image, with redactions—straight-edged for cases' and contacts' initials and last names, round-edged for case numbers—to preserve confidentiality, shows Darrow working to organize the relationships of the men he has linked to the cluster. The image suggests some of the many challenges facing researchers: the multiple geographic locations of the CDC's cases (New York, Los Angeles, San Francisco, and Philadelphia, for example); the existence of sexual partners who linked cases but who were not themselves reported as sick (the individual above case 226, for example, who had sexual contact with Patient 57 in 1978); and the impossibility of linking those cases, such as the one at the bottom left of the drawing, who refused to take part in the study. It becomes clear how important Patient 57's records of his contacts and his cooperation with the CDC investigators were to the completion of the cluster study and to the central role he would acquire as "Patient 0."

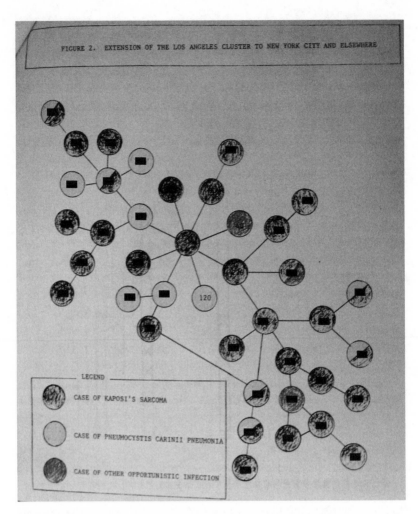

FIGURE 2.8 "Extension of the Los Angeles Cluster to New York City and Elsewhere."
Numbered cluster diagram, hand-colored with crayon, 21.6 × 27.9 cm, 1982, Professional
Papers of William Darrow. Courtesy of William Darrow. The original caption accompanying this image has been retained to provide context for the reader. This image, which accompanied figure 2.6 in Darrow's September 1982 trip report, shows the cluster diagram
reaching its near-final state. The image was hand-colored to indicate types of illness and
included each individual's CDC-assigned case number, allocated roughly in order that the
cases were reported to the CDC (with redactions to preserve confidentiality).

to demonstrate a sexual network of individuals whose contacts with each other were deemed unlikely to occur by chance, given their geographic dispersal.

It appears that an aesthetic decision was made to keep the image "clean" by retaining a significant amount of white space, which meant that other pertinent information was left out. Dates and frequency of sexual contact for each connected pair were excluded from the graphic (though some of this information would have been available to Darrow's colleagues through previous correspondence and additional information attached to his reports), as were the specific dates for the onset of their illnesses. Again, in the initial circumstances of production, the diagram that would become the iconic signifier of the cluster study was interwoven in a library of other diagrams and documentary evidence that gave it support and meaning. As the image moved farther from the initial workings of the task force and was selected, it seems, as the best representation to "illustrate" the study, the accompanying information and assumed knowledge required to interpret and interrogate the diagram diminished. It became difficult, if not impossible, to determine from looking at the image the dates at which patients fell ill and whether there was any directionality to the spread of infection. Thus, the farther observers were situated from the inner workings of the task force, the less information they had to contextualize their interpretations of its representation and the greater their chances of interpreting it through other means and assumptions.

Another feature missing from the image—perhaps not surprisingly, given the representational challenges it would have brought—was the number of total partners each patient had reported. Most of the cases in the cluster had hundreds of contacts that had potentially infected them with the posited transmissible agent. The diagram's clean circles, straight lines, and white space all work to artificially fix these cases and their interconnections within a single frame of space and time, removed from the messiness—and reality—of their lives. Many viewers would focus on the connections depicted, rather than the thousands of undepicted connections that had more likely infected these individuals, which had taken place outside of their memories, or without the necessary confirmation by a second party or a friend, and thus outside the allowed representation of reality framed by the image. In other words, many viewers assumed that the connections depicted in the diagram denoted the spread of a transmissible agent within the cluster that subsequently caused the patients in question to develop AIDS. In all likelihood, however, these sexual liaisons occurred *after* the men had been infected—again, outside the clean arrangement depicted by the diagram.

For several decades, sociologists had made use of images known as *sociograms* to represent the social relationships they studied.[131] While undertaking his PhD in sociology at Emory University, Darrow had been taught by one of the former research assistants of James Coleman, a sociologist renowned for his study of the relationships between teenagers in high schools during the 1950s.[132] Coleman had made use of numbered circles, squares, and triangles linked by lines to represent the alliances and groups that made up the student populations in the schools he studied. The elaborate diagrams he created clearly influenced Darrow's representation of the sexual relationships he included in the cluster (see fig. 2.9).[133] Representational conventions had developed over the years to standardize sociograms and to develop a shared visual knowledge among research professionals. The "most chosen individual" in a network was typically placed in the center of the image; nodal points (in this case representing individuals) were to be arranged for maximal clarity and minimal line overlapping; and individuals were to be depicted in their "'natural' groupings of diads, triads, and so forth"—the real-world relationships being modeled.[134]

Whether consciously or not, Darrow followed these established visual conventions by placing "Patient 0" at the center of his cluster diagram. From a geographic perspective, there was some logic to this positioning— the placeless "Patient 0" serving as "the missing link" between cases in Los Angeles on the left and New York on the right (though this geographic structure disintegrates with cases from other cities). The flight attendant's superior ability in recalling the names of former contacts led to his being the "most chosen individual" in the network, an arbitrary status which was then naturalized and reinforced through visual means. Later research, which indicated that individuals may mistakenly attribute more importance to a centrally positioned node in a representation

131. Alden S. Klovdahl, "A Note on Images of Networks," *Social Networks* 3 (1981): 197–214.

132. This research assistant was sociologist Martin Levin; William Darrow, e-mail to author, August 8, 2013.

133. James S. Coleman, *The Adolescent Society: The Social Life of the Teenager and its Impact on Education* (New York: Free Press, 1961), 175–82.

134. Klovdahl, "Note on Images," 199.

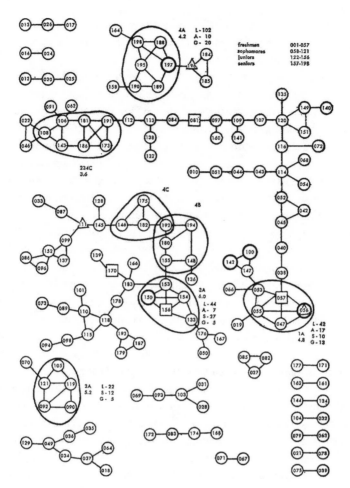

FIGURE 2.9 Sociogram titled "Network of Reciprocated Friendships among Marketville Boys," in James S. Coleman, *The Adolescent Society: The Social Life of the Teenager and its Impact on Education* (New York: Free Press, 1961), 175; 13.0 × 18.5 cm. Reprinted with the permission of Free Press, a Division of Simon & Schuster, Inc., from *Adolescent Society* by James S. Coleman. Copyright © 1961 by The Free Press. Copyright © renewed 1989 by James S. Coleman. All rights reserved. Coleman's research assistant, Martin Levin, taught Darrow at Emory University in the 1970s and introduced him to the use of sociograms to represent human relationships. In these representations of teenaged boys in a small, coeducational high school in autumn 1957, the bolded circle represents the boy most mentioned in interviews as the best athlete in each year group, the square shows the most scholarly, and the triangle the boy most often mentioned as most attractive to members of the opposite sex. The larger rounded shapes represent social cliques. The reciprocated relationships between the school's girls were depicted separately, and attempts to show relationships between the two sexes were abandoned due to the technical challenges of analyzing such a high quantity of relationship data.

of a network, suggests that this combination—of visual conventions and subsequent viewer interpretation—served to amplify the perceived significance of "Patient 0."[135]

The initial importance of the study—as reported in the June 1982 *MMWR* article—was the evidence it seemed to offer that AIDS was caused by a sexually transmissible agent. Later that year, as the interviews of the New York cases offered more details, it offered the possibility of estimating a preliminary incubation period for the condition. Both of these developments focused on the role of the "Out-of-California case," and the excitement he generated is captured by his prominent role in the cluster diagram. As these conclusions made their way up the chain of command in the US Department of Health and Human Services, a fixity to the results developed. In a message outlining the activities undertaken by the National Institutes of Health in response to AIDS, Edward N. Brandt Jr., the assistant secretary for Health, described the investigation as such: "Investigators traced a case from one individual which was spread to nearly a dozen sexual contacts."[136] This conclusion, that AIDS had "spread" from the "out-of-California" patient to his sexual partners, had been communicated by James Curran as recently as December 1982. It was, however, in conflict with the evolving conclusions of the cluster study. Shortly after Brandt wrote his message, a prepublication draft of the extended cluster study was circulated for feedback; it urged caution in interpreting any directionality in the cluster. "A cluster of AIDS patients linked one to another by sexual contacts does not necessarily imply," the authors noted, "that an infectious agent was directly transmitted from an infectious host to a susceptible partner." They also acknowledged that "most of the patients included in this cluster were exposed to another member of the cluster during a single sexual encounter or during periods of sexual contact that lasted for several days or weeks."[137] This finding represented another potential weakness in the

135. Cathleen McGrath, Jim Blythe, and David Krackhardt, "The Effect of Spatial Arrangement on Judgments and Errors in Interpreting Graphs," *Social Networks* 19 (1997): 223–42.

136. AIDS events and actions undertaken by the National Institutes of Health, chronology attached to letter from Edward Brandt to Henry Waxman, 4 March 1983, AIDS TRACER M 1983 Jan–June (1 of 2), AIDS Correspondence (TRACER) archives, 1982–1990, Office for the Assistant Secretary for Planning and Evaluation, US Department of Health and Human Services, MS C 607, National Library of Medicine, Bethesda.

137. Auerbach et al, "Cluster of Cases," 7–8.

diagram. The uniform straight lines between circles, which indicated the sexual connections in the diagram, did not allow readers to distinguish between the relative "strength" of these sexual connections, which suggested that a single sexual encounter was as likely to transmit the suspected agent as a relationship spanning several months.[138]

As we shall see in chapters 3 and 4, Randy Shilts was one of the most influential consumers of the cluster study to misconstrue (or at least misrepresent) its findings, and the diagram featured strongly in his skewed reading. "At the center of the cluster diagram," he wrote, "was Gaetan Dugas, marked on the chart as Patient Zero of the GRID epidemic," making use of the acronym for "gay related immune deficiency," an early term coined for the syndrome. Shilts appears to have viewed the diagram as a sort of closed sexual network with infection radiating out from the center. "At least 40 of the first 248 gay men diagnosed with GRID in the United States . . . either had had sex with Gaetan Dugas or had had sex with someone who had," he wrote, incorrectly, apparently not noticing the additional degrees of separation between Dugas and patients on the outer edges of the cluster. "The links sometimes were extended for many generations of sexual contacts, giving frightening insight into how rapidly the epidemic had spread before anyone knew about it." Shilts went on to describe these sexual connections in a fashion that was distinctly reminiscent of the example of Voltaire's Pangloss presented in chapter 1:

Before one of Gaetan's Los Angeles boyfriends ["LA 3"] came down with *Pneumocystis*, for example, he had had sex with another Angelino ["LA 2"] who came down with Kaposi's sarcoma and with a Florida man ["FL 1"] who contracted both Kaposi's and the pneumonia. The Los Angeles contact ["LA 2"], in turn, cavorted with two other Los Angeles men ["LA 1" and

138. Later research would provide a much better understanding of the relative risk of contracting HIV per sexual exposure and per type of exposure. Recent estimates place insertive and receptive oral sex as very low risk, and per-act transmission rates for insertive penile–vaginal intercourse at 4 per 10,000 exposures to an infected person, receptive penile–vaginal intercourse at 8 per 10,000 exposures, insertive anal intercourse at 11 per 10,000 exposures, and receptive anal intercourse at 138 per 10,000 exposures. Factors such as concurrent genital ulcers and high viral load can increase the risks of transmission, while using condoms and taking antiretroviral medications (as preventive or as treatment) can reduce these risks. See Pragna Patel et al., "Estimating Per-Act HIV Transmission Risk: A Systematic Review," *AIDS* 28 (2014): 1509–19.

"LA 4"] who later came down with Kaposi's, one of whom ["LA 4"] infected still another southern California man who was suffering from KS ["LA 5"]. The Floridian, meanwhile, had sex with a Texan who got Kaposi's sarcoma ["TX 1"], a second Florida man who got *Pneumocystis* ["FL 2"], and two Georgia men, one of whom got *Pneumocystis* ["GA 2"] and another who soon found the skin lesions of KS ["GA 1"]. Before finding these lesions, however, the Georgian ["GA 1"] had sex with a Pennsylvania man ["PA 1"] who later came down with both *Pneumocystis* and KS.

He summarized: "From just one tryst with Gaetan, therefore, eleven GRID cases could be connected."[139] Interpreting the cluster image without access to information about each case's dates of sexual contact and symptom onset, Shilts drew a false assumption based on his perception that "Patient 0" was the most important individual in the cluster and that certain cluster patients had infected others. Judging by his later comments, Shilts may also have interpreted a public health official's disclosure—which linked a French Canadian flight attendant to the first two reported symptomatic AIDS patients in New York or to their lovers—as a statement suggesting that the cluster's patient numbers indicated the earliest cases in each city.[140] This too was erroneous—this numbering was not absolute but rather relative to the cases linked to the cluster. Earlier reported cases existed, particularly in New York, but Darrow and his colleagues had not been able to link them to the men in the cluster, and thus these were left out of the ordinal series employed in the study.

Some of these misconceptions would be clarified when the cluster study later reached a welcoming audience in the related field of network dynamics in the mid-1980s, albeit after a slightly bumpy start.[141] When Alden Klovdahl, a sociologist with experience in network analysis and computer-aided graphic design, published a letter criticizing some of the cluster study's limitations, Darrow recruited him to expand on his work.[142] In an article published in 1985, Klovdahl used the study's information to demonstrate the strengths and weaknesses of a network approach to the spread of infectious diseases; in the process, he revisualized the cluster

139. Shilts, *Band*, 147 [cluster labels added].
140. Sipchen, "AIDS Chronicles," V9.
141. Douglas A. Luke and Jenine K. Harris, "Network Analysis in Public Health: History, Methods, and Applications," *Annual Review of Public Health* 28, no. 1 (2007):77.
142. Darrow, e-mail to author, August 8, 2013.

in a way that destabilized the conventional centrality of "Patient 0."[143] To manipulate the cases in the cluster diagram, Klovdahl employed ORTEP—short for Oak Ridge Thermal Ellipsoid Plot—a computer program which had been designed in the mid-1960s as a means of representing crystalline structures in three dimensions. (Fittingly, the internal newsletter that announced the program's creation began with the phrase "A picture is worth a thousand words."[144]) Using ORTEP, Klovdahl arrayed the cases by date of symptom onset, rather than the roughly geographic approximation depicted in the original diagram, to demonstrate what he called "time sequence anomalies" (see fig. 2.10). With the inclusion of an axis for time in the model to account for symptom development, cases LA 1, NY 1, NY 2, NY 3, and NY 4 near the bottom of the diagram take on a new prominence. When one considers that the average number of partners reported by these patients was 227 per year (with a range of 10 to 1,560), one begins to realize the very likely absence of important links to earlier cases.

To explain the "time sequence anomalies," Klovdahl noted that the "possibility was that there were 'missing nodes' in this network, for example, individuals who were exposed to an infectious agent by LA1, who had not developed symptoms at the time of the original CDC study, and who transmitted an infectious agent to '0' directly, or to others who did. It follows that good network data can signal the existence (and identity) of individuals with subclinical infections."[145] Others would not be as diplomatic. In addition to Andrew Moss's 1988 letter, Duncan Campbell, a British journalist, published strong critiques of Randy Shilts's use of the cluster study in response to the author's British book tour for *And the Band Played On* that year. In his work Campbell included excerpts from a recent interview he had conducted with Darrow, in which the CDC sociologist stressed that the 1982 hypotheses of incubation could no longer be maintained. This statement was taken by some observers to suggest that he dismissed his earlier work, and many would later clumsily interpret the cluster study out of its original context. For example, on Octo-

143. Klovdahl, "Social Networks," 1206.

144. Bill Felknor, "Laboratory Scientist Draws 'Atoms-In-Depth' Using Computer-Oriented Graphic Technique," *The News* [Oak Ridge National Laboratory], April 2, 1965, 1, accessed November 3, 2014, http://www.umass.edu/molvis/francoeur/ortep/ortepnews .html.

145. Alden S. Klovdahl, "Social Networks and the Spread of Infectious Diseases: The AIDS Example," *Social Science and Medicine* 21, no. 11 (1985): 1208–9.

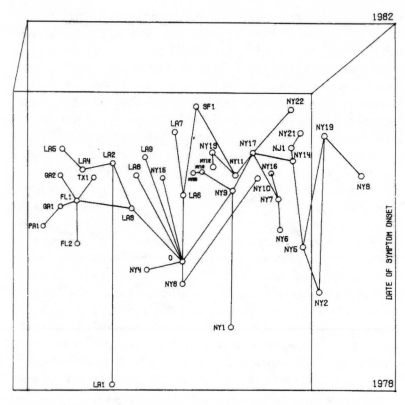

FIGURE 2.10 A rotated reconfiguration of the "AIDS cluster," using the Oak Ridge Thermal Ellipsoid Plot Program (ORTEP), with date of symptom onset represented on the z-axis; 11.6 × 11.0 cm. Reprinted from Alden S. Klovdahl, "Social Networks and the Spread of Infectious Diseases: The AIDS Example," *Social Science and Medicine* 21, no. 11 (1985): 1206, © 1985, with permission from Elsevier. With "0" off-center and cluster patients arrayed from bottom to top by date of symptom onset, other individuals are able to assume more visually prominent roles in Klovdahl's diagram. "LA1" and "NY1," for example, both reported having more than one hundred partners in the year before they experienced symptoms, yet their inability to recall many names for the investigators means that they are surrounded by white space. This diagram suggests the new directions being pursued by network analysis researchers and foreshadows the far more complex representations of sexual networks that would be made possible with the assistance of computers.

ber 31, 2007, in the light of recently announced scientific work which suggested that HIV had first arrived in the United States via Haiti in 1969, two journalists for the *Miami Herald* wrote that the new evidence "debunks the original 'Patient Zero' theory that said the HIV virus came to Los Angeles via a gay Canadian flight attendant named Gaetan Dugas.

That theory was created by Dr. William Darrow and others at the CDC and turned into the 1987 book *And the Band Played On,* by journalist Randy Shilts. Darrow later repudiated his own study."[146] It would appear that the journalists had briefed themselves by consulting one of several online articles that offered this misleading history.[147] In response, Darrow—who by this time had left the CDC and was a public health professor at Florida International University leading community-based AIDS prevention programs—wrote his own letter of frustration regarding the cluster study in 2007 to the *Miami Herald,* complaining that

> I have never repudiated the findings of the L.A. Cluster Study. Nor, to my knowledge, has anyone else.
>
> Some people who have never taken the time to read our initial report in Morbidity and Mortality Weekly Report (June 18, 1982), subsequent articles published in the American Journal of Medicine (and other peer-reviewed journals), and chapters (that have been published in books about AIDS) have misinterpreted the purpose of the L.A. Cluster Study, methods, findings, and conclusions. To be counted among those who have misrepresented the significance of our work and our conclusions are two reporters for the Miami Herald.[148]

Darrow's letter was never published.

* * *

The cluster study that gave rise to the epidemiological phrase "Patient 0" in the early years of the AIDS epidemic must be understood in the context of a longer history of shifts in epidemiological practice and venereal disease control. Framing the discussion in this way allows us to see how the US federal government's response to VD from the 1950s onward laid

146. Fred Tasker and Jacqueline Charles, "Disease Research: Scientists Trace AIDS through Haiti; Findings Draw Anger," *Miami Herald,* October 31, 2007, 1A. The reporters quoted a professor of medicine who, while expressing his doubts on the study's findings, pointed to the topic's perpetual intellectual appeal: "People love to play history, and it would be great to figure out who Patient Zero was."

147. Their history bears a strong resemblance to the one available on Wikipedia.com, the free encyclopedia website, at that time: *Wikipedia,* s.v. "index case," October 28, 2007, http://en.wikipedia.org/w/index.php?title=Index_case&oldid=167559312.

148. William Darrow, "Re: Disease Research—Scientists Trace AIDS through Haiti, Stirring Ire," unpublished letter to the editor, n.d. [2007], Darrow Papers.

the groundwork for the training and working culture for the VD Branch at the CDC, and in turn for some of the early investigations into AIDS. Public health investigators were taught to think of themselves as detectives, to suspect homosexuality in cases of syphilis, and to trust the cluster method of contact investigation to allow them to reach the source of an outbreak. Such a working style laid the groundwork for potential conflicts with their colleagues working on chronic disease, some of whom appear to have viewed contact epidemiology as a quaint, outmoded approach from a simpler past. In communicating their research for the cluster study, Darrow and his colleagues faced significant challenges in terms of representing complex human relationships. Linguistic and visual choices unintentionally served to inflect the cluster study with overtones of origins, connotations that were later adopted and elaborated by other scientists, the media, and members of the public.

As we have seen, further developments in understanding the natural history of AIDS eventually led to the gradual receding of the cluster study's importance in most scientific circles. Because the main thrust of the study—that a sexually transmissible agent caused AIDS—was on the "winning" side of history and helped redirect research efforts toward this consensus, the outmoded hypotheses that underpinned it would escape more careful reevaluation at a later date. In 1982, it had seemed reasonable to hypothesize that sexual contact could transmit an infectious agent that would result in an illness appearing within nine to twenty-two months. This belief, which was necessary to convey the significance of the network being represented by the cluster, was increasingly difficult to sustain over time. Later, when investigators were interviewed for a popular history of the epidemic, they would recall the study's importance for the work it accomplished—reorienting a research consensus—rather than scrutinize how well its constitutive elements had withstood the test of time. Thus, as part of the edifice that sustained this consensus, "Patient 0" and the cluster study that generated this phrase would continue to retain their explanatory power for popular audiences for many years to come.

CHAPTER THREE

"Humanizing This Disease"

As a gay person myself I wasn't thrilled about Gaetan's behavior. I don't see him as any more typical of a gay man than Jack the Ripper was of the heterosexual—but it did happen.
—*Randy Shilts*, 1988[1]

On the afternoon of March 15, 1986, Randy Shilts addressed an audience of Canadian journalists at a conference in Vancouver, British Columbia. The Ottawa-based Centre for Investigative Journalism (CIJ) was holding its annual conference at Vancouver's Pan Pacific Hotel, and Shilts, on the strength of his AIDS reporting for the *San Francisco Chronicle*, had been invited to join four other panelists for a discussion on AIDS in the media. The reporter had accepted the invitation, though it was not the sole reason for his Vancouver visit. A month later, the Vancouver-based conference coordinator wrote to thank Shilts for his participation, adding that she hoped "your other business in Vancouver worked out well."[2] She could have had little idea of how successful his research expedition had been. During his twenty-four-hour Vancouver stay, Shilts had managed to gather nearly all of the background information he would need to tell his version of the "Patient Zero" story, a tale that would ultimately bring the author and his history of the American AIDS epidemic to international attention.

In front of his peers at the conference, Shilts delivered what would become his standard criticism of the mainstream media's response to

---

1. Philip Young, "Patient Zero: Man Who Gave the World AIDS," *Northern Echo* [High Wycombe, UK], April 9, 1988, 6.

2. Anne Mullens to Randy Shiltz [*sic*], 24 April 1986, folder 23, box 34, Shilts Papers.

AIDS, complaining about the lack of coverage the disease had received
when it had appeared to affect mostly homosexuals and about the "most
shameless press release journalism that's existed since the Vietnam war."
In addition to outlining the Freedom of Information requests that he
had filed to interrogate the US government's response to the epidemic,
Shilts explained that "the other focus of, of the reporting that I was interested in, was in terms of *humanizing this disease.*" He slowed his typically rapid delivery to emphasize these last three words, before picking up his pace once more: "I mean these people are, who we're dealing
with, are human beings, and, and, and I am not so cynical as to believe
that the fact that these people, that, that because these people are gay or,
or where essentially all we have this number of a percent of gay men in
San Francisco getting it, I think that people can relate to anybody if you,
if you present who these people are." [3] In his presentation, Shilts conveyed how important he believed it was to render human the people behind the statistics, in a bid to promote understanding and to garner support for efforts to tackle the spread of the AIDS epidemic.

This is the conundrum that this chapter attempts to explain. How is
it that Shilts, despite his publicly stated goal of helping people relate to
those with AIDS, spent his weekend in Vancouver gathering as much
information as he could about Gaétan Dugas? And that he would use
this information to create a personification of the early AIDS patient
that would lead many readers of his work to believe that the French Canadian man was a monster? How is it that a journalist who worked for
years to develop his craft and was a vocal advocate of his profession's
ethical code may have misled his sources, relied on unsubstantiated information, and defended his depiction of Dugas from critics by pro-
claiming that it represented "very good investigative journalism"?[4]

Douglas Crimp, a cultural theorist, AIDS activist, and one of Shilts's
most vocal critics, has suggested that Shilts's claims of being "not ideo-

3. I draw my verbatim quotations of his presentation from a sound recording made
of the panel, reprinted with permission from the Canadian Association for Journalists (CAJ): [Media Coverage of AIDS], March [15,] 1986, copy consultation numbers
167573–1990–0395–39-S1.mp3 and 167573–1990–0395–39-S2.mp3, item number 167573,
accession number 1990–0395, Canadian Association of Journalists fonds, Library and Archives Canada, Ottawa.

4. Crimp, "Randy Shilts's Miserable Failure," in Crimp, *Melancholia and Moralism*,
120–21; see also Tim Kingston, "Controversy Follows Shilts and 'Zero' to London," *Coming Up!* April 1988, 11.

logical" and wanting to "get the whole story out" represented either a "dangerously naive or cynically disingenuous ideological position," particularly when Shilts defended his reporting of the "Patient Zero" story on the basis that it had actually happened. Crimp points out that Shilts himself acknowledged that he chose to tell Dugas's story not because it was representative but because it was "fascinating." Of the 6,079 people included in the official statistics for US AIDS deaths by the end of *And the Band Played On*'s coverage, Shilts chose to write a story about Dugas, which, to Crimp, "makes his story about one six-thousandth of the 'truth.'" Crimp ponders what *"unconscious* mechanisms . . . would account for this very selective will to truth" before concluding that the story's truth mattered "not one whit," given that the fantasy of the deliberate disease disseminator had already existed in the public's mind before Shilts had penned it.[5]

Similarly, the cultural critic Priscilla Wald questions Shilts's motivation in her skillful scrutiny of the "Patient Zero" story. In an analysis of Shilts's comments to a reporter regarding the irony of the media's focus on "Patient Zero" in the face of his larger policy stories, Wald comments that "it is hard to imagine that Shilts really did not recognize the importance of his character."[6] Furthermore, in contemplating Shilts's statement that researchers would later "try to fathom the bizarre coincidences and the unique role the handsome young steward performed in the coming epidemic," she writes, "It is hard to know exactly to what 'unique role' refers; for in Shilts's narrative Dugas plays more than one."[7] The criticisms of both Crimp and Wald suggest the utility of having a better understanding of what may have guided Shilts in depicting this character.

To understand Shilts's claims and, perhaps more important, his unstated ideas about Dugas and the character of "Patient Zero," it is helpful to investigate what may have motivated the reporter, not only in his ambitions for the book but also in the years leading up to his work as a journalist covering AIDS. To this end, the author's extensive personal and professional papers provide a useful opportunity to understand the forces that influenced his thinking and reporting—particularly in the absence of any published biographical material of depth—as well as a

5. Crimp, "Miserable Failure," 122–24; emphasis in original.
6. Wald, *Contagious*, 231.
7. Shilts, *Band*, 23; cited in Wald, *Contagious*, 233.

means of establishing the development of the fictional character, "Patient Zero."[8]

The chapter has four main sections which, taken together, allow us to build a more nuanced picture of Shilts and a crucial context for his best-selling book on AIDS. The chapter's first section draws on material from Shilts's personal papers as well as interviews he gave throughout his career to contextualize Shilts's deep-seated motivation to be a successful journalist and his developing writing style. The second outlines Shilts's growing interest in AIDS as a story which would eventually define his professional career, and it follows him up to his decision to write a book on the history of the American AIDS epidemic. It is important to consider how Shilts's self-perceived role as a cultural interpreter between the gay and straight communities shaped his approach to writing *Band:* he wrote, as was his custom, for a heterosexual audience.[9] The third section scrutinizes Shilts's interview notes to reconstruct the manner in which he uncovered the "Patient Zero" story and outlines the journalist's growing fascination and self-described obsession with the dead flight attendant. The chapter's final section examines the way in which Shilts made sense of his source material and guided it through the draft phases toward publication. It also draws on another journalist's suggestion that Shilts was a skillful observer of everyone except himself as a means of explaining how his strong personal opinion would color his statement of the "facts," in spite of his aspirations to the highest professional standards of objectivity.[10] Shilts's journal entries, the interviews he gave while promoting *Band*, his letters, and his story

8. Apart from some obituaries published at the time of his death, there is little biographical work on Shilts—perhaps a sign of the divisions he raised in the gay communities he profiled. The entry for the author in the *American Dictionary of National Biography* is currently the best short sketch; see Ralph E. Luker, "Shilts, Randy Martin," in *American Dictionary of National Biography*, Oxford University Press, 2000–2010, article published 2000, http://www.anb.org/articles/16/16–03326.html. For an excellent description of Shilts's AIDS reporting, see James Kinsella, "Chronicler of the Castro," in *Covering the Plague: AIDS and the American Media* (London: Rutgers University Press, 1989), 157–84.

9. Mike Weiss, "Randy Shilts Was Gutsy, Brash and Unforgettable. He Died 10 Years Ago, Fighting for the Rights of Gays in American Society," *San Francisco Chronicle*, February 17, 2004, D1, http://www.sfgate.com/cgi-bin/article.cgi?f=/c/a/2004/02/17/DDGGH50UAU1.DTL. As the article demonstrates, many observers interpreted his stance as that of an "assimilationist."

10. John Weir, "Reading Randy," *Out*, August–September 1993, 46.

drafts all offer evidence that Shilts's personification of Dugas rests to a certain extent on an external projection of the reporter's own fears and insecurities. The journalist's excitement about uncovering the identity of the "Patient 0," about whom he had read, combined with both his drive to become famous and his legitimate concerns about the consequences of AIDS led him to produce a skewed—and thus even more compelling—characterization of Gaétan Dugas for the straight audience he held in his mind.

"Typewriter Therapy"

The 1986 CIJ Conference was not Shilts's first time in Vancouver. The reporter had visited the city in late 1975 during a different and difficult period of his life, one marked by wanderlust and personal frustration. Shilts had recently graduated from the University of Oregon with a double major in English and journalism, and he was encountering significant difficulty finding employment as a journalist at a mainstream paper. To make ends meet, he freelanced as the Northwest correspondent for the *Advocate* and pitched ideas for story after story to the magazine's editors. His frequent letters in 1975 to Sasha Gregory-Lewis, one of the *Advocate*'s senior editors, demonstrate an eagerness to develop his writing style as well as a hardworking, entrepreneurial attitude.[11] The Vancouver trip was for an article in a series of travel pieces on North American gay destinations. In a journal entry, Shilts described the experience of visiting the foggy, rainy city in early December as "rather depressing." He found the local politicos "boring," so he took to the streets and settled for "three consecutive nights of tricking" with a local man.[12] Even the ambitious Shilts would likely not have been able to imagine the more triumphant circumstances of his next visit to Vancouver a decade later. Similarly, his path to becoming a journalist had not been clearly signposted either.

11. Folder 5: Advocate, 1975, box 11, Shilts Papers.
12. "Seattle—December 14, 1975," folder: Journal '75-'76, carton 2, Alband Collection. Shilts kept a number of journals, copies of which are held in the San Francisco Public Library LGBTQIA Center's Shilts Papers as well as in the GLBT Historical Society's Linda Alband Collection.

Randy Martin Shilts was born in Davenport, Iowa, on August 8, 1951, and grew up in a conservative, Methodist household in Aurora, Illinois, third eldest of six brothers. His parents both drank heavily, and although Shilts would grow to appreciate their better qualities at a later age, dedicating his first book to them, his feelings for them were characterized by hatred during his childhood, when he received regular beatings at the hands of his mother, and his adolescence. Katie Leishman, Shilts's friend and a manuscript editor for *Band*, has suggested that his propensity for writing grew from these near daily instances of violence and that, after years of wrestling with multiple addictions, he had realized that writing was "the only anesthesia that lasted."[13] Shilts himself would refer to his "typewriter therapy" in his periodic journal entries during the 1970s, as well as to his frequent use of sex, alcohol, and a variety of drugs to cope with his troubles.[14]

The teenaged Shilts did not have the conceptual framework to categorize his early sexual experiences with other young boys on Eagle Scout campouts; he would not hear the word *homosexual* until he was eighteen.[15] Described by his local newspaper as a "hard-boiled conservative" at age sixteen—and one who "doesn't expect to be out-talked"— Shilts founded an Aurora chapter of Young Americans for Freedom, a nationwide conservative youth organization, before experiencing a profound shift in political beliefs during his senior year of high school.[16] Caught up in antiwar protesting—spurred in part by the receipt of a low draft number, representing an earlier induction into the army—Shilts earned the title of "class nonconformist" in the final weeks of his high school career by organizing antiwar rallies and handing out black armbands at school assemblies.[17] He would later remark that "it's impor-

13. Randy Shilts, "The Summer of '74," pp. 5–6, journal, carton 2, Alband Collection; Randy Shilts, "April 4, 1978," "Green" Journal [1977–1978, 1984, 1986], carton 2, Alband Collection; Katie Leishman, "The Writing Cure," *New York Times*, March 5, 1994, 23.

14. "January 3, 1976," folder 3: Jobs, box 11, Shilts Papers.

15. Ken Kelley, "The Interview: Randy Shilts," *San Francisco Focus* 36, no. 6 (1989): 108.

16. Ron Krueger, "He Eats, Thinks and Drinks Ideas: Randy Shilts and Young Americans for Freedom," *Beacon-News* [Aurora, IL], January 23, 1968, 2; "Shilts: 'Incredible Programs We Could Do,'" *Oregon Daily Emerald* [Eugene], March 30, 1973, 6.

17. Charlotte Bercaw, "Author Bemoans AIDS Travesties in Best-Seller," *Beacon-News* [Aurora, IL], November 15, 1987, A1; Charlotte Bercaw, "Shilts Gets Grip on His Being, Then Worldwide Epidemic," *Beacon-News* [Aurora, IL], November 15, 1987, A5.

tant to have seen the extreme right and left—to realize there are well-intentioned people on both sides of the political spectrum and no one has a monopoly on the truth. As a journalist, you have to have that basic open-mindedness."[18]

Encouraged by a Thanksgiving trip to New York City just months after the influential Stonewall riots, and a Ritalin-fueled conversation with a friend on Christmas Eve 1969, Shilts made the decision to leave home—and his first year of college in Aurora—in early January 1970 and embarked on several months of hitchhiking around the United States as a hippie.[19] An employment history detailed on an application to the Pulliam Journalism Fellowship in 1975 reveals that by September 1970, Shilts had settled in Portland, Oregon, and was working as a security guard for the campus of Portland Community College while he took courses in anthropology and English. Shilts also proudly noted on his application form that he did not receive any financial assistance from his parents between 1970 and 1975.[20]

While a student at community college, Shilts came to terms with his sexuality, making the decision to come out of the closet at the end of 1971. By this point he had met a number of older closeted men and, encouraged by the emerging gay liberation movement, decided that he did not want to share their fate by allowing the fear of others discovering his secret to ruin his life. It was in one of his college anthropology classes that Shilts would come out more publicly on May 19, 1972, using the opportunity of a course assignment to invite a group of gay friends to join him in making a presentation on homosexual life in America.[21]

Shilts then moved to Eugene, Oregon, having transferred to the University of Oregon to continue his studies in English in the fall of 1972. He

18. Bercaw, "Shilts Gets Grip," A5, A8.

19. "December 25, 12:30 AM—1979," "Green" journal, Alband Collection. See also "Train to New York City, January 31, 1978," in the same journal.

20. "Application; the Pulliam Journalism Fellowship," 1975, folder: Shiltsmas + X-mas Cards/Mem, Personal Stuff + Humor + Misc. Things, Alband Collection. Unlike a later employment history that he filled out for St. Martin's Press, Shilts did not mention his work as a gay bathhouse attendant during the summer of 1974 at Portland's Majestic Baths. See Authors' Questionnaire, 2, folder: Shilts, Randy. [The] Mayor of Castro [Street], box 843, St. Martin's Press Archive (SMP-2000), John Hay Library, Brown University, Providence, RI. See also Shilts's disgust at being seduced by his single-testicled employer at the Majestic: "The Summer of '74," Alband Collection.

21. Bercaw, "Shilts Gets Grip," A5.

believed that studying English had taught him to read but not to write, and at a roommate's suggestion, he enrolled in a journalism course to rectify this imbalance. "I sort of stumbled into my calling," he would later remark.[22] Shilts found that he enjoyed writing news stories, perhaps because the straightforward nature of "factual" news reporting appealed to his developing political self-identity. He viewed himself as having ventured to both ends of the political spectrum before settling, in his mind, somewhere in the "objective" middle. He also found that through journalism he could marry his creative writing to his desire to bring about social change. From this early period, Shilts would maintain that reporting about gays to the straight community could achieve such a change, and "without violating the ethical standards of a professional journalist." He argued that "an unbiased, objective account of the situation of gay people, whether written by a straight, gay, or whatever, will work in our favor—the facts are on our side. Most people are prejudiced simply out of ignorance. They've never heard our side of the story because the current media usually won't touch us with a ten foot pencil."[23]

At this embryonic stage in his career, Shilts would also express the concerns that he would carry with him for years: doubts that a predominantly heterosexual profession would accept a homosexual reporter. "'I'm a little skeptical,'" he admitted, in an article profiling his role as managing editor of the University of Oregon's student newspaper, a position he held for a year beginning in May 1974. "'The journalistic world is very conservative,'" the twenty-three-year-old Shilts opined. "'No matter how qualified I am, I might get the shaft. They'd rather have an alcoholic than a gay.'"[24]

A mix-up following the 1975 National Writing Championship of the San Francisco–based William Randolph Hearst Foundation only exacerbated the young writer's fears of unfair treatment for being gay. Several newspapers had named Shilts, who had written articles for the contest alongside competitors from various American journalism schools, as the winner of the annual competition's second prize of $1,000. The

22. Ibid.

23. "Northwest Personality: Randy Shilts," *Northwest Gay Review*, December–January 1974, 7.

24. Ibid., 7. Ironically, Shilts would later fear losing his job at the *Chronicle* because of his heavy drinking.

foundation's secretary wrote Shilts later that month to inform him of an "unfortunate error": the competitors' entries had been coded when they were sent to the judges for anonymous evaluation, and two of the entries had had their codes transposed on the results sheet. Thus, the secretary explained, Shilts had been incorrectly identified as the second-place winner, when he had actually placed fourth.[25]

Shilts was convinced that he had placed second for the pieces he had written in San Francisco. Furthermore, he was of the opinion that his prize had been taken away when the Hearst Foundation had discovered that the second-place winner had been the candidate who had qualified for the finals by writing about gay issues (one of Shilts's articles covered drag queens in Portland, while the other dealt with closeted gay professionals). In an account he sent to Nathan Blumberg, a friend's father who was a professor at the University of Montana's journalism school, he voiced his suspicions that the Hearst Foundation had staged the clerical error to cheat a candidate thought to be "too flamboyant" by foundation employees. Rigidly faithful to his ethical training, though, Shilts conceded that "as a journalist, however, I cannot say it was due to prejudice unless I have black and white proof."[26] In the accompanying letter, in which Shilts also wrote of his frustrations in being rejected in his applications to newspapers, he admitted the possibility that sometimes he might come on too strong: "I acted aggressive because I thought that would be a trait which a managing editor would appreciate. (Journalists are supposed to be aggressive aren't they?)."[27] With similar brashness, the budding journalist wrote to the director of the Hearst Foundation threatening legal action if they did not restore to him the original $1,000 award.[28]

The aforementioned experiences compounded the sense of frustration Shilts felt with the job he began that summer as a freelance writer for the *Advocate*. "My articles mostly were done with disembodied

25. Amy Fink to Randy Shilts, 29 May 1975, folder 9: Hearst [W.R. Hearst Foundation, Journalism Awards Program], box 11, Shilts Papers.

26. Randy Shilts to Nathan Blumberg, memo, 21 July 1975, pp. 2, 4, folder 9, box 11, Shilts Papers.

27. Randy Shilts to Nathan Blumberg, cover letter, 21 July 1975, p. 2, folder 9, box 11, Shilts Papers.

28. Randy Shilts to Ira Walsh, 25 August 1975, folder 9, box 11, Shilts Papers. It appears that he eventually backed off from that demand.

voices over the phone," he reflected a few months into the work. "My
Advocate job itself was a disembodied one as I merely had an enve-
lope relationship with the paper augmented by an occasional phone
conversation."[29] Although he was able to gain success, first as the magazine's Northwest correspondent and then, following a move to San Francisco in early 1976, as a staff writer, he still longed for bigger projects and
the professional prestige of employment at a "straight" newspaper. Writing in one of his journals in June 1976, Shilts confided that "I really don't
put my energy into having high status in the gay community. I definitely
want status in the American journalistic community, but I don't want it
among gay 'leaders.' I think because that is an empty status which few
recognize. I want 'real' more objectifiable success and status."[30]

Indeed, success and status were the stuff that Shilts craved, and he
recorded these yearnings repeatedly in his journal entries. Yet he was
plagued with insecurity about his social abilities, his looks, and, when
he was later working in television, his voice. In early January 1976,
Shilts was in a dejected state after having decided to move from Portland to San Francisco on Christmas Eve 1975. He had then spent a desperate New Year's Eve there, searching for a place to stay. The passage
he typed at that time is worth repeating at length and unedited, for it ex-
presses the depths to which Shilts had sunk. It is also worth considering
the resemblance between the description of Chris Stone, a good-looking
Advocate writer, and Shilts's depiction of Gaétan Dugas ten years later:

January 3, 1976
Halm Moon Bay, California
He walked into the room. A loose shirt unbuttoned to his navel, exposing a
narrow, hairy chest and waist. . A set of gold chains dangling loosely from his
neck. . His hair cut in the latest style and his mustache trimmed evenly—of
that uncertain age which is somewhere in the '20s though the haircut and
well-kept bodyx may disguise an early '30s. An expensive leather coat draped
over his shoulders.

Into the room he walked with Robert McQueen and the editor's 'Significant Other.' He was charming, dapper, handsome—eyed by all the men in the

---

29. "Moscow, Idaho, November 30, 1975," p. 2, folder: Journal '75-'76, Alband Collection; *occasional* misspelled as "occassional" in original.
    30. "June 1 '76," folder: Journal 76, Alband Collection.

room. Favorite of the publisher who paid his way up. . He was Chris Stone. And I was nothing.

In a large sense, he seems to represent that p eer group which I so dearly want to have and yet lack. . While I really can't say I dislike myself or my trip, I always find it and myself somewhat inadequate when= I measure it up against such charmer standards. And he was the pet of the editor.

Three days agao that same editor knew of my situation. . He knew that I was taking to the streets to find places to stay. He knew the predicament in which I found myself to the point that he felt obliged to make some phony excuse about his bed being to narrow. . Yet when dapper Mr. Stone walks in, he is treated by a king.

Shilts continued, confiding to his typewriter for comfort:

As a matter of traditional typewriter therapy, I might as well say to the keys what I want to say to my beloved editor.

Does he know what it is to stand like a slut, like a whore on a street coener, somehow hoping that one of the Castro Street tramps will pick you up for that place you so desperately need. . He left me like a whore on a street corner, tricking my way through a subsistance while giving the handsome and finely dressed public relations writer a warm bed in which to sleep. I*m not god's gift to journalism, but I'm good and the best that The Advocate has . . I graduated with an arm full of awards and honors . . I turn in some good copy, serious copy. . And y et I'm left to be a whore while the public relations, entertainment writer gets treated like a king. Someone who probably can't think beyond the next name he can drop or the next cocktail party he ca n go to. I should clarify that I have no rational feelings of hostility against Mr. Stone. . He may be a fine person and I may soon be a friend of his for all I know. To some extent I resent the fact that he can move so easily among the people I can only stumble hrough.

I do my best. I try and work at my job. But that is not enough in this world of status and illusions. . He has a well-honed, image of handsome sexua lity. . While I am only a clutz, a more-or-less unattractive misfit who can find a nich only through an intense dedication to my work—a dedication which I carry through in lieu of anything meaningful social interact on. .

And I am left like akprostitute on a street and this person—who is so much of everything I am not—is treated as royalty by the people for whom I sweat over my typewriter. .

The lump in my throat has gone big enough that breathing is somewhat difficult. I'm closer to crying than in any time in the past dozen or so years. Here I am—the nobody whore. Alone again.

[Signed]

Randy Shilts[31]

In this brutally frank and self-loathing entry, written only weeks after his disappointing Vancouver visit, Shilts admits his despair at the injustices he perceived to be at play in the world of gay journalism—a "world of status and illusions"—where, to him, talent mattered far less than appearance. The extent to which Shilts abases himself in his comparisons to Stone will be important to bear in mind in the context of the journalist's later presentation of Dugas.

This self-abasement also finds expression elsewhere in his journals, when he reflects on his frequent sexual connections with "hundreds" of other men and finds in them a lonely search for love. Commenting on his "insatiable sexual appetite" while traveling through the Northwest, Shilts decided that "I have to cut down the time which I spend on sex or at least integrate it into my normal life." He reflected that this might be easier to do in San Francisco or another large city, "as I would be living a gay lifestyle in a gay world."[32] He linked his lack of success in love to his lack of confidence and his use of alcohol. "I think that it's just that I get drunk + horny + will sleep w[ith]/the most available person who seems least likely to reject me," he wrote in January 1978, while on the road. "Thus, I get dip-shits that don't satisfy me in any sense. . . . What's wrong w[ith]/me? Is there no one in the world to look into my eyes and say I love you—so I can look back and say the same?"[33] And later, in Boston, "When will the loneliness ever end. I seem to have suffered this loneliness all my life. Will there be only more pain?"[34] A serious bout of hepatitis B in San Francisco in 1976 had not helped matters. The sickness, he wrote later, "would put me out of full-time work for 15 weeks, wreck

31. "January 3, 1976," typed journal entry, folder 3: Jobs, box 11, Shilts Papers.
32. "Moscow, Idaho," p. 3, typed journal entry, November 30, 1975, folder: Journal '75-'76, Alband Collection.
33. "Portland, Maine," January 24, 1978, "Green" journal, Alband Collection.
34. "Boston, Massachusetts," January 29, 1978, "Green" journal, Alband Collection.

me financially, disrupt career plans and . . . leave me with only a fraction of my normal energy."[35] The experience made him confront the possibility of an early death from liver failure as a result of a sexually transmitted disease: "all because I had slept with the wrong person sometime last Spring."[36] Throughout these periods of loneliness, depression, and despondency, Shilts turned to his "typewriter therapy." He wrote and wrote, taking solace in words and ideas, and dreaming of the right story opportunities to which he could apply his talents. "I only want to wake up in the morning with an exciting project to look forward to," he declared. "I want to sit exuberantly at my typewriter and thrill at the construction of a new thought—and a new way to say it."[37]

Mindful of an earlier suggestion from Sasha Gregory-Lewis to investigate how gay groups were responding to VD, Shilts turned his experience with hepatitis into an article for the *Advocate*.[38] In it, he interviewed a number of health experts, including Selma Dritz, the San Francisco Department of Public Health physician, whose comments on carriers of hepatitis may have laid the groundwork for Shilts's eventual understanding of Dugas: "A person walking around with hepatitis—even though they may not be jaundiced—can give fatal hepatitis with jaundice to someone else." Ironically, given what he would later write about Dugas, Shilts also noted that the "two- to six-month incubation period for hepatitis B makes it epidemiologically impossible to find the source of a sexually transmitted case of hepatitis in a sexually active male."[39]

Although Shilts would continue to wrestle with his insecurities, his professional fortunes improved, by virtue of his drive to network, ability to spot opportunities, and willingness to work long hours. In January 1977 he successfully auditioned for a TV reporting position with KQED, San Francisco's public broadcasting station. He began to present TV news stories for them the next month, working one day a week for

35. Randy Shilts, "The Decade's Best-Kept Medical Secret: Hepatitis Doesn't Come from Needles," *Advocate*, January 12, 1977, 23.

36. Ibid, 24.

37. "Moscow, Idaho," p. 4, typed journal entry, November 30, 1975, folder: Journal '75-'76, Alband Collection.

38. Sasha Gregory-Lewis to Randy Shilts, 21 July 1975, folder: Advocate, box 11, Shilts Papers.

39. Ibid, 25; *hepatitis* and *epidemiologically* misspelled as "heptitis" and "epidemeologically" in original.

TV and spending the rest of his time working for the *Advocate*, the magazine having offered him the role of contributing editor shortly after his depressed journal entry in January 1976.[40] As his friend and mentor Ken Maley recounted in 2007,

> At KQED Randy found what he had been unable to find as a print journalist, and that was *celebrity*, because his face was on the camera but wasn't a byline. He was now a face on the screen, so when Randy went to the bars, when Randy went out it became a very powerful tool for Randy in meeting people. Because Randy was always very unhappy with the fact that he perceived in those days that sex was based on the beauty that he did not possess. So his next option was attraction by celebrity, that if he was recognized and was a celebrity, oh that was a *powerful* aphrodisiac. That brought boys around. . . . That was an addiction Randy could not resist. It was too powerful and too successful, because it gave him the recognition and the contextual fame that Randy always sought. That was the goal of his ambition and it's what drove him, I think, in my view unfortunately, through most of his career and most of his life.[41]

Maley was a well-connected San Francisco man who had built important networks of contacts ranging from Los Angeles to New York through his background in political organizing and consulting. In him, Shilts found someone who believed in his abilities and had the connections to give Shilts the opportunities the reporter believed he deserved. "I'm launching ever more ambitious projects," Shilts wrote in a March 1978 journal entry, "largely because Ken Maley has been pushing and encouraging me . . . and so I'm proud of myself that I've started reaching for goals that I'm good enough to reach for, but yet I'm generally too insecure to attempt."[42] A month later, he reflected with some confidence: "Certainly I've been getting big," and "I'm finally edging into those big markets I've always wanted to break."[43] With new opportunities in hand, Shilts resigned from the *Advocate*, leaving the publication

40. Tony Ledwell, Associated Press newswire, March 3, 1977, Nexis UK.

41. Ken Maley, interview with author, San Francisco, July 28, 2007, recording C1491/13, tape 1, side A, BLSA; emphasis on recording. See also Weiss, "Randy Shilts," D1.

42. "March 31, 1978," "Green" journal, Alband Collection; "too insecure" written as "to insecure" in original.

43. "April 19, 1978," "Green" journal, Alband Collection.

in March 1978. He had been dissatisfied for some time about his prospects there but was finally disgusted when David Goodstein, the magazine's publisher, undertook political fund-raising through the magazine. This action, an outraged Shilts told a regional gay newsletter, "undermines my professional standing as a reporter to be part of a political group."[44] The projects he subsequently pursued included magazine articles for *New West* (a stinging critique of a self-realization course run by the *Advocate*) and *Village Voice*, work for an ultimately unpublished *Rolling Stone* magazine article, and a book he intended to write about the Castro Street neighborhood, as well as his ongoing TV reporting.[45] He maintained himself as a freelance writer, helped along, Maley contends, by constantly asking himself the question: "How do I roll this experience over into the next experience?"[46]

Through Ken Maley, Shilts was beginning to gain access to the circles to which he had long aspired. However, there is evidence that Shilts felt some competition with the other, more famous gay San Franciscan media star in Maley's group of friends: Armistead Maupin. Maley had helped launch Maupin's local celebrity and the author's subsequent career, and Maupin's success was what Shilts yearned for while working for the *Advocate*. Recalled Daniel Detorie, Maley's partner from 1977 to 1987:

He and Armistead were both kind of gay icons at the time and Ken was friends with both of them but they were totally rivals with each other, because Armistead had other jobs other than writing and Randy was *very* cocky, and his thing was that he'd never ever had a job out of college other than writ-

44. Jim Marko, "'Advocate' Employee Claims EST Training Refusal Led to Firing," *Arizona Gay News*, April 21, 1978, 1.

45. Shilts wrote to Sasha Gregory-Lewis and Robert McQueen on January 1, 1976, with a story submission about Castro Street, and provided suggestions for an editorial note: "I think I'm going to be writing my first book on Castro Street and . . . this story and the quotes are gleened [*sic*] from the research I am doing on a book. (Mentioning this will make the article look all the more impressive and show that the Advocate hires *serious* writers that do *serious* things like write books)" [emphasis in original]. By this point, Shilts had undertaken two months of research for the article, which was eventually published in February 9, 1977, issue of the *Advocate*. The experience likely presented him with his earliest encounters with Harvey Milk, the local politician whose political career and assassination Shilts would later fuse with his neighborhood history of the Castro in his first book. See Randy Shilts to Sasha [Gregory-Lewis] and/or Robert, January 1, 1976, folder: Castro St., Mecca or Ghetto, Adv. 77, Alband Collection.

46. Maley, recording C1491/13, tape 1, side A.

ing. . . . So we spent a lot of time together, we smoked *a lot* of pot together, drank a lot of wine, and then he got the job at the *Chronicle* which was pretty much a first. [47]

Shilts confided to a journal (given to him as a Christmas gift by Detorie in 1977) that he was working hard on his writing skills, which could help "make me famous and successful like Armistead."[48] This professional rivalry inevitably led to tensions, with Maley remembering that "Armistead was afraid that Randy could not resist his journalistic temptations to maybe report on stuff that Armistead did not want reported on. So there were certain parties or events that we had that Randy was welcome to, and others that Randy was not."[49] This approach may have been wise, as Shilts wrote in his journal in October 1978, after Maupin had been in the media spotlight in relation to the city's mysterious Zodiac killer: "Armistead believed in nothing but publicity, unaware that his story was entirely within the realm of journalistic investigation. But [he] didn't know what journalism was, so didn't know how to defend. Destroyed by craving for publicity, though the reality of situation [*sic*] was far different than imaginary scenario. A tremendous lesson about the double edges of fame."[50]

Reviewing his journal in 1986, while he was hard at work on *Band*, Shilts remarked on some notable absences from his personal chronicle: "Jesus, what a trip to read all these entries. It seems all I ever thought about was career *and* sex. Here I've got all those entries on 76 + 77 and I never talk about Harvey Milk or all that idealism—just whether I'll be a success or not—now that I have achieved so much of that success I have a hard time recall[ing] the times when I was so driven—Was that really me?"[51] Indeed, Shilts rarely mentioned Milk in his journals, despite the powerful impact the gay politician had in shaping the young journalist's idealistic dreams of driving social change. The politician's assassination on November 27, 1978, was a devastating blow for Shilts but served

47. Daniel Detorie, interview with author, San Francisco, July 12, 2007, recording C1491/04, tape 1, side A, BLSA; emphasis on recording.

48. "April 19, 1978," and "December 25, 12:30 AM—1979," "Green" journal, Alband Collection.

49. Maley, recording C1491/13, tape 1, side B.

50. "SF, October 7, [1978]," "Green" journal, Alband Collection.

51. "April 6, 1986, SF," "Green" journal, Alband Collection; emphasis in original, *career* written as "carreer."

to galvanize his energies. As he wrote early on Christmas Day in 1979, looking back on a decade of Christmases since leaving home, "Xmas 1978—at home again—Miserable about Harvey's assassination. Miserable. Working on Harvey story."[52]

The "Harvey story" would provide the impetus Shilts needed to help him reach his ultimate goal of working as a reporter at a mainstream newspaper. Immediately after the assassination, the New York–based publishers of *Christopher Street* magazine, Michael Denneny and Charles Ortleb, decided that they ought to publish a biography of Milk and that Shilts, with whom Denneny had become acquainted through Maupin, was the best person to write it. Denneny recalled that the magazine "put up four thousand bucks for Randy to write a twenty-thousand-word piece for *Christopher Street* that I could then use as a book proposal to try and get a biography signed up at St. Martin's [Press, where Denneny worked as an editor]. Which is what we did. It was very useful to have a magazine and a newspaper if you were a book publisher."[53] The book proposal eventually proved to be successful, and Shilts found himself with a contract for his first book.

Shilts had taken on a second TV reporting job in 1979, working for the commercial TV station KTVU as a correspondent for the nightly news broadcast to cover city hall politics. This position, however, did not prove to be sufficient for his earnings when KQED canceled his main show in 1980. Shilts was subsequently told by other stations he contacted that viewers would not respond well to a gay anchor. Unable to find work, he went on unemployment insurance and then into debt to write a book about Harvey Milk's life and death, incorporating many of the stories he had covered over the previous five years.[54] Shilts admitted that he was highly influenced by James Michener, having read *Hawaii* around this time. "That gave me the concept of doing books where you take people and have them represent sort of different forces in history and different social groups. I realized that is how I could do *The Mayor*

---

52. "December 25, 12:30 AM—1979," "Green" journal, Alband Collection.

53. Michael Denneny, interview with author, New York, April 8, 2008, recording C1491/22, tape 1, side B, BLSA. Ortleb and Denneny would go on to publish the *New York Native* newspaper beginning in December 1980; Denneny, recording C1491/22, tape 2, side B; Rodger Streitmatter, *Unspeakable: The Rise of the Gay and Lesbian Press in America* (Boston: Faber and Faber, 1995), 248.

54. Laurie Udesky, "Randy Shilts," *Progressive* 55, no. 5 (1991): 30–34. See also David J. Thomas, "An Interview with Randy Shilts," *Christopher Street* 6, no. 1 (1982), 28–35.

of Castro Street, with a cast of characters who represented different elements of the community, and then just weave their stories together the
way that Michener does."[55] Shilts would develop what became his signature style of book writing on this project, blending his accumulation of
details from hundreds of interviews into reconstructed scenes and the
imagined thoughts of his characters. When he was not able to use an
on-the-record interview to support his factual claims, he noted that he
would rely on a "standard rule of reporting" and "corroborat[e] possible
points of contention with at least three unnamed sources."[56]

His book received moderately positive reviews in the gay and straight
press, with Shilts proudly noting that "the straight press is saying that
this is the first gay book that straight people can read. That's what I was
hoping to do."[57] Amid the publicity for his book, which went into publication in the summer of 1981, Shilts was offered a job as a general assignment reporter at the *San Francisco Chronicle*'s City Desk. He started
his dream job in early August 1981, as stories of "gay pneumonia" were
beginning to catch his attention.

"I Was Convinced They Were Going to Let Us All Die"

In June 1989, Shilts was in Montreal, Canada, to deliver a plenary address at the Fifth International Conference on AIDS. The journalist began his speech with a reminiscence: "It was eight years ago this week
that I was at a cocktail party in San Francisco and somebody said that
the Centers for Disease Control claimed there was a gay pneumonia. I
remember saying it wasn't bad enough that they were trying to blame gay
people for the deterioration of the American family; now we were causing pneumonia too. It seemed patently absurd. Needless to say, a lot has
happened since then."[58]

55. Garry Wills, "Randy Shilts: The Rolling Stone Interview," *Rolling Stone*, September 30, 1993, 49.

56. Shilts, *Mayor of Castro Street*, xiii.

57. Thomas, "Interview with Randy Shilts," 33.

58. See Shilts's RSVP message, April 19, 1989, and printed speaking script: "Beyond
Compassion: Remarks by Randy Shilts," June 9, 1989, p. 1, folder: Int'l AIDS Conference,
1989, Alband Collection; *pneumonia* typed as "pneymonia" in original. Acknowledging
his divisive public reputation, Shilts warned the conference organizers that his invitation
might spark controversy in many quarters: "There are people who feel my book was not

Though AIDS was originally a story given to David Perlman, the *Chronicle*'s science writer, Shilts soon reached out to the contacts he had forged while writing about gay health issues for the *Advocate* in the 1970s. On August 18, 1981, he wrote to Dr. Marcus Conant, a local dermatologist who was organizing a multidisciplinary clinic to investigate Kaposi's sarcoma and opportunistic infections, and who had sent Shilts some information about KS.[59] The journalist suggested that he hold off writing a "local angle story" until Conant had managed to put together the necessary public education materials regarding the then rare skin condition. "That way," he wrote, "we'll be alertin[g] people in the medical community and the general public won't be banging down the public health department's doors with questions that can't be answered." Shilts closed cheerily with a reference to his new job at the *Chronicle*: "I'm gainfully employed at last."[60]

Despite these early intentions, Shilts would not produce an AIDS article for the *Chronicle* until May 1982, when he penned "The Strange, Deadly Diseases That Strike Gay Men."[61] The piece, a single article out of the 120 he wrote between August 20, 1981, and June 30, 1982, profiled the KS clinic at the University of California–San Francisco (UCSF) and the weekly support group for gay related immune deficiency (GRID) patients.[62] Interviews with Dritz and Dr. Harold Jaffe from the CDC provided a factual basis for the article, to which Shilts added a political flavor, highlighting Congressman Henry Waxman's criticisms of the slow

---

pro-gay enough while some scientists feel the book was not kind enough to certain researchers; conservatives felt the book was too liberal while some liberals felt the book was not liberal enough." Nonetheless, he gratefully accepted the offer. As he explained, "the pursuit of truth is not always applauded from all quarters."

59. For an overview of the history of the San Francisco KS Clinic, see Sally Smith Hughes, "The Kaposi's Sarcoma Clinic at the University of California, San Francisco: An Early Response to the AIDS Epidemic," *Bulletin of the History of Medicine* 71, no. 4 (1997): 651–88.

60. Randy Shilts to Marcus Conant, 21 August 1981, folder 3, box 1, K-S Notebook—Chronological Files, Conant Papers.

61. Randy Shilts, "The Strange, Deadly Diseases That Target Gay Men," *San Francisco Chronicle*, May 13, 1982, 6–7. Shilts had left the *Chronicle* for a six-month period, during which he promoted his book; this delay was compounded by an initial reluctance on the part of the *Chronicle*'s editors to cover the disease; see Kinsella, *Covering the Plague*, 166–67.

62. This count is based on the clippings of Shilts's articles in the bylines folders of the SFPL collection. See folders 18 and 19: Shilts, Randy Bylines, box 23, Shilts Papers.

federal response. It demonstrated Shilts's willingness to go to multiple sources for his facts and that by 1982 he had already established useful contacts at both the CDC and the San Francisco Department of Public Health, on whom he would rely over the next five years. Of the 37 stories that Shilts filed during the rest of 1982, only one additional piece dealt with AIDS, a short article outlining avenues of support for AIDS patients.

It was in 1983 that Shilts was first able to make his mark in AIDS coverage, spurred on by the January diagnosis of Gary Walsh, a psychotherapist friend whom he had dated in the 1970s and whose experience he portrays in *Band*. It is instructive to note the way in which Shilts later described what made AIDS real to him. "Suddenly I saw that someone like me—a middle-class professional—could get this disease," Shilts explained, apparently unaware of what this remark conveyed about his class-based assumptions about sexual activity. "The image had been that it was just someone who had 2,000 sexual contacts."[63] Again, we see Shilts constructing an oppositional image between himself and the character of Dugas in *Band*, drawing the sort of imaginary line between "good" and "bad" sex that one of his San Francisco contemporaries, the activist and writer Gayle Rubin, was critically articulating at exactly that time.[64]

With the disease striking close to home, Shilts pushed harder for increased coverage of AIDS at the *Chronicle*. He was permitted to devote more time to covering the disease, and of the eighty stories he wrote for the *Chronicle* in 1983, twenty-four dealt with AIDS.[65] Shilts upset several community workers with an article in which he questioned their response to a UCSF study which suggested that the number of gay men with AIDS in the Castro district was much higher than previously thought—a story which received national network television

63. Johnette Rodriguez, "AIDS: Reporter Randy Shilts Chronicles the Deadly Epidemic," *NewPaper* [Providence, RI], February 3–10, 1988, sec. NewSection, 1. See also Shilts, *Band*, 229–31.

64. Gayle S. Rubin, "Thinking Sex: Notes for a Radical Theory of the Politics of Sexuality," in *Culture, Society and Sexuality: A Reader*, ed. Peter Aggleton and Richard Parker (London: UCL Press, 1999), 152. First published in Carol S. Vance, *Pleasure and Danger: Exploring Female Sexuality* (Boston: Routledge and Kegan Paul, 1984).

65. Shilts would later recall that he had been covering AIDS full-time since 1983. Refer, for example, to CAJ, [Media Coverage of AIDS].

coverage.[66] Angrily confiding to his video display terminal the day after the story was released, Shilts complained that "I had just endured 36 of the most pressured hours of my career—hours in which gay leaders and researchers had worked feverishly to cover up the story of the dramatic proportions that the fatal AIDS epidemic had reached in the city's gay neighborhoods." Shilts continued, stating that he was reluctant to use the first person, "a reticence exacerbated by my decidedly old-fashioned view of the role of a reporter in contemporary society," and noted that he was not going to use the names of the individuals involved "in an uncharacteristic act of mercy." He did not believe that the individuals involved deserved this leniency, since they were "[rank] amateurs playing games of life and death for other people." Defending his actions to himself, Shilts rationalized that "as a reporter, my duty is not to ponder or even consider the consequences of a story. My job is to disseminate information, not withhold it. The UCSF study clearly was a good story, containing information that the public had a right to know."[67] Contemplating the issue of having community "leaders" whose actions might not be in the best interest of those they claim to represent, Shilts concluded, "Thankfully, it's the job of reporters to ask questions, not to answer them."[68]

66. Randy Shilts, "Study of S.F. Neighborhoods: Startling Finding on 'Gay Disease,'" *San Francisco Chronicle*, March 23, 1983, 2.

67. Shilts exuded a confidence in being able to instinctively know "a good story" that was common to the journalistic profession at the time. An authoritative guide to the industry described the task of writing the lead to a story as "finding the phrase, the quotation or the fact that reaches the essence of the story"; see John Chancellor and Walter R. Mears, *The News Business* (New York: Harper and Row, 1983), 16. Such a view, which suggests that each story has a quintessence, downplays the role of the reporter in the construction of a single, authoritative view.

68. "3/24/83," folder 8: March 83, box 21, Shilts Papers; the word *rank* is added as a handwritten correction to the printed type. See Shilts, *Band*, 255–56, for more on this episode and where he names the individuals involved. Although in this book excerpt the journalist partially acknowledges the gatekeeping process involved in journalism—"AIDS stories still needed a careful marshaling of editorial support to clear the various hurdles toward publication"—he seems less aware of the socially constructed features that made "a story" interesting to an "old-fashioned" reporter. Also, one reviewer of *Band* later suggested, based on a visit he (the reviewer) had made to San Francisco at that time, that Shilts overexaggerated the initial secrecy of the data: Tim Burak, "Books," *Seattle Gay News*, November 27, 1987, 28.

Gary Walsh's diagnosis, verbal and written attacks from members of the gay community regarding his reporting, and the death of his mother from a stroke all combined to make 1983 a particularly difficult year for Shilts. He continued to push for more coverage of AIDS at the *Chronicle* and was a significant contributor to the newspaper's "This World" special weekend edition released in January 1984, which focused on the syndrome.[69] A Freedom of Information Act request yielded his first evidence that the federal government was resisting spending additional funds on AIDS. Shilts first released this material in an article for the *Chronicle* and then expanded it for the *New York Native*. It would form the foundation of his national-level coverage of the federal response to AIDS in *Band*.[70] Leah Garchik, a colleague of Shilts at the *Chronicle*, was the editor of the AIDS edition of "This World." She recalled that Shilts was a "hot dog" reporter and kept on developing ideas and directions for the special edition. At one point, she had to remind him that she was the editor and he one of the contributors. "He started crying," Garchik remembered, the stress of the reporting on the devastation of his community having become too much to bear.[71]

At that stage, Shilts's alcoholism "went into a final tailspin," a situation which was compounded by the death of Gary Walsh on February 21, 1984, and attacks from the gay press for his AIDS reporting relating to the city's bathhouses. "I went out the day after Gary died and drank like crazy," he revealed in a 1989 interview. "I was working a swing shift and had six double shots of Jack Daniels back to back and then went back to the *Chronicle*." One of the editors suggested that he go home. At this point, he decided to join Alcoholics Anonymous: "I struggled so hard to get that job at the *Chronicle* after years of discrimination, and I was finally on a story that I felt was important. And here I was blowing it for this cheap high."[72] The criticism he faced in his reporting on the delays in closing the bathhouses in San Francisco through the rest of 1984 was

69. "AIDS OUTLINE—For December 11 Issue of THIS WORLD," October 20, 1983, folder 6: AIDS 83, box 21, Shilts Papers.

70. Randy Shilts, "House Panel's Ideas on AIDS Research Financing," *San Francisco Chronicle*, December 6, 1983; Randy Shilts, "Memos Show Administration Falsified AIDS Funding Needs," *New York Native* (hereafter cited as *NYN*), December 19, 1983, 18–19, 64.

71. Leah Garchik, interview with author, San Francisco, January 6, 2009.

72. Kelley, "Interview: Randy Shilts," 108–10; Kinsella, *Covering the Plague*, 176.

challenging, yet, combined with his relative sobriety, fulfilling too.[73] After a four-year hiatus from introspective journal writing, he made an entry on March 22, 1984, one month into being alcohol-free:

> I can see now the dramatic changes which I hoped would come in my life. Boy, I thought I was trapped in a rut forever—and then things started falling into place—*just when* I stopped drinking. I have new confidence (too m[u]ch dr[u]gs, h[o]w[e]v[e]r) . . . even though I have fight ahead—maybe I should be more concerned with my physical safety and I hope those fears will pass. But I don't want to feel bad now—I feel I'm blossoming, things fall into place.[74]

By the autumn of 1984, however, he had become convinced that nationally, despite his local accomplishments in reporting on AIDS in San Francisco, the government and the media were not interested in the mounting deaths of mostly gay men: "I was convinced they were going to let us all die."[75] Shilts made the decision to write a book on the emergence of the AIDS epidemic in the United States, hoping to raise the profile of the issue in the media and "rephrase the debate about AIDS" in a way that his newspaper reporting could not. "Here I was doing all these stories and the national press wasn't paying any attention. . . . I had the sense that there was no way to capture the attention of the national media, especially in New York, unless I did a book."[76]

Several publishing houses passed on the project. A book on AIDS was viewed as doubly problematic, since it would be both treading on sensitive ground with leaders of the gay community and of limited appeal to straight readers.[77] Half a dozen publishers declined interest

73. For a discussion of the controversy surrounding the closing of the San Francisco bathhouses, see Ronald Bayer, "AIDS, Privacy, and Responsibility," *Daedalus* 118, no. 3 (1989): 79–99; Christopher Disman, "The San Francisco Bathhouse Battles of 1984: Civil Liberties, AIDS Risk, and Shifts in Health Policy," *Journal of Homosexuality* 44, no. 3–4 (2003): 71–129.

74. "March 22, 1984," "Green" journal, Alband Collection. Shilts's fears about safety almost certainly refer to the escalating tensions around the city's bathhouse crisis of that year and the controversial stance of his reporting.

75. Kinsella, *Covering the Plague*, 181.

76. Patrick O'Neill, "Gay Reporter's AIDS Exposé Vents Anger over Epidemic," *Oregonian* [Portland], November 18, 1987, B4.

77. "AIDS: At the Heart of an Epidemic," *Pittsburgh Post-Gazette*, March 28, 1988, 14. A national poll conducted for ABC News and the *Washington Post* in September 1985 indicated that only 6 percent of Americans knew anyone, living or dead, who had contracted

before Michael Denneny agreed to submit a proposal at St. Martin's Press.[78] Denneny recalled the difficulty he encountered having the book approved at an editorial meeting in the spring of 1985:

> I had a lot of problems with it. I mean I had an eighty-page proposal, it was an incredibly good proposal. I'd already had some friends die, which people knew about in work. So they knew that this was a fairly sensitive topic with me. And I made every single editor read the proposal, something like sixteen editors at the time. And I remember [St. Martin's Press CEO] Tom Mc-Cormack went around the table, *t, t, t, t, t, t* [*counting*] all sixteen. Because I'd laid down the law. I'd said to everybody, "This is of major importance to me. You all have to read this." And every one of them essentially said it was one of the best book proposals they'd ever read, but they all voted against it. They said, "First of all there's no ending." Which there wasn't. . . . Everybody was afraid—'83, '84—that they might find a cure tomorrow, so there would be no reason for the book. I said, "You know, I can't guarantee that they're not going to find a cure tomorrow, but I'll bet you two years' salary on it." . . . While it wasn't in the news that well, we were fighting very hard to get coverage of AIDS in any media whatsoever. [*Pause*] There was a lot of fear that the story would just disappear. Finally it came around to Mc-Cormack, and this long silence and finally he said, "Okay, I want to point out three things to you people." He said, "One, virtually every one of you have said this is the best book proposal you've ever seen. Two, all of you have voted against it, and three, Michael's going to kill all of us if we don't sign up this book." So we signed it up, for sixteen thousand dollars, which was not a huge advance.[79]

Notes from Shilts's papers, scrawled in Shilts's quick handwriting on *Chronicle* stationery, appear to document a decreasing amount of money being offered for the book advance, foreshadowing a decrease in the originally intended scope:

$25,000 start
down to $20,000

AIDS; see Eleanor Singer, Theresa F. Rogers, and Mary Corcoran, "The Polls—A Report: AIDS," *Public Opinion Quarterly* 51, no. 4 (1987): 584.

78. David Streitfeld, "Book Report," *Washington Post*, January 24, 1988, BO15.

79. Denneny, recording C1491/22, tape 1, side B.

travel to:

-Atlanta

-Haiti

-NYC

future

9 months

concept novel

    interwoven

    straight audience

. . . 60,000 words – 240 pp

100,000 words – 400 pp[80]

The book's proposal clearly stated Shilts's objectives for writing the book. He intended to write a book with heroes and villains, to explain to a "straight audience" how "a disease unheard of just four years before—and without a name until 1982—had swept through every corner of the nation, seizing 10,000 lives." "How," Shilts asked, "did such a deadly epidemic . . . spread so thoroughly through America before it was taken seriously?"[81] The journalist clearly highlighted the areas that he believed ought to have worked better: "the world's most sophisticated medicine and the most extensive public health system, . . . an amply financed scientific research establishment, . . . the world's most aggressive media institutions, . . . [and] a substantial political infrastructure" built by the gay community.[82] Given that the book was structured around "the lives of a core of characters," Shilts promised that "AIDS at last will leave the realm of dry science writing and become firmly enmeshed in the lives of flesh-and-blood people," resulting in "provocative conclusions about

80. Randy Shilts, undated handwritten note, folder 6: Research Materials "Ambulance," box 42, Shilts Papers.

81. Randy Shilts, "Overview," 1985, pp. 1–2, folder 9: "2nd book proposal," box 41, Shilts Papers. This is a draft proposal for the book "BRAND X" that Shilts worked on during the first two weeks of May 1985. In the archival records, the first two pages are missing from the revised copy of the outline, the copy of the book proposal from which most of the subsequent quotes are drawn; see "Book Proposal," n.d. [1985], folder 1: Book Proposal, box 36, Shilts Papers.

82. Shilts, "Overview," 2.

how AIDS became so entrenched in America."[83] "Put simply," he wrote, "these will be the heroes in a conflict with—and to some extent triumphant over—the book's villains."[84] The journalist suggested that, by the end of the book, "the reader will find in the range of human responses to the epidemic much of what there is to loathe and to love in the human animal . . . cowardice and courage, bigotry and compassion, venality and inspiration, despair and redemption." He finally noted that the book's aim "will not be altogether distinct from the goal of Albert Camus' fictional Doctor Rieux in *The Plague*." Rieux, Shilts explained, had tried to "bear witness" to the "plague-stricken," to commemorate "the injustice and outrage done them," and "to state quite simply what we learn in a time of pestilence: there are more things to admire in men than to despise."[85] In this description, we can begin to understand one aspect of this chapter's central question: Shilts's interpretation of the task of "humanizing." Rather than making the coverage more "humane," or civilized, his intention was to characterize the history of AIDS with the best—and worst—of human traits.

Though the action would center on San Francisco, Shilts imagined an international scope for his book, with stock settings providing a backdrop for his allegorical characters. He saw his history "following the epidemic from the jungles of Africa, to the slums of Haiti, the Bethesda laboratories of the National Institute[s] of Health, the cramped Atlanta offices of the Centers for Disease Control, the august corridors of the Pasteur Institute in Paris and the gay neighborhoods of San Francisco and Manhattan."[86] By contrast, at this stage, the journalist did not specifically envisage a role for Canada or Canadians. He explained that "the characters have been chosen to represent the book's various institutional and social themes." Significantly, in an earlier book proposal draft, this sentence was followed with, "There probably will be some rearranging as the final research of the book uncovers people who have stories that are more dramatic or better emblematic of the book's central

---

83. Shilts, "Book Proposal," 3, folder 1: Book Proposal, box 4, Books/Band, Shilts Papers.

84. Ibid., 6.

85. Shilts, "Book Proposal," 7. For more about the similarity between *Band* and Camus's *The Plague*, see Steven G. Kellman, "From Oran to San Francisco: Shilts Appropriates Camus," *College Literature* 24, no. 1 (1997): 202–12.

86. Shilts, "Book Proposal," 8.

ideas." [87] In this way, we can see how in 1985 Shilts was keen to find people with interesting stories that fit the aims of his book and that, consequently, he would have been particularly attuned to learning the identity of the medical literature's "Patient 0."

In the final proposal, Bill Kraus was to be the "central homosexual character of the book," Cleve Jones "the personification of the Gay Everyman," while Gary Walsh "reflect[ed] the best aspects of how many gay people heroically responded to an AIDS diagnosis in the first years of the epidemic."[88] Some characters, including Marcus Conant, Selma Dritz, and—most important—Gaétan Dugas, are not mentioned. These figures evidently overtook and replaced other characters who were planned but never appeared in the final manuscript. This latter group included Dr. Thomas Ainsworth, the "typical gay community doctor"; the Bauer Family, a working-class family in the suburbs who must deal with transfusion-associated AIDS and the heterosexual transmission of HIV; and Clarence Ridle, a Haitian immigrant living "in the squalor and poverty of Belle Glade, Florida." Shilts noted that "through Ridle, who contracts AIDS in 1981 and dies in 1983, we examine the curious role of Haitians and impoverished drug users in the AIDS story."[89] There is no mention of "Patient Zero" or of Dugas, the identity of whom Shilts would not discover until at least six months later. Significantly, though, at this stage the writer included "THE EPIDEMIC" in his outline's cast of characters. "To a large extent," he wrote, "the disease itself is the major character. In the beginning of the book, the spreading infection lurks insidiously and mysteriously, appearing in manifestations which few understand. Quietly, the infection proliferates—to a large extent, before it is even detected. As the book progresses, the masks that have hidden the face of this enemy fall away as more becomes known about AIDS."[90]

As Shilts's work on the book progressed and he learned more about Dugas, it seems that the journalist began to equate the flight attendant with the character of "THE EPIDEMIC" and, to a lesser extent, "the curious role of Haitians."[91] The medical historian Charles Rosenberg has

87. Ibid., 10. See also "Proof of Story '21880,'" May 21, 1985, folder 2: "2nd book proposal," box 41, Shilts Papers.

88. Shilts, "Book Proposal," 10–13.

89. Ibid., 14–18.

90. Ibid., 19.

91. Compare this description with "the unique role the handsome young steward performed" in Shilts, *Band*, 23.

suggested that Dugas's narrative function in the book resembles that of the rat in Camus's *The Plague*, though he points out that the moral implications are significantly different when an author does so using a human vector.[92] It is possible to go further: to Shilts, Dugas came to represent the plague itself.[93] This view supports the suggestion of other observers that, through his characterization of Dugas, Shilts invested the virus with agency.[94]

The proposal also shows that Shilts intended to begin the book in 1980 with the San Francisco Gay Freedom Day parade, noting that "the major San Francisco characters of the book are all assembled at the parade that day."[95] The opening section of the book would offer "ominous vignettes of women and men falling ill of strange cancers and pneumonia in San Francisco, New York, Haiti, Zaire and in European cities with close contacts to Africa." He wrote that doctors would "later recall 1980 as a year of grim foreshadowing and the section documents how the virus spread rapidly across America even while amusement parks whirled and gays celebrated their new liberation."[96] As Shilts would discover, the last few years of Dugas's life would fit uncannily well into the book that the journalist had already decided to write.

"I Got So Obsessed with Him"

Shilts later claimed that Dugas "was the one person in the book I wasn't looking for. He just appeared. Everywhere I turned in doing the research, his figure arose." Some might view this statement as a late attempt to downplay the importance that many readers would eventually place on Dugas. These readers might be interested in learning at what point Shilts, in his own words, "got so obsessed with him."[97] On the one hand, Shilts's original book proposal did indeed start with the San

92. Rosenberg, *Explaining Epidemics*, 287.

93. The Halloween party scene in *Band*, where Jack Nau picks up a masked blond who turns out to be Dugas, bears a striking resemblance to the aforementioned description of "The Epidemic." See Shilts, *Band*, 41.

94. Wald, *Contagious*, 215–17. See also Hans Zinsser, *Rats, Lice, and History* (London: George Routledge, 1935), where the author undertakes a biography of the disease typhus.

95. Shilts, "Book Proposal," 25.

96. Ibid., 30.

97. Bluestein, "Cries and Whispers," 65.

Francisco Pride Parade in 1980, and his discovery of Dugas's life fit perfectly into an already established framework. On the other hand, the author believed that AIDS could have been prevented. He combined his search for heroes and villains with a tendency to glorify epidemiology, confident that this discipline—like the journalistic profession—could observe, report on, and establish an objective reality. Significantly, he did not question the initially suggested incubation rate of several months, even though he had himself written an article in 1985 about the lengthening incubation period for "HTLV-III, the suspected AIDS virus"—up to fourteen years.[98] All of these factors contributed to the generation of the mythical and negative portrayal of Dugas.

In an undated first interview with Selma Dritz, Shilts was told about a "Montreal case" with "8 contacts—all had AIDS." This man moved from "SF→LA→Montreal," and apparently Dritz and her colleagues "were hoping he had died," since he had been "going to baths." She noted that he had a diary with "176 names," including "many famous NYC names," and that "3 [were] already SF patients." Though it was a time when a variety of causes were being considered, "8 confirmed he was contact"; therefore, it "had to be infection."[99] Shilts would recall that he had written a story about AIDS patients who continued to go to the baths. As he told an interviewer in 1993, "I had known there was a guy [with AIDS] knowingly having sex in the bathhouses, and I did a *Chronicle* story on that in November of '82, and I also knew that there was this study that had linked a lot of the early cases, but I didn't know that the person in that study was also the person who was having sex in the bathhouses. And it was only through people dropping comments that I was able to piece that all together."[100] Shilts would have been aware of the cluster study in 1982, and in 1983 have heard local AIDS researchers talking about a Canadian man who traveled frequently between coastal cities of the United States, and who was diagnosed with AIDS, as were some of his sexual partners.[101] He may also

98. Randy Shilts, "Longer Incubation Period Reported: New Fears about Spread of AIDS," *San Francisco Chronicle*, April 18, 1985, 4.

99. "Dr. Selma Dritz [I]," interview notes, n.d., pp. 9–10, folder 19: Dritz, Selma K., box 33, Shilts Papers.

100. Wills, "Rolling Stone Interview," 48. Shilts made an error regarding the year in which he wrote this story; see Shilts, "Some AIDS Patients Still Going to the Baths," *San Francisco Chronicle*, November 15, 1983, 4.

101. April, "Doctors Brief," 3.

have been aware of a rumored version of this tale that was circulating in New York in 1983, in which another member of the flight crew was posited to be one of the first affected cases and whose example supported the notion of an asymptomatic period of infectiousness. "An airline pilot who shuttled between New York and Los Angeles apparently passed the illness on to four lovers in each city," a magazine explained. "In a three-month period, all eight lovers died."[102] In her interview, Dritz may have been hinting that the two separately told stories were linked through this Canadian man. Later in the interview, she recounted her interaction with the "Montreal case." "It's none of your goddamn business. It's my right to do what I want to do with my own body," Shilts's scribbled notes read. "It's their duty to protect themselves," declared "Montreal." When Dritz replied "not at baths," the man from Montreal retorted, "They all know what's going on there." According to Dritz, he then declared, "I've got it. They can get it too." Shilts recorded that Dritz had not been able to "prove anything" and had contacted the attorney general for guidance.[103]

It seems that Marcus Conant gave Shilts a similarly tantalizing version of the story on January 8, 1986. The notes from this interview speak of "the Canadian case" hailing "from Toronto." Shilts wrote:

big dick, handsome
blond
slim

wounded puppy faces
brought tremendous empathy
seductive in movements, spe[e]ch
affect
could get anyone he wanted

take home, after sex,
turn on lights

102. Michael Daly, "AIDS Anxiety," *New York* [Magazine], June 20, 1983, 25.
103. "Dr. Selma Dritz [I]," 12. Shilts's handwritten notes of this section of the interview read as follows: "Montreal 'Ts none f yr gddm [/] busns. Ts my rt t do [/] wht I wnt to do w/my [/] own bdy.' [/] SD→ Your right [/] Mon: Ts tr duty to prtct tmslvs [/] SD→ not at baths [/] Mon: Ty o knw wt gg on [/] there [/] Ive got it. [/] Ty cn get it true."

"See t[he]s[e] bumps. [I']V[e] g[o]t gay
cancer."

Conant noted that people were "calling [the KS] hotline" to report that
this man "would screw (anal intercourse)." Conant recalled that he had
phoned Dritz, and he noted that the man had apparently "already threatened to sue Friedman-Kien." The dermatologist finished by pointing out
that the man had had 250 partners in 1979 before he was symptomatic
(five of whom had been confirmed as AIDS cases), and another 250 in
1980 when he had lymphadenopathy, which had produced another five
AIDS cases. In 1981, he had displayed KS lesions, and of his estimated
250 partners from that year, two AIDS cases had been discovered.[104]
Shilts pestered Dritz and Conant for the name of this Canadian,
which they both refused to give him. Conant recalled that

> when Randy Shilts found out that there was such a patient, Randy went nuts
> trying to get the name out of me as to who the patient was. Randy and I by
> that time had become close friends, and of course, I was trying to give him as
> much information as I could. But I wouldn't give him Gaetan Dugas's name.
> I can remember calling Randy one day and he said, "You don't have to tell
> me. I've got it." So I don't know where he finally got the name from, but he
> got the name.[105]

Shilts found out the name within a week of his interview with Conant,
while he was interviewing a longtime person with AIDS (PWA) and activist, Dan Turner, on January 13, 1986. After asking Turner what it was
like to have AIDS in 1982 and inquiring about his experiences as a PWA
at the Fifth National Lesbian/Gay Health Conference in Denver in 1983,
Shilts may have asked Turner about an early Canadian case.[106] On the
last page of the interview notes, Shilts recorded:

104. "Dr. Conant [II], Jan 8 '86," pp. 11–12, folder 14: Conant, Marcus, box 33, Shilts
Papers. This was an approximate recounting of the cluster study's data.
105. Marcus A. Conant, "Founding the KS Clinic, and Continued AIDS Activism,"
oral history interview conducted in 1992 and 1995 by Sally Smith Hughes, in *The AIDS
Epidemic in San Francisco: The Medical Response, 1981–1984, Volume II*, Regional Oral
History Office, Bancroft Library, University of California–Berkeley, 1996, Online Archive
of California, 2009, http://ark.cdlib.org/ark:/13030/kt7b69n8jn.
106. The Denver conference would later become viewed as the birthplace of the PWA

Canadian steward—treated
    chemo since 1980—(Gayton)–
    2 friends died
    airline steward
    sandy colored hair—cute
    treated at SFGH
        has KS
    Laubenstein treats Gayton[107]

From here, Shilts was led, following the clue of Dr. Linda Laubenstein, to New York City, a destination to which he had recently booked travel for a research trip in late January and early February. Following this interview with Turner, in his notes from his second interview with Dritz on January 15, 1986, Shilts uses the name "Gayton."[108]

Shilts's realization that he was on the trail of "Patient Zero" appears to have struck him in early February 1986, when he was conducting interviews in New York City. While he was there, he found out from a New York City public health official that the first two patients in that city had sexual links to a French Canadian flight attendant.[109] This official, judging from Shilts's list of interviewees during this trip, was most likely Mel Rosen, a former executive director of Gay Men's Health Crisis (GMHC), by then the director of the AIDS Institute within the New York State Department of Health.[110] Shilts later explained dramatically, "The worst day . . . which I'll never forget, was the day I discovered that Gaetan Dugas was Patient Zero and was conceivably the person who brought the disease to the United States." Shilts related that on the night that he

---

movement. These activists decried the use of the term "AIDS victims," or "patients," preferring instead to be called "people with AIDS." See Grover, "AIDS: Keywords," 26–27; Silversides, *AIDS Activist*, 43.

107. "Dan Turner 1–13–86," interview notes, January 13, 1986, p. 12, folder 32: Turner, Dan, box 34, Shilts Papers.

108. "Dr. Dritz II," interview notes, January 15, 1986, p. 8, folder 19, box 33, Shilts Papers.

109. See Sipchen, "AIDS Chronicles," V9. Shilts seems to have interpreted this description of the first two patients in absolute terms, rather than as first among the early reported cases in New York's gay community.

110. Shilts's New York to-do list laid out his intended interviewees, including Mel Rosen, Michael Callen, and Paul Popham, in that order: "New York, 1986," handwritten list, folder 11: New York, Trip, box 35, Shilts Papers.

discovered "Dugas's role as Patient Zero," he interviewed a dying Paul Popham, the former president of GMHC. "I'd decided to ask everybody I was interviewing if they knew Patient Zero, and Popham said very casually that sure, he knew him, and he told me that his former lover, who had died of AIDS, once went out with Gaetan."[111]

Shilts's interview notes from his meeting with Popham are headed with a boxed inscription: "Gayton [/] is [/] Patient Zero."[112] Popham told him how, as Shilts noted, on "Halloween, 1980," "Gayton met Jack at Flamingo" and that Popham had "met Gayton at Trilogy [and] suggested he see Laubenstein."[113] Shilts appears to have been reminding himself to ask more questions about Dugas while he listened to Popham talk about his experiences with GMHC and being diagnosed with AIDS, as the word *Gayton* appears twice more in the margins of his notes, until he arises with more detail once again on page 15. The flight attendant is described as "blond curly" and having a "trace of a Fr[ench]-Canadian accent." Apparently Dugas had promised Popham that he would visit Jack Nau in hospital. Popham later "told Linda [Laubenstein] to get in touch w[ith]/him."[114] On the last page of notes, Shilts recorded Popham's recollection that in 1983 he had seen "Gayton" in Vancouver, his "hair thin from chemotherapy." Dugas was "angry" and demanded, "How could this happen to me[?]" The notes conclude with the ominous note that "Gayton had airline tickets after he went on disability."[115]

It would appear from his New York interview list that, after visiting Rosen and before seeing Popham, Shilts interviewed Michael Callen, the prominent New York AIDS activist. On page 7 of the reporter's notes is written, "Gayton— Patient Zero of cluster."[116] This could be a written attempt to process the information from the recent Rosen interview, as the realization was sinking in to Shilts's mind. Alternatively, the

111. Bluestein, "Cries and Whispers," 65.

112. "Paul Popam [*sic*]," interview notes, 1986, p. 1, folder 25: Popham, Paul, box 34, Shilts Papers. This interview appears, subsequently, to have been incorrectly labeled "II," although it occurred in February 1986 and before the archived notes for the interview dated "Apr 17 '86," which has been labeled "I."

113. "Paul Popam," 2.

114. Ibid., 15.

115. Ibid., 17.

116. "Michael Callan [*sic*]," interview notes, 1986, p. 7, folder: 12: Callen, Michael, 1983–1986, box 33, Shilts Papers; box and emphasis in original.

notation might represent a corroboration offered by Callen, an acquaintance of Dan Turner's, that "Gayton" was the same French Canadian flight attendant as the one Turner had mentioned in San Francisco.[117] The entry is followed by a description of a member of a support group Callen had attended whose actions and attitude Shilts began to map onto his rapidly solidifying impression of the flight attendant:

mid-30s, professional
    arrow shirt man
    lived for sex
    dark hair, mustache
    identity threatened

doctor guiding group said
civil liberties have right
to choose

The tone for the rest of the interview, however, was perhaps even more influential. Callen spoke at length about what he viewed to be the decline of "ethical constraints" in the sexual activities of the gay community, which had been "breaking down since 1975." He related to Shilts a story of a man who came out of the closet and soon became a hepatitis B carrier. When asking the "clap doctor" about any precautions he should take, the doctor replied pessimistically, "'If they don't get it from you, they'll get it from somebody else.'"[118] Callen noted that "ethically—after syph[ilis]—no sex for week." If one was infected with amoebas, "ethically 6 weeks no sex," while after hepatitis, a disease with which Shilts was intimately familiar, "ethically [one] can't have sex for months." Given the high numbers of anonymous sexual contacts one could have in bathhouses—establishments which Callen dubbed "death factories" in the interview—one could not "contact partners if [one] wanted" if a sexually transmitted infection was diagnosed; in any event, "it was every man for himself."[119] Callen also spoke of the concern he

117. Turner and Callen had both been members of the PWA forum at the 1983 Denver Conference.
118. "Michael Callan," 4.
119. Ibid., 2; reference to bathhouses on p. 14.

experienced at an AIDS support group meeting in the late summer of 1982, when he realized that "1/3 [of the members were] having sex—no bones[,] 1/3 having sex—confused[, and] 1/3 no sex from illness."[120] Callen's concerns would lead him to write, along with Richard Berkowitz, "We Know Who We Are," for the *New York Native* in November 1982 and subsequently the pioneering safe sex guide *How to Have Sex in an Epidemic*.[121] Recalling this time in his interview with Shilts, the activist pessimistically reflected that "AIDS destroyed [the] myth that there was a community."[122]

Following this discussion with Callen, it is difficult to imagine Shilts being in a more receptive mood to picture Dugas as an angry gay man not heeding the danger his condition might pose to others in the bathhouses. It becomes easier to guess at the journalist's state of mind during his interview with Popham later that same day. To one journalist, he later stated, "That was when the entire scope of the AIDS tragedy just hit me like a bullet between the eyes. Gaetan had slept with somebody on Oct. 31 of 1980 and now I was looking at somebody in 1986 who was dying."[123] To another, he explained that "I realized that Paul, who had visible lesions on his face, was dying from a virus from this guy. It was like I was seeing the legacy of this person and his virus."[124] In these statements, Shilts posits Dugas's significance as "Patient Zero," the original outsider bringing in disease and threatening the American public's health. When one combines this role with scenes from *Band* in which Shilts depicts Dugas as deliberately infecting other men, the result is a horrific portrait of an apparent sociopath leaving, as Shilts put it, his "legacy" all over the United States through "*his* virus."[125] From this stage, I argue that Shilts became convinced of Dugas's importance to the

120. Ibid., 3.
121. Michael Callen and Richard Berkowitz, with Richard Dworkin, "We Know Who We Are: Two Gay Men Declare War on Promiscuity," *NYN*, November 8, 1982, 23, 25, 27, 29; Richard Berkowitz and Michael Callen, *How to Have Sex in an Epidemic: One Approach* (New York: News from The Front Publications, 1983). See also Brier, *Infectious Ideas*, 26–44; Richard Berkowitz, *Stayin' Alive: The Invention of Safe Sex; A Personal History* (Oxford: Westview Press, 2003), 135–39, 151–82.
122. "Michael Callan," 5.
123. Sipchen, "AIDS Chronicles," V9.
124. Bluestein, "Cries and Whispers," 65.
125. Emphasis added.

spread of the epidemic, of the flight attendant's immorality, and of the titillating factor inherent in the "Patient Zero" story. The information he gathered after this point would serve as supplementary details to make his depiction of Dugas more compelling.

It appears that Shilts did not interview Linda Laubenstein during his New York City visit, but he managed to do so at some point before the Vancouver journalism conference in March, probably by telephone. Shilts learned that Laubenstein had heard from one of her first KS cases: "'Y[ou']v[e] g[o]t t[o] meet Gayton.'" Apparently, "he had it too." The nurses "called him vector of disease," and he had a "'little bl[ac]k book' [that] wasn't little."[126] After he became a patient, he would fly "to NYU [New York University] for monthly chemo."[127] He had been one of a number of patients, a group which included health care professionals, with whom she had discussed "g[oin]g to baths" and the "Mineshaft," a sado-masochism sex club. Laubenstein thought that it was "very clear early on that everybody had been there," assembled in New York and exposed to "whatever it was—physical agent or microbe."[128] Laubenstein informed Shilts that Dugas had "died of progressive KS" in 1984, though he first "moved to Vancouver" and then "to Quebec to die in hospital."[129]

Having returned from New York, Shilts sent a typed thank-you note to Selma Dritz. His research on the East Coast had impressed on him "how much of human history relies on a few people" willing to carry out "unrewarding work," and he thanked her for having established a "unique relationship" between her office and gay doctors even before the AIDS epidemic. He also warned that he would "nag" her "about Patient Zero since he has such a unique role both in the epidemic and by epitomizing (in one body) so many of the public health issues which defied a knee-jerk response. (What to do about a Patient Zero remains something the gay community has yet to face up to. . . . and such pa-

---

126. "Dr. Linda," interview notes, 1986, p. 2, folder 10: Laubenstein, Linda, box 34, Shilts Papers. Shilts documents two interviews with Laubenstein in his book notes, one in January and the other in June 1987; see *Band*, 608. It seems likely that he would have telephoned her following his mid-January interview with Dan Turner. The nurses at New York University called Dugas "The Vector," a point corroborated by Dr. Christos Tsoukas, interview with author, Montreal, July 9, 2008, recording C1491/30, tape 1, side A, BLSA.

127. "Dr. Linda," 4.

128. Ibid., 4–5.

129. Ibid., 4.

tients will certainly arise again.)"[130] Shilts's developing fixation on Dugas would no doubt have made him even more eager to dig around for additional information about the man in Vancouver.

As it turned out, he would not have to look far. As Shilts later recalled in a *Rolling Stone* interview, "I was speaking in early '86 at an investigative reporters' conference at Vancouver, British Columbia, and on the panel on AIDS reporting, there was the head of the People with AIDS group in Vancouver, and when I mentioned to him that I was interested in finding friends of Gaetan's, this man's grief counselor was Gaetan's best friend."[131] Unable to believe his good luck, Shilts moved with his characteristic speed. His one-hour panel session had ended by 4:15 in the afternoon; by 6:12 that evening he had interviewed Kevin Brown, the PWA representative, and received a message back from "Frank," Brown's grief counselor, to arrange a meeting for the following morning.[132]

Brown provided Shilts with a sympathetic depiction of Dugas—and corrected Shilts's persistent misspelling of Gaétan's first name. He recounted the discrimination that Dugas faced as an early AIDS patient ("told of how one of 1st in N. Amer."), that he was the target of rumor and conjecture, but that "p[eo]pl[e] who knew him—Dr. [Brian] Willoughby [for example]—only had greatest respect."[133] Shilts set up an interview with "Frank" for 10:00 a.m. the next day; and most likely Shilts received the phone number of Gordon Price, a founder of AIDS Van-

130. Randy Shilts to Selma Dritz, 25 February 1986, Selma K. Dritz Papers, Archives and Special Collections, UCSF Library and Center for Knowledge Management (hereafter cited as Dritz Papers).

131. Wills, "Rolling Stone Interview," 48.

132. "Room 1016, Message," hotel reception clerk's note to Randy Shilts regarding missed call, March 15, 1986, folder 23: Patient Zero, box 34, Shilts Papers. "Frank" and another interviewee, "Simon," requested that Shilts not use their names, so I have created pseudonyms to refer to the notes Shilts made when interviewing these individuals to help protect their privacy. Kevin Brown would go on to play an important role in early Canadian treatment activism, drawing attention to the government's inadequate provision of drugs for PWAs and lobbying for the eventual release of the antiviral drug AZT in Canada as an experimental therapy. See Silversides, *AIDS Activist*, 142–45; Arthur D. Kahn, *AIDS, The Winter War* (Philadelphia: Temple University Press, 1993), 77–79.

133. "Kevin Brown," interview notes, 1986, folder 23, box 34, Shilts Papers; quotation on p. 2, correction of name spelling on p. 7.

couver, from "Frank" at this time.[134] The journalist contacted Price to set up for an interview and to look for documents from the AIDS Vancouver meetings of 1983. Price later recalled that the journalist "was disappointed that there really wasn't very much. There was hardly anything in the minutes."[135] In the end, Shilts took a copy of the meeting minutes from April 1983.[136] He also managed to obtain a phone number for Michael Maynard, one of the AIDS Vancouver members and one of Dugas's former physicians, as well as for the health writer of *Fine Print*, a regional gay paper in Edmonton. There is no evidence in Shilts's files to suggest he attempted to contact Brian Willoughby, the physician Kevin Brown mentioned who would defend Dugas against innuendo-based accusations, with whom the journalist would never speak.[137]

It was likely that Shilts was out late that night chasing leads, as a message was left for him at the hotel, shortly after midnight, asking him to call a man who could offer "more information on Mr. Dugas." It seems that this individual eventually provided Shilts with the names of two additional flight attendants, whom he would try to interview by phone later, and informed him that Dugas had "lived in Toronto, [and] Halifax."[138] Shilts later described his meeting with one of Dugas's best friends the next morning: "So the next day I was sitting with him, and he is the guy in the opening scene of *Band*, who was asked to dance with Gaetan. It was just luck that I had opened the book on that specific day, Gay Freedom Day 1980, and he remembered what they were doing. He had a great big photo album with all kinds of pictures, he had flown with Gaetan, he was a flight attendant, too, so it was just totally serendipitous."[139] "Frank" provided Shilts with a detailed description of his times with Gaétan and some psychological insight to Dugas's feelings, though, as I will argue in the following section, Shilts did not reflect the full range of this insight in *Band*. The reporter would have had to rush to catch his 12:30 p.m. flight

134. "Pan Pacific Vancouver, 10AM," Shilts's appointment notes, 1986, folder 23, box 34, Shilts Papers.

135. Gordon Price, interview with author, Vancouver, August 28, 2007, recording C1491/17, tape 1, side A, BLSA.

136. Shilts, *Band*, 262.

137. Brian Willoughby, interview with author, Vancouver, August 31, 2007, recording C1491/18, tape 1, side B, BLSA.

138. Printed hotel telephone message sheet with Shilts's handwriting, 16 March 1986, folder 23, box 34, Shilts Papers.

139. Wills, "Rolling Stone Interview," 48.

back to San Francisco. By that evening, he was tirelessly typing up his notes from a productive weekend, spending about an hour on each of the accounts of "Frank" and Kevin Brown to develop them. That evening his typed notes assumed a form similar to the way they would eventually appear in *Band*.[140]

To this information he would add a later interview, most likely conducted by phone, with another flight attendant friend, "Simon," who knew Dugas well.[141] Shilts also interviewed Bob Tivey, former executive director of AIDS Vancouver, later in March as well. Tivey had originally intended to attend the Vancouver journalism conference but was in Washington for another meeting, so Kevin Brown had taken his place. Tivey later declared that Shilts had misrepresented his intentions for gathering the information and that the reporter had promised not to use Dugas's name if Tivey agreed to tell him "what it was like to be friends with one of the first AIDS patients in Vancouver."[142] The journalist also conducted a follow-up interview with Popham, in which the dying man reemphasized his view of Dugas as a disease spreader: at the March 1983 forum, Popham "could tell he was trying to establish it was OK for PWAs to have sex."[143]

On May 14, 1986, Shilts wrote to Marcus Conant to pass on the reference details for an article. "By the way," he added proudly, "I've researched out Gaetan's whole life story. Great stuff—." In his handwritten letter he thanked Conant for the offer of Conant's cabin in Russian River, noting that he would probably look to make use of it in early June, almost certainly for writing.[144] Two months later, Shilts wrote to Conant

140. Shilts's printed video display terminal entries bear automated user information indicating, for example, that he worked on the entry for "Frank" from 18:06 to 18:54 (by the 24-hour clock, meaning 6:06 to 6:54 p.m.) and that of Kevin Brown from 19:00 to 20:09 (7:00 to 8:09 p.m.). See various printed copies in folder 23, box 34, Shilts Papers.

141. "Simon" requested that Shilts not use his name, thus I have given him a pseudonym. His interview notes in the Patient Zero folder are headed with the boxed phrase "raised in [name of province]."

142. Roger Ross, "Media Finds Easy Target in Dead Man: Friends Angry That Gaetan Dugas Is Labelled Patient Zero," *Q Magazine* [Vancouver], December 15, 1987, 5; copies of this short-running Canadian periodical are available at the British Columbia Gay and Lesbian Archives.

143. "Paul Popham, Interview—April 17 '86," interview notes, p. 5, folder 25, box 34, Shilts Papers.

144. Randy Shilts to Marcus Conant, 14 May 1986, folder 60, box 1, K-S Notebook—Chronological Files, Conant Papers.

once more, explaining that he was ready to write up some sections and, in addition to other details, would like to know "anything about Gaetan Dugas."[145] It appears, somehow, that the writer was able to obtain some medical information about the flight attendant from the doctor's office, as two pages of information in Shilts's records list the flight attendant's social insurance number, insurance provider, former doctors, illness and treatment history, and the date of one visit to Conant.[146] More important, however, the next phase of the development of the "Patient Zero" story was under way: over the next few months, Shilts wrote up his book, and Michael Denneny prepared its release.

"I Wait for a Pulitzer Prize"

A few weeks after returning to San Francisco from Vancouver, Shilts wrote a weary yet upbeat entry in his journal, reflecting on changes from his old self: "Then I wanted a job—Now I wait for a Pulitzer Prize. Then I wanted sex—now I still want a life-long relationship—A big change— It's been 2 years w[ith]/out alcohol and, in 9 days, one year without *Any* drugs. No pot. No coke and that has helped [me] see how success is my drug too and how I've been trying to have an applauded today replace a childhood in which I was beaten and emotionally abused—." The journalist was feeling "a little under the weather," a feeling which he attributed to working too hard on his second book, so he kept the entry short, noting in conclusion that "somewhere, I hoped to have a hand in making a better world and (most lately) in saving some lives. Life gets so much more serious than we ever expect it to be and all our youthful scheming can look pretty petty in retrospect—I hope I do a better job of all this life business in my second 34 years. Randy"[147]

The writing of his second book, *Band*, would drain Shilts emotionally and financially. After getting a green light from Denneny, Shilts reduced his work at the *Chronicle* to part-time in September 1985 to work on the book.[148] He took to writing during the day and working the night

---

145. Randy Shilts to Marcus Conant, 31 July 1986, p. 1, folder 14, box 33, Shilts Papers.
146. "Gaton Dagus [*sic*]," Shilts's handwritten notes, folder 23, box 34, Shilts Papers.
147. Shilts, "April 6, 1986 / SF," "Green" journal, Alband Collection.
148. Mark A. Perigard, "They Fiddled While Rome Burned—A San Francisco AIDS Reporter's Wide-Ranging Critique," *Bay Windows* [Boston], November 12–18, 1987, 6.

shift at the newspaper before eventually taking a leave of absence from the *Chronicle* to concentrate on the book full time. In addition to the difficulties of conducting interview after interview with dying PWAs, the expenses of research travel and telecommunication took their toll. He later stated that the publisher's advance just covered the cost of his long-distance phone calls and that he needed an additional $4,000 "to pull him through a personal financial crisis."[149] He borrowed the maximum amount on his credit cards and went $30,000 into debt.[150] An undated note in his papers for *Band* indicates that at one point Shilts "filed bankruptcy" and was "on foodstamps."[151] He also borrowed money from three of his brothers, whom he thanked in *Band*'s acknowledgements.[152] As Denneny recalled, "Randy went totally broke writing the book. Borrowed from all his friends, from his family. Finally, he's one of these people who has one of these great big glass jars that he'd throw his pennies and nickels into. He had to take that to the bank, to pay his rent."[153]

A letter written in late September 1986 from Shilts to his editor demonstrates the author's determination to complete the book despite setbacks. Shilts was enclosing the first half of the book, which would have included the Patient Zero segments, and nervously awaited feedback: "Of course, I'm neurotically sitting around until you call me up and tell me what you think, so read it. I don't think you'll be disappointed." Shilts mentioned that he was due to return to work at the *Chronicle* on January 4, 1987. Shilts continued, "That is when I want this book completed as well. It simply was impossible to even work part-time while I did this. Frankly, I was getting extremely stressed out toward the end of the summer, my dreams haunted with horrible nightmares about people trying to inject me with AIDS virus and the like." He warned of impending dire financial circumstances: "I left The Chron on the faith that somehow, somewhere, the money would come up to support me. I can take care of myself, probably, through October. In November, however, I must have money. I'm not posturing around this; I mean that I'll need money to pay rent and that kind of thing. I'm praying we can get what-

149. Steve Taravella, "'A Story of Prejudice': Author Chronicles Politics behind AIDS Policies," *Modern Healthcare*, January 1, 1988, 76.

150. "Heart of an Epidemic," 14.

151. Handwritten note, folder 6, box 42, Shilts Papers.

152. "Heart of an Epidemic," 14.

153. Denneny, recording C1491/22, tape 1, side B.

ever money deal we can worked out in October; we must get it worked out in October. I hate to have these kinds of worries dogging me when I'm working on such a massive project."[154]

The journalist also described the political context of his writing, which imbued his task with even greater urgency. "It's possible I never will write something this important again. I can't describe what it's like to be in California with the debate over the LaRouche Initiative raging." A far-right political leader, Lyndon LaRouche, and his associates had assembled enough signatures to place a referendum on public health policy onto the California state ballot, with the vote to take place in November 1986. Proposition 64 asserted that HIV could be spread through casual contact and insect bites, demanded mandatory testing for anyone suspected of being infected with the virus, and called for the quarantine of all those infected. "I assure you," Shilts continued, "Proposition 64 is the start, not the end, of such proposals. Behind it is an anger at AIDS. I think the anger is warranted. However, we are not the people to be mad at. I think this book sets the record straight. Hopefully it will also save our collective asses when the real numbers start to mount and the real anger, still nascent, begins to arise in full force."[155]

Shilts's use of "we" implies his self-identification with the gay community, wrongfully facing the anger and blame for AIDS, fury which, he believed, should be directed toward the Reagan administration's inaction. His word choice also prepared the ground for an act of scapegoating, an expulsion of an undesirable whom he deemed unworthy of community membership and on whose head the perceived collective sins of the group could be placed. The writer recycled long-held tropes about superficially attractive but deadly disease spreaders in his "othering" of Dugas; his acknowledgment of his own vulnerability to these external charms underscored their dangers. Speaking later of the flight attendant, a contemporary whose physical beauty he admired, Shilts admitted, "He was totally beautiful. I would have gone to bed with him in a minute. . . .

154. Randy Shilts to Michael [Denneny], 25 September 1986, folder: *Band* Letters, Reviews 87–88, Alband Collection; the first instance of *October* is typed as "Octobere" in original, and *these* typed as "theses" in the final sentence.

155. Ibid. See also Christopher P. Toumey, "Conjuring Medical Science: The 1986 Referendum on AIDS/HIV Policy in California," *Medical Anthropology Quarterly* 11, no. 4 (1997): 477–97.

Maybe that's why I got so obsessed with him and tried to find out every-thing I could about him. Winsome, sandy hair, mustache, very thin, not overly tall, well-defined torso with light hair all over it—Gaetan was the kind of man you'd see dancing shirtless at a disco, and everybody would fall for him."[156] Shilts became convinced, however, that there was a dark side to this beauty. In an interview with his hometown newspaper, Shilts gave a clue to the framework within which he viewed Dugas, speaking of his belief "in moral absolutes. To me, what is morally wrong is not being kind to your fellow man and ignoring situations in which you can help out."[157] Dugas, from Shilts's perspective, utterly failed in this respect.

Shilts would later be unrepentant about his depiction of Dugas, vari-ously comparing the flight attendant to a sociopath, a psychopath, and, in an interview published by the *St. Paul Pioneer Press Dispatch*, a se-rial killer. "He's no more representative of people with AIDS than Rich-ard Speck is representative of the typical male heterosexual. There are others who were infected and who behaved responsibly and heroically."[158] Similarly, for a British paper while on his UK book tour, he said, "As a gay person myself I wasn't thrilled about Gaetan's behavior. I don't see him as any more typical of a gay man than Jack the Ripper was of the heterosexual—but it did happen."[159] When asked by an interviewer from the *Advocate*, his old employer, to explain how Dugas could have done what Shilts wrote he did, the journalist deployed some armchair psychology: "I think the key line in the book that gives away every-thing about Gaetan is when he's watching Jerry Falwell on TV and he says maybe Falwell is right, maybe we are being damned. I think that Gaetan was someone who had never accepted himself as a human be-ing, hated the part of himself that was gay, hated other gay people, exter-nalized that self-hatred, and became what in effect was a psychopathic killer. Every city has its Gaetan Dugas."[160] Denneny recalled that he and Shilts had long discussions about boyfriends and ex-lovers who contin-

---

156. Bluestein, "Cries and Whispers," 65. Shilts seems to be completely unaware of the assumptions of race and class informing his construction of what "everybody" desired.

157. Bercaw, "Shilts Gets Grip," A8.

158. Jacqui Banaszynski, "Reporter Calls Accounting of AIDS a 'Mission,'" *St. Paul Pioneer Press Dispatch*, November 10, 1987, 4A. Richard Speck raped and murdered eight nursing students in Chicago in 1966.

159. Young, "Patient Zero."

160. Bluestein, "Cries and Whispers," 65.

ued to go to the baths after they were sick and apparently did not use protection. Though the two were not in a position to determine whether these were attempts to spread the AIDS-causing agent deliberately or a form of carelessness, or even how often such instances occurred, they agreed that it was important to document such actions, which they viewed as morally indefensible. Although Denneny would later concede that Shilts's characterization of Dugas as an individual was perhaps mistaken, he would remain adamant that the behavior that Dugas's character stands in for did happen.[161]

As some critics were horrified by the presentation of Dugas in the book, and particularly the scene from November 1982 in the San Francisco Club Baths, they might have been outraged by an earlier draft.[162] This earlier version is extraordinary for the extent to which it enlarges Shilts's view of Dugas as a sociopath. Almost identically to the final manuscript, Shilts described how Dugas chose a cubicle to enter in the bathhouse "and waited for the ritual nod that indicated he would be welcome. Without speaking a word, the assignation was set and Dugas pushed the door shut." At this point, the final manuscript stops, a result of an editorial decision to strike through the following lines: "~~Gaetan could barely restrain a giggle as the thought once again arched across his mind and a certain glint crossed his mischievous eyes. Maybe he would play his little joke with this one.~~"[163] In Shilts's version of 1982, there was no room for competing etiologies of "gay cancer," or for moral ambiguity.

Dugas's friends in Vancouver who were interviewed by Shilts would have been interested in other information that did not make it into the book. Bob Tivey, for example, had described a lighthearted day when Dugas had called him up for a picnic. They drove on Dugas's motorcycle to North Vancouver, where they spent the afternoon walking around, eating, and drinking from little airplane bottles of champagne. The isolation within the gay community that Dugas was facing was apparent to

161. Denneny, recording C1491/22, tape 1, side B; tape 2, side A; tape 3, side A. Additional recollections provided in e-mail to author, May 24, 2013.

162. Shilts, *Band*, 196–98; Guy Babineau, "The Prettiest One: Gaetan Dugas and the 'AIDS Mary' Myth," *XTRA! West* [Vancouver], November 29, 2001, 13–15; James Miller, "AIDS in the Novel: Getting It Straight," in *Fluid Exchanges: Artists and Critics in the AIDS Crisis*, ed. James Miller (Toronto: University of Toronto Press, 1992), 258.

163. Draft of *Band*, p. 456, folder: Draft (511p), n.d., p. 317–511 (3 of 3), box 37, Shilts Papers.

Tivey when, at the end of the day, Dugas dropped him off and gave him a kiss, saying, "T[han]k you for g[ivin]g me a normal day."[164] In writing the book, Shilts skipped over this anecdote in favor of one that reinforces the image of Dugas angrily resisting medical cautions to refrain from sex completely.[165]

Kevin Brown also shared a story with Shilts that did not get included in the final manuscript of *Band*. Brown and Dugas had gone on a date to the Conservatory, a beautiful restaurant in Vancouver's Stanley Park. When Brown admits he is interested in Dugas sexually, Gaétan hesitates before answering, "We can't. It won't work out. I can't say any more."[166] This page-long section, completely written up and included in an early draft, was cut. It is possible that this was done to tighten the pace of a long book, though its excision also removed any ambiguity from Dugas's motivations and strengthened the image of the flight attendant as a deliberate disease spreader. Shilts omits the recollections of "Frank" that Dugas was "always in love [and] needed [an] emotional bond, even if for a few days," and that he was "considerate, generous, would share anything." Also left out was the more humanizing point—to which Shilts could almost certainly relate—that Dugas "was once chubby—got weight down—hated old pictures."[167]

Shilts also left out humorous anecdotes about Dugas, diminishing the warm sense of humor remembered by the flight attendant's friends, who in their interviews with Shilts described Dugas as a clown. The flight attendant would twist his English words around in a humorous way that would make his friends laugh. Dugas would also make light of his condition: "If you find me dead, just bury me in the backyard." He "always had p[eo]ple laughing," Shilts's notes indicate, "he could charm a rattlesnake."[168] Dugas's charm would enter the book, but generally in a detached, coldhearted way. Shilts depicted the flight attendant making use of it to single-mindedly pursue his own aims. To a certain extent, some observers might say that the author deployed the information he had gathered about the dead flight attendant in much the same way.

164. "Bob Tivey," interview notes, 1986, pp. 6–7, folder 23, box 34, Shilts Papers.
165. Shilts, *Band*, 246–47.
166. Draft, 1986, p. 30, folder: Draft, box 36, Shilts Papers.
167. "Frank," interview notes, 1986, pp. 3, 10, 11, folder 23, box 34, Shilts Papers.
168. "Simon," interview notes, 1986, pp. 6, 9, folder 23, box 34, Shilts Papers.

* * *

In summary, Randy Shilts was an exceedingly driven reporter, one who had worked very hard to overcome insecurities relating to his looks, his talent, and his addictions, and had achieved significant successes in the process. On balance, he was dedicated and hardworking, with a natural talent for framing stories to suit the tastes of the heterosexual reading public whose appreciation he valued. At the same time, his self-professed "old-fashioned" view of the journalist's role in society—knowing what makes a good story and simply reporting the facts for the public—speaks to a distinct lack of awareness of how he, as a reporter, shaped his stories and how they, in turn, molded the public's social reality. Shilts was desperate to write an important book, not only to secure the fame he had long craved but also to help protect the gay community from the ever-growing threats—both pathological and political—posed by the AIDS epidemic. While he was constantly at pains to point out his ethical responsibilities as a journalist serving the public interest, the pressures that he was facing—death of friends, apparent lack of concern from authorities, and personal bankruptcy—played a significant role in coloring his view of anyone he believed was not working to fight the epidemic. In this state of mind, he learned the identity of the scientific literature's "Patient 0" and over time decided that this man was a sociopath and to blame for much of the epidemic, and that it was in the public's interest to know his name.

Shilts's view of the reporter's role centered around the idea that he was in search of black-and-white facts and stories—which added up to an objective and morally clear view of the world—to be communicated to his readers. While the more subtle aspects of his own subjective biases as a writer seem to have escaped him, he did understand the dangers of having his integrity compromised by appearing to be financially or politically connected to the groups he investigated. His commitment to this more explicit, professional ideal of bias-free reporting extended to a personal refusal to learn the results of an HIV test his doctor had ordered while he wrote his book, in case it might color the way he wrote his history. In March 1987, Shilts finished the final draft of the main text of *Band* and visited his doctor the same day, apparently having forgotten this previous test.[169] During his appointment he learned

169. Wills, "Rolling Stone Interview," 122.

that he was HIV-positive—carrying the same virus he had written so much about and whose widespread existence across North America he blamed on the flight attendant. Apart from telling his employer and a few close friends, Shilts kept this information to himself as he and Michael Denneny worked to make his book into a best seller.

Giving a Face to the Epidemic

The book is *massively* an attack on the Reagan administration. The media was not going to review an attack on the Reagan administration—they simply were not, in 1986. They were not going to pick up the failures of the medical research establishment, or the government. That wasn't a sexy story to them. But the man who brought AIDS to America, especially because he's *a fag*, and *a foreigner*? That was a sexy story to them. — *Michael Denneny*, Randy Shilts's editor at St. Martin's Press[1]

Randy Shilts had begun working on his history of the epidemic at a time when AIDS seemed far from the news headlines. Matters had changed by the spring and summer of 1987, however, when the book's release was being planned. After years of sporadic coverage that oscillated between disinterest and alarm, the North American news media was suddenly paying more attention to the epidemic—spurred on especially by the actor Rock Hudson's AIDS diagnosis in the summer of 1985. Increasingly, journalists sought to show their readers "the Face of AIDS," a phrase commonly employed in the second half of the decade.[2] Throughout 1986, the LaRouche Initiative focused the attention of millions of Americans onto the potential—and misstated—risks posed by people with AIDS (PWAs). Although the initiative's Proposition 64 did not pass at the state ballot box, it received 29 percent of the votes cast, drawing support from more than two million California voters. Such

1. Denneny, recording C1491/22, tape 1, side B; emphasis on recording. Unless otherwise indicated, Denneny's quotations in this chapter are drawn from this April 8, 2008, interview, conducted in New York City, with italics denoting emphases on the recording.

2. See especially *Newsweek*'s cover story on August 10, 1987, entitled "The Face of AIDS: One Year in the Epidemic."

fears circulated widely: a national survey conducted the following year showed that 41 percent of respondents believed that it was "'very or somewhat likely" that a person with AIDS could transmit the causative virus through coughing or sneezing.[3] Issues of criminal law were debated as well, following the publicity, in June 1987, of a court martial of a military man accused of knowingly transmitting the virus.[4] That month, under increasing pressure to appear decisive, the two houses of Congress agreed to policy changes that imposed mandatory testing for immigrants and prison inmates and excluded HIV-positive immigrants from entering the United States. While the developing consensus that the origins of AIDS lay in Africa formed part of the rationale for this shift—despite widespread views in many African countries that the United States was the source of the disease—long-lasting concerns about the role of homosexual travelers also continued to play a role (see fig. 4.1).[5] Intense social anxiety about deadly germs combined with heightened unease about an increasingly interconnected global community, leading at least one historian to conclude that the last fifteen years of the twentieth century saw the rise of a sustained "germ panic" in the United States.[6] Meanwhile, across North America most people did not personally know anyone with the disease. Thus, they relied on the news media for much of their information about the epidemic.[7]

By 1988, recently formed treatment activist groups had begun challenging the service-focused approach of many community-based AIDS

3. Thomas G. Rundall and Kathryn A. Phillips, "Informing and Educating the Electorate about AIDS," *Medical Care Review* 47, no. 1 (1990): 5.

4. Robert O. Boorstin, "Criminal and Civil Litigation on Spread of AIDS Appears," *New York Times*, June 19, 1987, A1, A16.

5. See Brier, *Infectious Ideas*, 104–10; Crimp, *Melancholia and Moralism*, 118. In figure 4.1, the planned flight path of a "foreign visitor" traveling between North American gay tourist meccas is rendered with imagery suggestive of Cold War paranoia. "Although atypical," the authors note, "this case clearly illustrates how an infectious agent might have been seeded in various urban populations in a relatively short period of time" (Darrow, Gorman, and Glick, "Social Origins of AIDS," 99). It seems that this itinerary was never completed— the man was admitted to a Florida hospital several weeks into his travels and died ten days later. Yet the vivid depiction of this potential threat is suggestive of the anxiety that was developing in the United States in the mid-1980s when this image was created and published, a trend which would soon result in the exclusion of immigrants and some travelers with HIV.

6. Nancy Tomes, "The Making of a Germ Panic, Then and Now," *American Journal of Public Health* 90, no. 2 (2000): 191–98.

7. Emke, "Speaking of AIDS in Canada," 259.

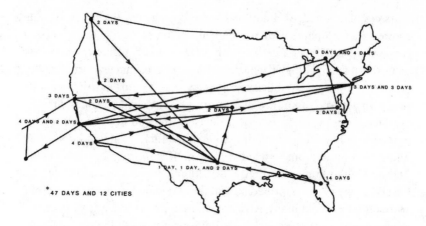

FIGURE 4.1 Map depicting a "Travel Itinerary (Forty-seven Days and Twelve Cities) for a Man with AIDS (PCP) from March 1983 to May 1983"; 16.3 cm × 7.6 cm (from Canadian border to southern tip of Texas). William W. Darrow, E. Michael Gorman, and Brad P. Glick, "The Social Origins of AIDS: Social Change, Sexual Behavior, and Disease Trends," in *The Social Dimensions of AIDS: Method and Theory*, ed. Douglas A. Feldman and Thomas M. Johnson (New York: Praeger, 1986), 102. The artist was an unnamed member of the CDC's graphics department. In contrast with the much slower spread of syphilis in the 1950s represented in figure 2.2, here the United States, again depicted in isolation, appears to be under attack by a rapid, almost missile-like force; the diagram's frenzied arrows reinforce its message of a swiftly moving "foreign" disease threat.

organizations. Groups such as the AIDS Coalition to Unleash Power (ACT UP) in the United States and smaller organizations including AIDS Action Now! and Vancouver PWA Coalition in Canada all demanded access to AIDS drugs and staged media-savvy protests that generated further news coverage.[8] Commemorative efforts—initially the NAMES Project AIDS Quilt and later more permanent physical structures such as the AIDS memorials in Toronto and Vancouver—served dually to remember the thousands of North Americans who had died in the epidemic and to draw attention in a dramatic fashion to the continued silence of the American and Canadian federal governments.[9] In

    8. Larry Kramer, *Reports from the Holocaust: The Making of an AIDS Activist* (New York: St. Martin's Press, 1989), 127–39; Gould, *Moving Politics*; Kahn, *AIDS, The Winter War*, 77–79.

    9. Marita Sturken, *Tangled Memories: The Vietnam War, the AIDS Epidemic, and the Politics of Remembering* (Berkeley: University of California Press, 1997), 183–219.

May 1987, US President Ronald Reagan delivered his first speech focusing on AIDS since he arrived in office more than seven years previously. Members of the audience responded with boos when he argued for the need for widespread HIV testing—including prenuptial HIV tests and mandatory screening for immigrants—since many public health experts believed that his proposed measures would do little to address the crisis.[10] In another attempt to signal his leadership, Reagan approved the formation of a presidential commission to investigate the impact of HIV on the United States and to formulate a national strategy, a move which guaranteed that the epidemic would stay on the media's radar.[11]

As early as 1983, health authorities had recognized that the Canadian epidemic appeared to be lagging behind that of the United States, by as much as two years. Nonetheless, Canada still had a high per capita number of cases and the world's third-highest reported incidence in the early 1980s.[12] Its federal government had also been hesitant to get involved in the response to AIDS, delegating the research and decision-making to an underfunded and often dysfunctional National Advisory Committee on AIDS (NAC-AIDS). The committee's chair would eventually resign in 1989 in protest of the continued inadequacy of the federal government's response.[13] With a hesitancy that resembled that of the American president, the Canadian prime minister Brian Mulroney waited until 1989—after nearly five years in office—before publicly mentioning AIDS, in front of booing protesters at the International AIDS Conference in Montreal. These activists—Canadians and Americans protesting together—were a testament to the strong networks of information and strategy distribution that flowed across the shared border and to other continents in the 1980s. These alliances benefited from previous connections established through gay liberation efforts in the preceding decades, ease of travel between the countries in question, and similarities in their gay cultures.[14]

10. Philip M. Boffey, "Reagan Urges Wide AIDS Testing But Does Not Call for Compulsion," *New York Times*, June 1, 1987, A1, A15.

11. Brier, *Infectious* Ideas, 91–101; Kahn, *AIDS, The Winter War*, 101–215; Kramer, *Reports from the Holocaust*, 149–61, 182–85.

12. Horace Krever, *Commission of Inquiry on the Blood System in Canada, Final Report*, 3 vols. (Ottawa: The Commission, 1997), 1:283.

13. Norbert Gilmore, interview with author, Montreal, July 10, 2008, recording C1491/32, tape 2, side A, BLSA.

14. Silversides, *AIDS Activist*, 190–98. As Silversides demonstrates in her book,

It was into this mélange of political developments and media coverage that Shilts's popular history made its first appearance, offering a compellingly readable—and at times dangerously simplistic—explanation of how the epidemic had begun. This chapter explores how North American audiences responded to *And the Band Played On* and, in particular, to the "Patient Zero" story that was used to sell it. The chapter focuses first on the yearlong period from the spring of 1987 to the spring of 1988, from the time that Shilts finished his manuscript to the peak of the book's success. It considers the marketing approach adopted by Michael Denneny, Shilts's editor at St. Martin's Press, and draws on newspaper interviews with Shilts over the fall and winter to evaluate Denneny's claim that he adopted the promotional strategy against the journalist's wishes.[15] The chapter turns next to how the story was imagined, adopted, ignored, and protested by various individuals and groups across North America and deployed for different aims. In particular, it shows how the idea of "Patient Zero" became embedded, with long-lasting consequences, in emerging discussions about the criminalization of HIV transmission in the United States. Throughout, the chapter emphasizes how the story displayed a widespread utility as it was recycled and reformulated for particular audiences. Here, with its recombination and recirculation of tales of disease origin and deliberate transmission, the North American AIDS epidemic bore a remarkable similarity to epidemics from centuries past.

Producing and Releasing *And the Band Played On*

By the time that Denneny commissioned Shilts's history in the spring of 1985, Denneny had been working in the publishing industry for fifteen years. The editor had developed a name as one of the few openly gay editors in a robustly closeted industry. Since 1981, he had also been closely linked to members of the New York lesbian and gay community who were leading the fight to respond to the emerging epidemic. Denneny

---

Michael Lynch was the quintessential border-crossing activist, forging and bridging responses in both countries.

15. In research that took place independently and in parallel to my own, Phil Tiemeyer covers similar ground in his book *Plane Queer: Labor, Sexuality, and AIDS in the History of Male Flight Attendants* (Berkeley: University of California Press, 2013), 168–93.

had begun as a part-time editor at the University of Chicago Press in the late 1960s, working there for two years while conducting research for his PhD in Social Thought under political theorist Hannah Arendt. Coming to New York City in 1971, he sought work in the publishing industry and secured a job as an editor at Macmillan, where he enjoyed a successful five years. With Charles Ortleb, Denneny founded the glossy gay magazine *Christopher Street* in 1976, an act that promptly resulted in his being fired from Macmillan following the first issue's release. Once again searching for a job, the editor impressed the CEO of St. Martin's Press and convinced him of the viability of an emerging gay market for which he wanted to develop books. Denneny soon brought forward a proposal for Shilts's first book, *The Mayor of Castro Street*. While working for St. Martin's, Denneny continued to collaborate with Ortleb in producing *Christopher Street*, a venture which drew perilously close to bankruptcy on several occasions. In a creative solution to solve the financial difficulties of their magazine, Denneny and Ortleb founded another publication, the *New York Native* newspaper, in December 1980 to generate revenue for their company.

In May 1981, this paper carried the first coverage of the condition that would become known as AIDS. Denneny proudly recounted, "So AIDS had hit. We were totally on top of AIDS. The *New York Native* carried the first public article on AIDS—we beat the *Morbidity and Mortality [Weekly] Report* from the CDC by eight weeks." The *Native*'s coverage of AIDS led the way for North American newspapers in terms of its early attention, in the form of measured articles by Dr. Lawrence Mass and in its sustained nature. For the first two years of the epidemic, its articles were read not only by many gay men but also by leading researchers looking for new leads in the crisis.[16] The coverage generated sustained debate and criticism among many members of New York's lesbian and gay communities, drawing attention to the emerging health crisis. As Denneny recalled, "Yes, they were really hostile and really agitated, but they were *really* paying attention. I think it must have been the *best-read* hated newspaper [*chuckling*] that ever existed in the gay community." Ortleb, who maintained the editorial stewardship of the newspaper, drew increasing criticism from 1983 onward for the *Native*'s promotion of theories of AIDS origin and etiology, including African swine

16. For more on the founding of the *Native* and its coverage of AIDS, see Kinsella, *Covering the Plague*, 25–47.

flu and other cofactor conditions. Though the newspaper may have increasingly lost credibility with mainstream researchers, it initially held a trusted status with many LGBT individuals for its guarded questioning of government intentions. Denneny described Ortleb as his best friend during this period; the editor was also well acquainted with Larry Kramer, a prominent playwright, writer, and AIDS activist. Thus, he was closely tied to the publishing industry and the forefront of AIDS political action in New York City between 1981 and 1985.

Describing the devastation brought by AIDS in the mid-1980s as "apocalyptic" and like "the Holocaust," Denneny was keen to distribute Shilts's book to a wide audience, and he later emphasized the challenges of releasing it. Before the era of centralized decision making, publishers would use the reactions of other salespeople at conferences to set their targets for a book's publication run, and it was crucial to have the support of a sales team for a large-scale book release. At a sales conference in early 1987, there was a powerful reaction to the sellers Denneny had selected to promote the book to their colleagues. Denneny knew that one was gay and the other lesbian, and he had counted on their being able to translate the book's importance to their colleagues, who were mostly straight. Both spoke to the sales floor about the deaths of their friends from AIDS and emphasized that each of them had canceled several days of work to read Shilts's book, such was the power of its prose. According to Denneny, the results of this conference led to the decision to increase the book's print run from five thousand to thirty-five thousand copies.[17]

Nonetheless, while the sales reaction drove up the editor's hopes for the wide appeal of the book, the mainstream media's reaction to the topic of AIDS presented difficulties. Denneny recalled, "We hit a blank wall. Everybody said, 'Oh, it's been covered. *Newsweek* did this huge story, it's been done.' I pushed at the *New York Times* and got a *very* snippy letter back, telling me that not only would the Sunday *Times* not review it, the daily *Times* would not review it. They figured the subject had been covered. We got turned down everywhere. There was going

---

17. More recently, Denneny discounted the figure of fifty thousand copies disclosed in "And the Band Played On: Politics, People and the AIDS Epidemic," *Publishers Weekly*, September 11, 1987, 72. In his message, Denneny wrote, "We always lied to PW and other media about print runs, all publishers do (or did)"; Michael Denneny, e-mail to author, April 4, 2013.

to be *no* publicity, in essence." Denneny explained that one Friday afternoon, the publicist met with him in desperation. He remembered her saying, nearly in tears,

> "We've got no radio, we've got no television, we've got no first serial, and *Time* has said they're not going to review it. *Newsweek* won't review it, the *Times* is not going to—we're hitting a total blank wall." So we spent an hour trying to figure out what to do. I had a lot riding on this because I had gotten the publishing house to go out on a limb on a book that a lot of people thought, while they respected Randy, et cetera, et cetera, they didn't think it was a book that would work. I had mobilized the sales force to the point where they really were going out on a crusade with it, and [*chuckling*] we were getting no publicity.[18]

In desperation, Denneny contacted a friend who worked as a publicist for advice and immediately sent him the manuscript.

> So he spent the weekend reading it and Monday we had lunch, and I said, "What do you think?" He said, "I can tell you how to make the book a bestseller, but you're not going to like it." And I said, "What?" He said, "Pull out the story of Patient Zero. I can sell that story. I can *tell* you. I mean I can guarantee that you can get the *Post*, the whole front page of the *Post*—the headline will be 'The Man Who Brought AIDS to America.'" Literally. Which of course I think was almost word for word what the headline was. And he said, "This is the only way the media is going to touch the story. But if you use this angle," he said, "*everybody* will pick it up. Everybody."[19]

The archival evidence supports this view to an extent. Shilts finished the book manuscript on March 16, in all likelihood just before the sales conference (which Denneny estimated to be about nine months before

18. With hindsight it appears that the August 10, 1987, *Newsweek* issue on "The Face of AIDS" may have given voice to a question—what is the face of AIDS?—which neatly set up an answer from the "Patient Zero" publicity. Denneny also had experienced the difficulties of media neglect with Shilts's first book in 1982 when the *New York Times* had come to an "editorial consensus" not to review *Mayor of Castro Street*; see David Rothenberg, "Unfit to Print," *NYN*, May 10–23, 1982, 11.

19. Denneny, recording C1491/22, tape 1, side B; emphasis on recording. The first extensive documentation of Denneny's explanation of the book's publicity strategy appeared in an LGBT community newspaper in Vancouver; see Babineau, "The Prettiest One," 13–15.

the book's release). It seems, however, that Denneny recognized the appeal of the "Patient Zero" story much earlier than he would later recollect. The editor wrote to Shilts just over a month after the manuscript's completion, on April 30, asking, "Do you have any photo of Gaetan? For second serial."[20] It may be that Denneny, though recognizing the salaciousness of Shilts's depiction of Dugas at an early stage, had not conceived of it as being sufficient to launch the book and was convinced otherwise by the advice of his publicist friend. In any event, the editor wrote back to Shilts on August 17, 1987, to inform him that the "first serial use of the patient zero story" had recently been sold for $3,500 as an exclusive to *California Magazine* for its October issue.[21]

According to Denneny, Shilts was against the use of the "Patient Zero" story as a promotional hook:

> I mean it took me most of a week of *really* hard fighting with Randy. He was appalled by the idea. And I said, "You don't do this we are going to sell four thousand copies of this book, and Larry [Kramer] says two hundred thousand people are going to die." And I said, "I don't know if his number's right, but a shitload of people are going to die. You know, I don't mind getting my hands dirty. I don't mind using yellow journalism. If this is the only way we can get this damn book on the agenda, we've got to do it. It would be immoral *not* to do it." And I said, "I understand it's tabloid journalism at the worst. I understand all your objections." The book is *massively* an attack on the Reagan administration. The media was not going to review an attack on the Reagan administration—they simply were not, in 1986. They were not going to pick up the failures of the medical research establishment, or the government. That wasn't a sexy story to them. Yeah, but the man who brought AIDS to America, especially because he's *a fag*, and *a foreigner*? That was a sexy story to them.[22]

20. Michael Denneny to Randy Shilts, 30 April 1987, folder 3: Editor's Corresp., box 40, Shilts Papers. A second serial is a reprint appearing after a work is first published.

21. Michael Denneny to Randy Shilts, with enclosure, 17 August 1987, folder 3: Editor's Corresp., box 40, Shilts Papers. This would be *California Magazine*'s October cover story.

22. Denneny, recording C1491/22, tape 1, side B; emphasis on recording. Larry Kramer consistently made use of the rising number of infections and deaths in the gay community to rouse support; see, for example, "1,112 and Counting," and "2,339 and Counting," in Kramer, *Reports from the Holocaust*, 33–51, 68–74.

Eventually, Denneny recalled, Shilts begrudgingly relented. "If you looked at the media," the editor explained, "he spent most of his time backing away from that and trying to refocus the attack on the government. But without that little piece of yellow journalism, we would never have gotten on to the national agenda. Absolutely no question in my mind. . . . They [the media] were *incredibly* recalcitrant for the first four or five years. They just didn't want to cover it."[23]

In any event, Shilts appears to have rebounded quickly. By August 22, 1987, the journalist had reviewed the edits for the *California Magazine* feature, which he thought were "terrific" and which left him feeling "very heartened." He made suggestions to one of the publication's feature editors about how best to present Dugas's final years. Shilts urged for the important insertion of a conversation from his book between William Darrow and Dugas "because it's the point at which somebody tells Gaetan he may be giving this to others—or that someone may have given it to him. (He obviously paid attention to only the latter part of the observation.)" Shilts suggested that it might be useful to foreshadow that Paul Popham was "getting AIDS too (more virus courtesy of Gaetan)." He also scribbled a point in the margin that "stresses the fundamental point I want to have totally covered: That there were many responsible gays, like Paul, who did good things, as opposed to the rare sociopath, like Gaetan [whose] viral legacy continued to haunt people."[24]

After Denneny had decided to generate more attention through the *New York Post*'s tabloid reporting, a well-oiled publicity machine ensured that the story got out, in the time leading up to and beyond the book's late October release. Shilts would be flown on a fifteen-city tour around the United States in October and November on a print, radio, and television promotional campaign that highlighted the role played by "Patient Zero." The publicity materials that were provided to the producers of TV and radio programs emphasized that Shilts was able to speak to a wide range of issues. Nonetheless, the order in which they were arranged suggested a priority of interest, and of apparent importance: "the identity of the first person to introduce AIDS to North American [*sic*]; how the government refused to provide funding before it was too late; how blood banks caused the needless deaths of hundreds of hemophili-

23. Denneny, recording C1491/22, tape 2, side A; emphasis on recording.
24. "RE: Patient Zero," Randy Shilts to Bob Roe, 22 August 1987, box 40, Shilts Papers.

acs; and how scientists and doctors sworn to save lives, did not."[25] The
strategy to get the book noticed worked precisely as planned. As Denneny recalled, "The week after that *Post* headline, which was *exactly*
word for word what [the publicist friend] had predicted, we got five stories in the *New York Times,* a Sunday *New York Times* review and a
daily *New York Times* review."

Despite Denneny's recollection, the book had generated a significant
buzz *before* the *Post* released its story on October 6, 1987—to the point
that Hollywood studios had made inquiries into acquiring the production rights. First *Kirkus Reviews* and then *Publishers Weekly,* two influential publishing magazines, both gave positive prepublication reviews to the book. The *Kirkus* reviewer noted the "incredible story of a
handsome French-Canadian airline steward named Gaetan Dugas (but
known as 'Patient Zero' in government studies)." The *Publishers Weekly*
review mentioned neither Dugas nor "Patient Zero" but emphasized that
the book's "importance cannot be overstated" and praised Shilts's ability to present "one alarming story after another without letting his own
passions—evident in the sheer enormity of the project—compromise
the excellent reportage."[26] A late September article in the *Hollywood
Reporter* indicated that the book had attracted interest from studios,
largely because of the strong *Kirkus* review.[27] Though some readers may
wonder whether the secondary publicity push from the *Post's* article was
in fact necessary, Denneny maintains that it was vital, in his and his publicist's professional opinions.

When asked about the use of a questionable story to launch a book,
Denneny recalled an interview from the mid-1990s with the newscaster
Robert MacNeil and his gay son.[28] The activist Larry Kramer had ac-
cused the father of avoiding coverage of AIDS on his popular MacNeil-
Lehrer news show, partly out of embarrassment over his son's homo-
sexuality. In the interview, MacNeil's son defended Kramer's actions,

25. Diane Mancher to Producers, n.d. [1987], untitled St. Martin's Press publicity
folder, box 1, Shilts Papers.

26. "The Man Who Gave Us AIDS: Triggered 'Gay Cancer' Epidemic," *New York
Post,* October 6, 1987, 1, 3; "Shilts, Randy, *And the Band Played On: Politics, People, and
the AIDS Epidemic,*" *Kirkus Reviews,* September 1, 1987, 1303–04; "And the Band Played
On," *Publishers Weekly,* September 11, 1987, 72.

27. Robert Osborne, "Rambling Reporter," *Hollywood Reporter,* September 25, 1987.

28. Georgia Dullea, "A Father and a Son, Growing Up Again: At Home with Robert
and Ian MacNeil," *New York Times,* May 5, 1994, C1, C8.

saying that "part of all that is to use any weapon anywhere to publicize the AIDS issue," and if that meant intruding on someone's private life as a means of raising awareness, then doing so was acceptable.[29] While admitting that he had not thought about the effect of the story on Dugas's family and friends, Denneny insisted that his decision to focus on Dugas was a "venial" rather than "mortal" sin and that it would have been far worse to take no action in the face of thousands dying from inaction, prejudice, and hostility: "It is like the Holocaust was going on, and so maybe you have to fight dirty. The world doesn't always give you the option to keep your hands clean. I mean had I not done that and we sold four or five thousand copies of the book and essentially resulted in silence on the national level, then I would feel real guilty. *That* I think would have been a *real* mistake."

"The Monster Who Gave Us AIDS": The North American Media Response

As Denneny and several critics have noted, the *Post*'s headline generated attention across North America and overseas, much of it sensational. The *New York Daily News* articulated the dangers of air-traveling disease spreaders with the article "The Man Who Flew Too Much." Other publications drew on the frequently rehearsed narrative of a disease introduced from abroad by a foreigner. "Canadian Said to Have Had Key Role in Spread of AIDS," headlined a *New York Times* story, and later the *National Review* nicknamed Dugas "the Columbus of AIDS," forging a link between AIDS and the suspected origins of the "French Disease" from centuries ago.[30] Internationally, the *Times* of London ran a story with the headline "Canadian Blamed for Bringing Aids to US," noting that CDC representatives refused to confirm nor deny Dugas's identity as "the hitherto anonymous 'patient zero.'"[31] The day the *New York Post*'s headline emerged, Shilts received thirty-four calls for inter-

29. Ibid., C8.

30. Michael McGovern, "The Man Who Flew Too Much: AIDS Traced to Sexy Steward," *New York Daily News*, October 7, 1987, 18; "Canadian Said to Have Had Key Role in Spread of AIDS," *New York Times*, October 7, 1987, B7; "The Columbus of AIDS," *National Review*, November 6, 1987, 19. These headlines were emphasized in Douglas Crimp's blistering critique of *Band*; see Crimp, "How to Have Promiscuity," 242.

31. "Canadian Blamed for Bringing Aids to US," *Times* [London], October 8, 1987, 11.

views from newspaper and television news reporters from across the United States.[32] It would not take long for headlines like "The Monster Who Gave Us AIDS" to appear. "Take a good look at this face," the authors of that article urged their readers, directing their gaze across the double-page tabloid spread to a nearly page-high reproduction of the photograph that had accompanied Dugas's 1984 obituary notice. "This is the man who brought the scourge of AIDS to North America.[33]

The book was released into a diverse and multisegmented North American audience, many members of which knew very little about the epidemic and relied extensively on the mainstream media for information about AIDS, people living with it, and the potential risks they might face. Others, drawing their understanding from the alternative media aimed at a range of readers—including feminists, racial and ethnic minorities, leftist and AIDS activists, and gay men and lesbians—made up a more informed and politically active minority. Generally speaking, the further one was removed from the alternative media, the less chance one would have of encountering articles that might be written by, or intended for, people with personal experience of the condition.[34] Unsurprisingly, there was a wide spectrum of engagement in terms of understanding AIDS and reacting to it. The responses to the idea of "Patient Zero" depended, to a certain extent, on where readers were situated along this continuum.

On the whole, reporters were quick to jump on the "Patient Zero" story, though Canadian newspapers such as the *Toronto Star* adopted a slightly dismissive tone, suggesting in one headline that "MDs Doubt Claim Canadian Carried AIDS to Continent."[35] "A Quebecois Man Responsible for Propagating AIDS in America?" *Le Journal de Montréal* asked its readers, in the first half of its headline, before answering em-

32. Patricia Holt, "Behind the Tragedy of AIDS," *San Francisco Chronicle*, October 18, 1987, sec. Review, 1.

33. Michael Stinton and Anne Eaton, "The Monster Who Gave Us AIDS," *Star* [Tarrytown, NY], October 27, 1987, 6–7. For all of its sensationalism, this tabloid appears to be one of the only English-language newspapers to give the Dugas family's perspectives any weight, translating statements from the interview published in *Le Soleil* earlier that month.

34. Treichler, *Theory in an Epidemic*, 88–89; Emke, "Speaking of AIDS in Canada," 415–76.

35. "MDs Doubt Claim Canadian Carried AIDS to Continent," *Toronto Star*, October 7, 1987, A2, LexisNexis News.

phatically, "IMPOSSIBLE TO CONFIRM."[36] This headline contrasts sharply with a follow-up headline in the *New York Post* on October 12, 1987: "Doc Confirms 'Patient Zero' Began Plague," the title referring to a confirmation provided by Marcus Conant, the San Francisco dermatologist on whose recollections and records the book drew frequently.[37] Shilts seems to have been surprised that his story received such a strong reaction in Canada. In an interview recorded several weeks after the story broke, he noted, "The Canadian press went crazy over that story. . . . It went all over on front pages in Canada, and Canadians . . . saw it as an offense to their nationhood."[38]

Certainly, Canadian news sources were scrambling to get on top of the story on October 7, the day after the *Post*'s bold headline set the scene. Radio-Canada, the French-language television network, led the coverage; it featured Dugas's story and apparently even displayed his 1984 obituary photograph in some areas. On *Montréal Ce Soir* (*Montreal This Evening*), the local evening news show for the largest city in French-speaking Canada, the program opened with the "absolutely breathtaking story that is literally travelling around the world today."[39] Two newscasters excitedly passed on Shilts's hypothesis that a Quebecois man was the CDC's *patient zéro*, that he had played an important role in the spread of AIDS at the end of the 1970s, and that he was at the origin of 20 percent of all cases reported in the United States in 1982. As one announcer read Dugas's name aloud, an animated background graphic showed a filing cabinet drawer—labeled with the red letters *SIDA*, the French acronym for AIDS—releasing a file entitled "G. Dugas." Giving a quick biography of first Shilts and then the flight attendant, her colleague incorrectly informed the audience that Dugas had died at the age

36. My translation of the French original: "Un Québécois responsable de la propagation du SIDA en Amérique? IMPOSSIBLE DE L'AFFIRMER—Des spécialistes," *Le Journal de Montréal*, October 8, 1987, 2.

37. "Doc Confirms 'Patient Zero' Began Plague," *New York Post*, October 12, 1987.

38. Margaret Engel, "AIDS and Prejudice: One Reporter's Account of the Nation's Response," *Washington Post*, December 1, 1987, sec. Health, Z10.

39. My translation of the French original: "Il y a une histoire absolument époustouflante qui est en train de faire le tour du monde littéralement aujourd'hui"; *Montréal Ce Soir* [nightly television news program], presented by Marie-Claude Lavallée, Philippe Bélisle, Réal d'Amours, and Charles Tisseyre, Radio-Canada, broadcast October 7, 1987, clip purchased by author from Radio-Canada, which furnished it on DVD.

of twenty-eight in 1984 and that Air Canada had recruited him as a flight attendant in 1978. "We also spoke today with people who knew Monsieur Dugas. They told us that he had an extremely active sex life and that he frequently traveled to Los Angeles, San Francisco, the West Coast, and to the Caribbean as well."[40] The presenter admitted that Radio-Canada had not managed to contact Dugas's surviving family members, who had, he said, instead communicated with colleagues at the English-language Canadian Broadcasting Corporation (CBC).

Citing a lack of unanimity in the scientific community, "where the story has obviously made a lot of noise today," the nearly nine-minute segment incorporated on-location interviews in Ottawa and Montreal.[41] An awkwardly edited video clip showed Greg (misspelled "Craig") Smith, the director of the Federal AIDS Centre, disagreeing with the reporter Réal d'Amour's suggestion that there might be other cases like this one in Canada. The director observed instead that in the United States there were several other examples where one individual had infected many other people. D'Amour smoothed over this disagreement by suggesting in his summary that the AIDS Centre had confirmed that Dugas was the first person to introduce the AIDS virus to Canada—and that although it was unclear, it was certainly possible that Dugas could have been the one to introduce it to the United States as well. The reporter quoted experts who suggested that it was not uncommon for such cases to report a list of sexual partners numbering up to three hundred. He concluded with a warning about the risks of "sexual tourism" and noted that in the United States, there were suspicions that more than a hundred male flight attendants had died since the epidemic had begun.

The program concluded with a taped interview with Dr. Robert Remis (misspelled "Remiss" in the captions), the director of Montreal's regional Infectious Diseases Bureau, who voiced his strong doubt about the allegations raised in the day's news. Asked what he, one of the people in charge of AIDS surveillance for the province, thought of the news,

40. Ibid. My translation of the French original: "Nous avons également parlé aujourd'hui avec des gens qui connaissaient monsieur Dugas. On nous a aussi dit que monsieur Dugas avait une vie sexuelle extrèmement active, qu'il voyageait fréquemment à Los Angeles, San Francisco, la côte ouest, également dans les Caraïbes."

41. Ibid. My translation of the French original: "C'est une histoire qui a fait évidemment beaucoup de bruit aujourd'hui dans les milieux scientifiques canadiens."

Remis emphasized that he had never heard of the gentleman in question and that he doubted that the flight attendant would have played a role of any importance, given that many others were infected at that time. Finally, since he worked regularly with the CDC, the official said that he would be surprised if the story was true because the CDC had not mentioned it to him. Asked what he thought the goal of the story might be, Remis closed by observing presciently that, though he could not guess at the motives of those individuals working behind the scenes, he doubted that it was for a scientific purpose.

Two days after the *Post*'s headline, a journalist who covered AIDS issues for *Le Soleil* (the *Sun*), the Quebec City daily newspaper, interviewed members of Dugas's family.[42] Their shock and outrage about the media circus was evident in the article published the following day. Largely sympathetic in its approach, the article offered readers the family members' perspectives, presenting them as unwitting victims of a mean-spirited media: "It was with consternation, sadness, and bitterness that the family of the deceased Gaétan Dugas, of Ancienne-Lorette, saw his photo projected nationally on the Radio-Canada TV newscast on Wednesday evening." The article gave space to Dugas's mother and sister to voice their anguished dismay with the media's "web of 'untruths'" and the family's exhaustion from the attention. Madame Dugas, Gaétan's widowed seventy-four-year-old mother, complained that such a story ignored the constant support her son had given to humanitarian efforts during his life—perhaps a reference to the flight attendant's assistance to AIDS Vancouver (an affiliation that will be discussed in greater detail in chapter 6). She also feared above all else that the story would cause irreparable harm to his surviving siblings.

One of Gaétan's married sisters, Hélène, told the newspaper that neither the author nor his publishing house had made any effort to contact the family and that the news stories and Radio-Canada's coverage had caught them completely by surprise. Pointedly, she felt it important to mention that no family member had spoken to the English-language

42. Roger Bellefeuille, "Propagation du sida aux États-Unis: La famille de Gaétan Dugas fort affectée," *Le Soleil*, October 9, 1987, A3. My translations of the French original: "C'est avec consternation, tristesse et amertume que la famille de feu Gaétan Dugas, de l'Ancienne-Lorette, a vu la photo de ce dernier projetée nationalement au téléjournal de Radio-Canada, mercredi soir"; and "un tissu de «faussetés»."

CBC, countering the claims broadcast on *Montréal Ce Soir* and published in *Le Journal de Montréal*. She emphasized that her brother had never hesitated in seeking treatment for his illness and that in the coming days the family would review their options, not only for protecting their private life but also whether they had any recourse in the event that Gaétan's confidential medical files had been breached. The reporter concluded the article with a confirmation from sources at the hospital where Dugas had died in Quebec City that the flight attendant had indeed been a patient seeking treatment there dating back to May 1980. It appears that the journalist was seeking to highlight the ease with which he was able to gain access to sensitive medical information.

Apart from raising the question of broken patient confidentiality at the hospitals where Dugas had sought treatment and at the CDC, and at times displaying more skepticism, the mainstream media coverage in Quebec appears to have mirrored the sensationalism present elsewhere in North America. There, as in most other places, the story appeared in the news for two or three days before falling into the background, resurrected occasionally by local responses or by further publicity efforts by St. Martin's Press. By the close of 1987, the idea had gradually saturated the media landscape. "I've got gay cancer. I'm going to die and so are you" was featured by *U.S. News and World Report* as a quote of the week for its late October edition, and this lurid focus could be seen as emblematic of the media's response.[43]

After visiting Washington, DC, in early October to cover the National March on Washington for Lesbian and Gay Rights, Shilts spent much of the fall of 1987 and spring of 1988 crisscrossing North America on publicity and lecture tours for St. Martin's Press. In its drive to sell copies of his book, the company sent him to New York, Boston, Philadelphia, Washington, DC, Atlanta, and Miami in October, then to St. Louis, Detroit, Chicago, Minneapolis, Houston, Denver, Los Angeles, Seattle, and Portland in November.[44] Penguin Books acquired the British rights for the history, and Shilts embarked on a two-week publicity tour in England and Scotland in February and March 1988, during which he also covered an English AIDS conference and encountered a hostile recep-

43. "Quotes of the Week," *U.S. News and World Report*, October 19, 1987, 7.
44. Shilts's book tour schedule, September–October [1987], folder 11 [untitled St. Martin's Press publicity], box 1, Shilts Papers.

tion from British AIDS activists at a book signing at London's Institute for Contemporary Arts.[45] The book's mainstream success led quickly to the fame and fortune of which Shilts had long dreamed, though he noted ironically to one interviewer, "This isn't exactly how I would've chosen to become rich and famous—by chronicling the decimation of my generation."[46] The attention given to *And the Band Played On* saw the author's profile in Hollywood rise, and by mid-October he had sold the feature film rights to *The Mayor of Castro Street*.[47] A bidding war over his AIDS history culminated in Shilts selling the rights to NBC in early November, for an amount his agent described as "in the high six figures."[48] He further benefited from a sale of the book's paperback rights in January to Penguin Books for $577,000.[49] Signing a lucrative public speaking contract with a New York–based literary lecture management company also contributed to both his visibility and his financial security. Shilts noted, in an aside to one reporter covering a Maryland conference exploring issues of criminalization relating to HIV transmission, that he could earn more in two weeks of lecturing than in a year on a reporter's salary at the *Chronicle*.[50] Such earnings allowed him to purchase a house in the Sonoma Valley region outside San Francisco in early 1988. Shilts's interviews with the press indicate that fame and fortune brought more challenges than he had anticipated. During nine months of interviews, from the fall of 1987 to the spring of 1988, the author would display a surprising lack of awareness—considering that he was a journalist—in his conversations

45. "Schedule [for UK book tour]," February 28–March 13, 1988, folder 13, box 1, Shilts Papers; Crimp, *Melancholia and Moralism*, 120–22.

46. Diane Eicher, "New AIDS Book Chronicles the Epidemic," *Denver Post*, November 13, 1987, 4E.

47. Liz Smith, "Movie Deal for Shilts' 'Mayor of Castro Street,'" *San Francisco Chronicle*, October 13, 1987, E1. Although the story had been made into a documentary film—the Oscar-winning *The Times of Harvey Milk* (1984)—the feature film project would languish in development for two decades before being produced and released in 2008 as *Milk*, garnering Academy Awards for Dustin Lance Black's screenplay and Sean Penn's leading actor performance as Harvey Milk, among other awards and honors.

48. Herb Caen, "Use 'Em or Lose 'Em," *San Francisco Chronicle*, November 10, 1987, B1. The rights eventually passed to Home Box Office, which released the television miniseries in September 1993.

49. Streitfeld, "Book Report," sec. Book World, 15.

50. Randi Henderson, "Speaking out on AIDS," *Baltimore Sun*, March 29, 1988, 3C.

with other reporters. He would talk about his earnings and large pur-
chases, seemingly without concern about how others might perceive his
comments. He would occasionally feel the need to justify his financial
success by emphasizing how far he had had to go into debt to complete
a book that had initially seemed an unlikely prospect for a best seller.[51]

In particular, Shilts was vocal in condemning the amount of attention
that the "Patient Zero" story had received. In one interview, for example, he turned to his publicist and groaned her name when a reporter inquired about Dugas, suggesting that he associated her publicity efforts
with this line of inquiry.[52] True to Denneny's recollection, in interviews
Shilts would attempt to steer conversation from the flight attendant to
what he believed were his book's more substantive elements of reporting. In an interview with the *Washington Post*, he lamented the "great
irony" of the reaction to his book. "Here I've done 630 pages of serious
AIDS policy reporting with the premise that this disaster was allowed to
happen because the media only focus on the glitzy and sensational aspects of the epidemic. My book breaks, not because of the serious public
policy stories, but because of the rather minor story of Patient Zero."[53]
In *Contagious*, Priscilla Wald suggests with regard to this quote that "it
is hard to imagine that Shilts really did not recognize the importance of
his character." [54] Clearly, Shilts was *bitterly* aware of how important Dugas was to his success. Given that his book was gaining attention before
Denneny activated the *Post*'s inflammatory coverage, the journalist may
have harbored hopes his book's potential to rise to national prominence on its own merits, without such promotional tactics. Constant
questions about the flight attendant would certainly have been irritating

51. "Heart of an Epidemic," 14.

52. Frank Spencer, "AIDS: A Failure to Respond," *Hartford Courant*, October 30,
1987, C1.

53. Engel, "AIDS and Prejudice," 10. Denneny noted in his 2008 interview that his doctoral supervisor had encountered a similar situation where the media obscured the importance of the author's whole work by focusing on a single part: "With Hannah Arendt's
Eichmann in Jerusalem, that book was published in [19]63. In it she has two paragraphs, in
a 320-page book, about the Judenräte, the Jewish councils in Eastern Europe and their cooperation with the Final Solution. And the Anti-Defamation League plus some establishment people in Israel launched a campaign against that book that was so effective that almost to this day people can't read the book straight."

54. Wald, *Contagious*, 231.

to Shilts, given his high career aspirations, his sense of his book's wider accomplishments, and the possibility that he felt somewhat guilty for agreeing to an act of "yellow journalism" to get his book on the agenda.

A Montreal TV station conducted an interview with Shilts in early October, within a couple of days of the story dominating the Quebecois airwaves. When asked whether the "Patient Zero" was simply a "cheap publicity stunt," Shilts immediately ended the interview and left the studio. That Shilts related this incident to another journalist suggests the seriousness with which he viewed his own reporting efforts and journalistic integrity. It may have given him cause for reflection, though, since he offered, via the reporter, an indirect apology to the Dugas family, saying that he was sorry if he brought them any pain.[55] Although he would continue to stand behind the technical truth of the statement that he had never unequivocally stated that Dugas had brought AIDS to North America, Shilts would nonetheless continue to offer a mixed view of the flight attendant's importance. In his interviews and public appearances, from Oregon to Vermont, from Colorado to Florida, Shilts would speak of Dugas as indicative of the "human factor" of why the epidemic had been able to take hold, though he took pains to point out that Dugas was not the norm. "I don't see him as any more typical of a gay man than Jack the Ripper was of the heterosexual," he told a British reporter, before adding, in defense of his view of the truth, "but it did happen."[56] Still, in Shilts's view, when unhindered by troubling questions about the Dugas family's reactions to his writing, the flight attendant was a psychopath.

While relieved at this dramatic change in his financial situation, Shilts would remain ruefully aware of the role played by the stories of the dead flight attendant and of other controversial historical players in his success. In 1991, he sent invitations for his fortieth birthday—Shiltsmas, as he would jokingly refer to these annual birthday parties—to be held at his new residence in Sonoma Valley. Tiny print on the back side of the invitation noted—perhaps as gallows humor, perhaps in a bid to address and deflect criticism of his relatively newfound wealth: "This invitation produced with resources provided by the Randy Shilts International Fan Club, Dr. Robert Gallo, Chairman. Further assistance was provided by

55. Craig Wilson, "The Chronicler of AIDS: Randy Shilts, Tracking the Epidemic," *USA Today*, October 12, 1987, sec. Life, 2D.

56. Young, "Patient Zero," 6.

the Northern California Bathhouse Owners Association, the Gay Cau-
cus of the French-Canadian Airline Flight Attendants Association and
the Investment Council of the American Bloodbankers Association."[57]

In summary, the sustained publicity efforts of St. Martin's Press to
bring Shilts's book to the national attention were remarkably successful and provided an efficient means for the "Patient Zero" story to be
mass-produced and to hold the popular imagination in North America
in late 1987. Shilts was billed as "the nation's premier AIDS reporter," a
role he eagerly adopted, though he would struggle somewhat more with
the rapid change in his personal fortune that came with the success of
his book.[58] Within a relatively short space of time, the idea of "Patient
Zero"—one which combined the suggestion of origins and gay promiscuity with the added deliberation of a serial-killing disease carrier—was
able to take hold over a geographically vast area.

Silences

In addition to locating and presenting sources that "speak," historians
are well advised to also seek out and pay attention to those that remain
silent.[59] Often it can be difficult to infer the existence of absences of
speech in the archive or in the media coverage of a story and to estimate
their contours amid the noise of the more straightforwardly expressive
sources. Beyond the material survival of records—a fact that crucially
shapes which stories may more readily be told—there are also distinct
types of silences in terms of the production of stories. For example, the
tactical decision to withhold comment is quite different from being prevented to speak. Some historians have characterized silences as vital and
manifold rhetorical "strategies" that run through discourses.[60] Others

57. "What becomes a legend most?" folder: Shiltsmas + Xmas Cards/Mem, Alband
Collection.

58. "Hear RANDY SHILTS, the Nation's Premier AIDS Reporter," flyer promoting
Shilts's talk at California State University, Northridge, April 11, 1988, folder 16: Apr. 1988,
box 1, Shilts Papers.

59. Historians seem to be paying more explicit attention to silence; see, for example,
Jay Winter, "Thinking about Silence," in *Shadows of War: A Social History of Silence
in the Twentieth Century*, ed. Efrat Ben-Ze'ev, Ruth Ginio, and Jay Winter (Cambridge:
Cambridge University Press, 2010), 3–31.

60. Foucault, *Will to Knowledge*, 27; see also Howard, *Men Like That*, 27–33.

have used silences to demonstrate how various social agents hold differing levels of power to produce history.[61] Indeed, some researchers have commented on the tendency of AIDS narratives to silence the voices of people living with HIV, a question that will be taken up in greater detail in chapter 6.[62] This section explores specific examples wherein the "Patient Zero" story was met with silence, to foster a more fine-grained understanding of these instances of exclusion and strategies of resistance.

In practice, it can be difficult to establish that historical actors were aware of an issue and then chose not to act or speak on it. Ironically, as the following example shows, it often requires that they later speak or write about these omissions to provide firm evidence of their existence. In the week following the "Patient Zero" story's rapid ascendance, Canada's national English-language broadcaster, CBC, aired the first episode of a radio documentary on its "Ideas" series, which explored the science and politics of AIDS.[63] An extended interview with Randy Shilts, taped at the Washington march in early October 1987, opened the documentary. The journalist spoke at great length about his new book, which detailed the failures of the Reagan administration, the news media, and the research establishment. There was a notable absence of a mention of the "Patient Zero" story. On the one hand, Shilts was probably happy not to focus on it; on the other, it would seem strange for the producers of the documentary to have been unaware of the story. In fact, they did know of the emerging narrative and practiced a strategic silence about it.

Max Allen, the *Ideas* series producer, was based in New York that September and became aware of the rumors about the flight attendant which were circulating in the wake of the first prepublication book reviews. Allen decided not only to omit any reference to the "Patient Zero" story in his documentary but also to alert a colleague of his, Ed Jackson, of the story's existence and of the "possible fall-out." Jackson,

61. Michel-Rolph Trouillot, "Silencing the Past: Layers of Meaning in the Haitian Revolution," in *Between History and Histories: The Making of Silences and Commemorations*, ed. Gerald M. Sider and Gavin A. Smith (Toronto: University of Toronto Press, 1997), 38.

62. See, for example, Patton, *Inventing AIDS*, 3; Brian Heaphy, "Silence and Strategy: Researching AIDS/HIV Narratives in the Flow of Power," in *Meddling with Mythology: AIDS and the Social Construction of Knowledge*, ed. Rosaline S. Barbour and Guro Huby (London: Routledge, 1998), 21–36; Emke, "Speaking of AIDS in Canada."

63. "Ideas," part 1 of eight-part radio documentary, hosted by Lister Sinclair, produced by Max Allen (CBC Radio, 1987), audiocassette recording of the original October 13, 1987, broadcast consulted in ACT Library, Toronto.

a former member of the Body Politic Collective, was now involved with the AIDS Committee of Toronto (ACT). On September 28, Jackson wrote a memo to the ACT media relations officer, Phil Shaw, and the organization's phone counselors:

> It may be of particular interest to Toronto journalists and gay men because it talks a lot about Patient Zero, the gay man who is identified by the CDC as the first AIDS patient in North America. He was the sexual link among the original Los Angeles group and was a Canadian airline attendant called Gaetan Dugas. He lived in Toronto and in Vancouver and slept with a lot of men after he had KS. This was before HIV was identified as the putative agent for AIDS and he used to say to people after he had had sex with them in the baths: see these spots, this is gay cancer. It's not clear whether he thought he was infectious.
>
> Max Allen thinks there is a sensational story angle here which could cause a real ripple to flow through the community if the media pick it up. Gaetan was well-known, I believe. I, for example, met him once ten years ago. So, Phil may get follow-up calls from the media and the phone lines could get calls from panicky people. Classic media stereotype: irresponsible gay man runs around infecting everyone. Is he not typical? (Or something to that effect).
>
> So, take note, for what it's worth. Whatever the fallout, Shilts is a very good writer. It should be a good read.[64]

In this case, a radio producer chose not to reproduce a story—for fear of its sensational consequences—but also alerted AIDS activists to prepare themselves for its eventual transmission.

In passing on his warning, Allen would not have known—nor, necessarily, would later readers of the memo—that Jackson had himself shared a sexual encounter with Dugas, when they "met" ten years previously, around the time of summer 1977. Jackson would later recall that the two cruised each other in the menswear department of the Bay department store before he returned to Dugas's hotel room to spend an

---

64. Ed Jackson, "To Phil Shaw and AIDSupport Phone Counsellors," memo, September 28, 1987, folder: Media Relations Officer: Memos In—1987, box 91–143/19, Records of the AIDS Committee of Toronto, Canadian Lesbian and Gay Archives, Toronto (hereafter cited as ACT Records); *attendant* spelled as "attendent," *Dugas* as "duGas," and *follow-up* as "followup" in original.

enjoyable night with a man he described as "sweet" and "an incredibly generous lover."[65] Jackson also recalled that Dugas subsequently provided moral support by attending court one day during the *Body Politic* trial. This court case, wherein the gay newspaper was charged with using the mail to distribute obscene material and in which Jackson was one of three defendants, was widely reported in Toronto and across Canada in January 1979.[66] These brief personal experiences he shared with the flight attendant impressed on Jackson the notion that Dugas had some sense of political awareness and solidarity with the gay movement, which in turn raised questions in Jackson's mind about Shilts's portrayal of the man he had met.

As it would turn out, while the "Patient Zero" story did make headlines as Allen and Jackson had feared, it did not translate into a barrage of panicked phone calls for ACT. The organization's media contact records for the month of October indicate that the story generated two specific inquiries out of at least ninety-nine media contacts.[67] Thus it formed only part of the landscape of questions reaching the organization, competing for attention alongside a dentistry conference dealing with AIDS as well as the case of the HIV-positive Nova Scotian teacher, Eric Smith, whose name had recently been leaked to the media and who faced a boycott from parents of students at the school where he taught. Indeed, the story about the boycott against Smith peaked in Canada at exactly the same time as the "Patient Zero" story broke.[68] Smith later suggested,

65. Ed Jackson, interview with author, Toronto, September 14, 2008, recording C1491/48, tape 1, side A, BLSA. In their recorded testimonies, two interviewees based in San Francisco reported single unprotected sexual encounters with Dugas between 1980 and 1982. At the time of interview in July 2007, one, Josh Lancaster (pseud.), was HIV-positive and angrily convinced that he had contracted his infection from the flight attendant and not his other San Francisco bathhouse encounters; interview with author, July 28, 2007, recording C1491/12, tape 1, side A, BLSA. The other man was HIV-negative and believed that his encounter with Dugas in Vancouver—after which he immediately began hearing stories of the flight attendant's "gay cancer"—may have helped him by raising his awareness of the risks associated with AIDS at an early date; Ross Murray, interview with author, July 29, 2007, recording C1491/15, tape 1, side A, BLSA.

66. Bill Lewis, "Case May Set Precedent, Decision Expected Feb 14," *Body Politic*, February 1979, 7–9.

67. Media contact record sheets, folder: Media Contacts: October 1987, box 91–143/11, ACT Records.

68. See, for example, Canadian Press, "AIDS-Fearing Parents Plot Boycott," *Vancouver Sun*, October 9, 1987, A6.

with good humor, that he had not been aware of the story about the flight attendant at that time: "If [*chuckling*] there was an AIDS story carried in Halifax, it was me, because two or three a times a week at least, some parent would be saying something idiotic, or the school board would be making an announcement, so they were getting their quota of AIDS stories just locally."[69]

In contrast to the hospital in Quebec City, which readily confirmed to *Le Soleil* that Dugas had once sought treatment there, the US Centers for Disease Control held a silence over Dugas's identity. Harold Jaffe, the former KS/OI Task Force member who spoke for the organization in an interview published in mid-October 1987, denied the idea that "Patient Zero" referred to a single individual who brought AIDS to "North America or California or Canada." It would be impossible to know this, he said, and besides, "For every individual we were aware of, there were probably 10 that we weren't aware of." He also refused to confirm or deny whether Dugas was "Patient Zero," saying that the CDC had never identified this man.[70] Given its long history of work in venereal disease control and its early history of gathering the names of individuals with AIDS, the CDC believed it was vital for its interests and credibility that a silence was kept on the identity of "Patient Zero."[71]

The Dugas family crafted another silence. Apart from their few spoken words to *Le Soleil*, family members refused to comment publicly.[72] Before the *New York Post* broke the story, CBS Television recruited a local Canadian reporter to gain the family's cooperation for a *60 Minutes*

69. Eric Smith, interview with author, Halifax, August 1, 2008, recording C1491/36, tape 1, side B, BLSA.

70. "'First AIDS Patient' Story Dismissed," A3.

71. This silence continues largely to the present day. In his 2008 oral history interview, Bill Darrow referred to this man consistently as "Patient O." When Harold Jaffe and the author began jointly drafting a collaborative article in 2013, the former requested that the flight attendant's name be removed and replaced with "Patient 0," preferring that the identification be held at arm's length through a citation of *And the Band Played On*.

72. This strategic silence, like that of the CDC, extended for decades. In October 2007 a reporter from *Le Soleil* had contacted Dugas's sister and sister-in-law to ask what they thought about reports announcing a recent scientific theory that HIV had arrived in the United States in 1969. They replied that it had brought the family some relief, but having had their name "blackened," they preferred to let the subject die, wishing to speak of it no more since they were fed up with "all this s—" (my translation); Ian Bussières, "Agent de bord exonéré d'avoir propagé le sida en Amérique: la famille de Gaétan Dugas soulagée mais amère," *Le Soleil* [Quebec City], October 31, 2007, 17.

episode. She recalled that "I was a journalist with CBC TV in Montreal and a researcher from *60 Minutes* contacted our newsroom looking for someone who'd translate between French and English on a 'secret' assignment to Quebec City. I picked up the researcher at the Montreal airport and she told me the chilling story on the drive to Quebec City. She'd made an appointment to speak to the Dugas family, to ask for access to family pictures and interviews." The Canadian reporter was struck by her own attachment to and sympathy for the Dugas family members, and she found herself contemplating how to protect them from the media's gaze:

> They were very decent people who'd adopted Gaetan Dugas and deeply loved him. There was a mass card with Gaetan's photo on their refrigerator door. His sister, a dental hygienist, had nursed him and was concerned that, if this was known publicly, she'd lose her job. I was able to give the family some options to cooperating with *60 Minutes* (in French) that the *60 Minutes* researcher was unaware of. The parents were very concerned about controlling the story in order to protect Gaetan's reputation. . . . I found myself profoundly protective of them and would not give out their address to my French or English colleagues when the story broke in Canada. The Dugas family did not cooperate with *60 Minutes* to the best of my knowledge. They did not believe the researcher's assurances that the story would not be sensationalized. Indeed it was, with Gaetan being called the "Typhoid Mary of AIDS" . . . I'm sure they were devastated. His mother told me he'd take her on trips and was very kind and loving to them. A good son.[73]

Indeed, the *60 Minutes* piece on "Patient Zero"—a long-awaited first piece of investigative reporting from that program on the epidemic—was deeply exploitative. It was allegedly focused on the Reagan administration's lack of attention to AIDS—a strategic nonresponse to the epidemic which ACT UP had begun to protest with the adopted battle phrase "SILENCE = DEATH."[74] Yet the first half of the segment, as the

73. Marie Wadden, e-mail message to author, June 6, 2008. This e-mail was sent in response to a nationally broadcast interview about my research on CBC Radio's *Sounds Like Canada*, June 4, 2008.

74. Douglas Crimp, "AIDS: Cultural Analysis/Cultural Activism," in Crimp, *AIDS*, 3–16. In early 1987, members of the SILENCE = DEATH Project, an activist design collective, mounted visually striking posters across New York City that carried this phrase. The slogan appeared in white capital letters beneath a pink triangle, all set against a black background. The collective's members, who shortly thereafter participated in ACT UP's inau-

cultural scholar Leo Bersani noted, was an examination of "the mur-
derously naughty sexual habits of Gaetan Dugas." This choice of content resulted in a report that was sensational from its beginning, Bersani
maintained, "with the most repugnant image of homosexuality imaginable: that of the irresponsible male tart who willfully spread[s] the virus after he was diagnosed and warned of the dangers to others of his
promiscuity."[75] While the program's producers did not add any new information to Shilts's version of the story, they managed to acquire several photographs of the flight attendant, and thus they were able to put a
face to the disease for their North American audience (see fig. 4.2).

Viewers were invited to gaze upon the shirtless torso of Dugas and
ponder his motivation as the camera zoomed in slowly to a close-up
(see fig. 4.3). The program's host, Harry Reasoner, matter-of-factly—
and without a trace of irony—explained, "Patient Zero is the name that
Dr. Dritz and the medical detectives used to describe this man, the airline steward, to protect his identity. Randy Shilts reveals that he was a
French-Canadian named Gaetan Dugas." A jump cut to a tight shot of
the flight attendant accentuated Reasoner's designation: "Patient Zero—
one of the first cases of AIDS." Finally, the last jump cut brought the audience face-to-face with an extreme close-up of Dugas's eyes: "the first
person identified as a major transmitter of the disease."[76] The program
also reproduced the cluster diagram in a misleading animated cartoon it
labeled "Cluster Study Patient Zero." The animation began with a sin-

gural activities, loaned their distinctive image to the new activist group for wide use in its
protest work; see Douglas Crimp, "AIDS: Cultural Analysis/Cultural Activism," in Crimp,
AIDS, 3–16; Christian Liclair, "Silence=Death-Project," *The Nomos of Images* (blog),
ISSN: 2366-9926, December 30, 2015, http://nomoi.hypotheses.org/198. Since the 1970s, a
transnational network of European and North American gay rights activists had adopted
the pink triangle—the emblem which male homosexuals were forced to wear in Nazi concentration camps during the Second World War—as a symbol to challenge cultural silences
around homosexuality and to promote gay pride; W. Jake Newsome, "Migrating Memories: Transatlantic Commemoration of the Nazis' Homosexual Victims in West Germany
and the United States" (paper presented at the annual meeting of the American Historical
Association, Atlanta, January 10, 2016).

75. Leo Bersani, "Is the Rectum a Grave?" in Crimp, *AIDS*, 202.

76. Lowell Bergman, "Patient Zero," *60 Minutes*, CBS, airdate November 15, 1987, online video, 14:10, https://www.youtube.com/watch?v=Sc7bYnH2Zpo. For a critical discussion of the media's use of images of PWAs to "reveal" what one British tabloid called "the
disturbing truth about AIDS sickness," see Martha Gever, "Pictures of Sickness: Stuart
Marshall's *Bright Eyes*," in Crimp, *AIDS*, 108–26, quotation at 115.

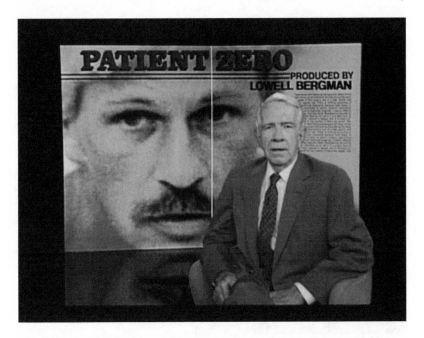

FIGURE 4.2 Host Harry Reasoner introducing "Patient Zero" segment on *60 Minutes*, CBS, broadcast November 15, 1987. With the name "Patient Zero" authoritatively stamped across Dugas's forehead, there is nothing in this message to indicate the contingent and unplanned route by which the designation came into being. This episode of *60 Minutes* was the fifth most watched television show nationwide that week (topped only by four sit-coms), according to the Nielsen Ratings service. The program reached twenty-one million households with television sets (Associated Press, "It's Waterloo Again for 'Napoleon,'" *Orlando Sentinel*, November 19, 1987, E8).

gle circle containing the numeral 0 filling an otherwise blank and grid-lined dark blue canvas. As the camera pulled back, the other cluster case connections, represented by spokes and unnumbered colored circles, popped outward from this central point, until the full cluster diagram filled the frame, rotated slightly counterclockwise so that the length of the network was now arrayed horizontally across the screen. This animation suggested an inexorable growth outward from "Patient 0," the only identified case. It represented a subtle yet powerful misinterpretation of the connections traced by Bill Darrow, one which further emphasized and naturalized Dugas's supposedly central role.

John Greyson, a Toronto artist and filmmaker who was involved with AIDS Action Now! (an Ontario-based activist group modeled on ACT UP), was struck by the intensity of the media's gaze on the flight atten-

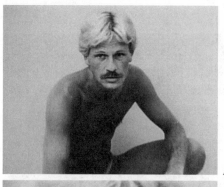

A

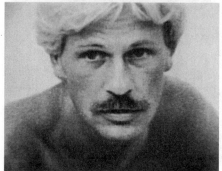

B

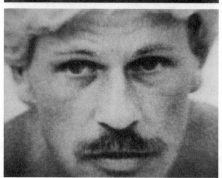

C

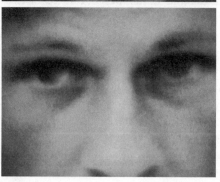

D

FIGURE 4.3 Gaétan Dugas, "the first person identified as a major transmitter of the disease," as described in voiceover by Harry Reasoner on CBS program *60 Minutes*, broadcast November 15, 1987. The sequence of images began with (*A*) a torso shot, zooming in slowly to (*B*) a close-up, jumping to (*C*) a tight shot, and finally jumping to (*D*) an extreme close-up. The program's editors employed jump cuts to bring millions of viewers up close with the man Reasoner described as "a central victim and victimizer."

dant and the family's studied silence. Before the Canadian Film Centre accepted him as a resident in the organization's three-year directors' program, he incorporated the media's handling of the "Patient Zero" story into two art pieces he produced in 1989. In one, initially published as "Requiem for Gaetan" in 1988, a viewer flips across several fictitious television channels searching for a documentary on the life of Dugas. On the last channel, the viewer catches the end of the documentary, and here Greyson conceptualized the reaction of the flight attendant's mother as one of defiance, resisting the commodification of her image as the mother of "Patient Zero" and shifting her strategy of silence to one of invisibility:

CLICK

CHANNEL 17: . . . close-up of Gaetan Dugas, the black and white photo from the *National Enquirer*. A disembodied voice, a woman, bitter and clipped, Québécois.

"Look, I've done a lot of research on my own. I've talked with maybe two dozen specialists, here, in the United States, in Europe. They all say there's no such thing as a Patient Zero, it doesn't make sense medically, the epidemiology is all wrong. The cluster groups around the continent, and the numbers, indicate no one person could have been responsible. Plus all the new stuff about co-factors. And I've told a thousand reporters—but do you think anyone has printed it? Not a chance. They just want a photo of Patient Zero's mother. So forget it."[77]

Elsewhere in the piece, Greyson employed the fictional Mallory Keaton—a teenaged character from *Family Ties*, a popular contemporary American television series starring the Canadian actor Michael J. Fox as Alex Keaton with Justine Bateman as his sister Mallory—to ventriloquize his critique of Shilts. "I want to explore the book's double messages," Mallory—a scatterbrained character cast here as a wise fool— tells Alex, "the simultaneous critiquing and validation of the mainstream

---

77. John Greyson, "Liberace's Music Helped Cure Me," in *Urinal and Other Stories* (Toronto: Art Metropole and the Power Plant, 1993), 268–69. Earlier versions of this work, which Greyson initially wrote to highlight a strong culture of lesbian and gay video production in Canada, were published in British and Canadian gay periodicals: see *Square Peg* 19 (1988): 28–29; *Rites*, September 1988, 12, 18; and the Vancouver-based *Video Guide* 10, no. 3–4 (November 1989): 8–9, http://www.vivomediaarts.com/wp-content/uploads/2015/06/VGUIDESno046small.pdf, accessed February 24, 2017.

medical establishment; the appropriation of gay liberation discourse to buttress deeply conservative positions; and finally, Shilts' dangerously reactionary views concerning sexuality and its regulation." Mallory continues, "Right now I'm working on how he constructs the Gaetan Dugas story, turning him into the dangerous, exotic Patient Zero, a latter-day Typhoid Mary." There is a dark irony at play when Greyson has Alex, backed up by the show's recorded laugh track, mock his sister and ask her if she is "on drugs." Greyson would continue pondering the mainstream success of the "Patient Zero" story. Needing to develop a feature film proposal for his fellowship at the Canadian Film Centre, Greyson's critique would evolve into an unusual film project, *Zero Patience*, which will be examined in greater detail in chapter 5.

Michael Denneny was concerned that if only five thousand copies of *And the Band Played On* were sold, the result would be a continued national "silence" on AIDS policy. His deployment of the "Patient Zero" story to hook the media's interest and generate discussion was powerfully effective. In these aforementioned examples, we can see how silence was used in a variety of ways: to deal privately with familial grief and anger, in the case of the Dugas family, and to reclaim a space of dignity. Employees of the Centers for Disease Control employed silence in an attempt to guard a dead man's identity and the agency's own reputation, as part of a wider necessity of safeguarding a long tradition of protecting confidential health information. Meanwhile, workers for the Canadian Broadcasting Corporation sought to employ silence for protection. One exploited the cloak of secrecy afforded by linguistic incommensurability to help guard a family's little remaining privacy in one case, while another withheld a story to shield lesbian and gay communities and AIDS organizations from potentially damaging rumors in another. The decision to stay silent may, in some cases, have been successful, while in others it may have deprived the wider public of useful, corrective information to counter the "Patient Zero" story. Ultimately, there may be too little evidence to suggest that these acts of silence— enacted by members of the media and the public in opposition to the widespread naming of Gaétan Dugas and dissemination of the "Patient Zero" story—made a significant difference to the narrative's impact, in view of the sustained efforts by St. Martin's Press to promote the book. They do, however, point to moments of individual agency and alternatives to the compulsion to disseminate information that appears to have underpinned the approach of Shilts and other reporters like him.

Reactions

As *California Magazine*'s exclusive rights to the "Patient Zero" story expired near the end of October 1987, St. Martin's Press licensed the excerpts from the book dealing with Dugas to be serialized and featured in newspapers across North America. In artwork accompanying one of these featured segments, a uniformed flight attendant's face was replaced with a fingerprint, in an allusion to Dugas's own personal stamp on the virus within him (see fig. 4.4). His gloved fingers are separated and tightly constricted in a clawlike, predatory manner suggestive of a vampire or other demon in search of a victim. The article's subtitle—"Wherever Gaetan Dugas paused, gay men began to sicken and die"—strongly reinforced this message.[78] Response in the form of letters to mainstream and gay newspapers reveals fears that the reported behavior of Gaétan Dugas—as a conscienceless monster—would tar the entire gay community.

Many readers certainly did take away that impression. A Florida man writing to his local newspaper, the *St. Petersburg Times*, used Shilts's work to buttress his claim that homosexuality was synonymous with promiscuity. With a muddled sense of the facts gleaned undoubtedly from a combination of the media's misleading reports and the serialized excerpts, the man explained that "Dugas picked up the disease in Europe through sexual contacts with Africans. He was diagnosed in 1980 as communicating a possibly fatal sexual disease and labeled 'Patient Zero' by medical researchers. Even then he refused to restrict his homosexual activity, which averaged some 250 partners per year and was spread from coast to coast through his airline travels." The letter writer signaled his disdain for the claims by gay AIDS organizations that they were being unfairly criticized: "If, as one letter writer claims, homosexuals 'have done more than any other group to combat the AIDS crisis,' then it is also an inescapable fact that these same homosexuals brought on the crisis in the first place and for the most part refuse to curtail the activity that is spreading it exponentially."[79]

Another reader wrote to *Time* magazine, nominating the flight attendant for the publication's annual "man of the year" award. "Unfortunately,"

78. *Chicago Tribune*, November 1, 1987, sec. Tempo, 1, Shilts Papers.
79. James V. Christy, letter to the editor, *St. Petersburg* [FL] *Times*, November 8, 1987, 3D, Factiva (stpt000020011118djb802326).

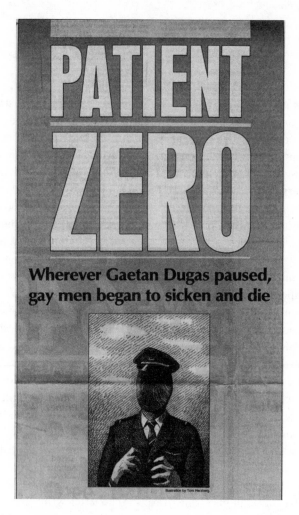

FIGURE 4.4 Artwork accompanying the serialized "Patient Zero" story, *Chicago Tribune*, November 1, 1987, sec. Tempo, 1, Randy Shilts Papers (GLC 43), LGBTQIA Center, San Francisco Public Library. Framed image of flight attendant measures 7.5 × 10.4 cm. © Tom Herzberg. Reproduced with permission from the artist. This image, by Chicago-based editorial illustrator Tom Herzberg, introduced the *Tribune*'s serialization of the "Patient Zero" excerpts from Shilts's book. At the bottom of this page, below the floating image of the uniformed air steward, a reader of the *Tribune* would have seen a pixelated, black-and-white photograph of a crowd of about twenty people walking toward the camera. Four of them had a fingerprint stamped on their faces, suggestive of the spread of one individual's virus. A photograph of Dugas from his 1984 obituary in *Le Soleil* lay buried in the section's fifth page, perhaps indicating the decreasing significance of Dugas's actual likeness to the development of the mythological figure of "Patient Zero." In a September 2016 e-mail to the author, Herzberg recalled being intrigued by the idea that AIDS could be traced to one person, and given the feature's emphasis on identifying Dugas, he developed the idea of featuring a fingerprint. Since the job was a rushed one and the technical process involved in rendering an artistic fingerprint was too time-consuming, he simply used his own. This image and the accompanying story were distributed to more than 1.2 million readers of the *Tribune*'s Sunday edition.

the woman noted dryly, "it appears he was man of the year for a number of years."[80] It would seem that *People* magazine took such a suggestion seriously: the publication featured Dugas as one of the year's "25 most intriguing people" in an issue released two weeks later, alongside Princess Diana and other luminaries of the period. The entry, which reused the *60 Minutes* photograph of Dugas, suggested that the flight attendant was a "human explosive" who "never fully understood or accepted his role as a major transmitter of the virus" and was "sexually active to the end."[81]

In Halifax, this magazine article infuriated those flight attendants who had been close with Dugas. As his friend and former colleague Desiree Conn recalled, it was an affront not only to Dugas's memory but also to their profession:

I remember reading that and being so angry, and I mean I'm not gay, but I was *so angry* about what they were accusing him of. And I thought to myself, "Okay, how many people before Gaétan—Gaétan, when I knew him, thought he had cancer—so how many people before him who thought maybe they had cancer didn't really have cancer at all but had AIDS?" So *how dare they* [*speaking slowly*] say that, and how dare they say that when he knew he *had* AIDS that he didn't care about other people and actually tried to spread it on purpose. . . . But when that particular issue of *People* came out, everybody was so up in arms, we were buying them to throw them out, [*pausing*] because we were just so, I don't know, ticked, I guess, with the article and the fact that it wasn't just a slight against Gaétan, it was a slight against all of us. And they were saying in the articles that basically we were a bunch of promiscuous fly people and that that's what we basically did for a living.[82]

Conn recalled many copies of the popular issue being left on planes after passengers disembarked: "We kept picking them up so that if people were reading them, we were taking those magazines and throwing them in the garbage, so that they didn't stay circulating."[83]

Some friends and colleagues, like Conn, were later adamant that the

80. Jeanne Padron, "Man of the Year?" letter to the editor, *Time*, December 14, 1987; this letter was also quoted in "Did You Hear . . . ?," *NYN*, December 21, 1987, 4.

81. "Patient Zero," *People*, December 28, 1987, 47.

82. Desiree Conn, interview with author, Halifax, NS, July 31, 2008, recording C1491/34, tape 1, side B; emphasis on recording.

83. Ibid.

man they knew had not "a mean bone in his body" and would never deliberately hurt another person in the manner suggested by Shilts and by media reports like the *People* magazine article.[84] Others held more complicated views. One queer-identified and HIV-positive male acquaintance recalled "a very popular saying back then, 'Stiff dick has no conscience.'" Though this man completely rejected the notion of apportioning any blame to Dugas, he believed it was likely that the flight attendant had engaged in "unprotected sex when he probably knew he shouldn't have."[85] Another colleague, while carefully stressing that she did not know Dugas well enough to interpret his specific experience, acknowledged what for her was an abstract plausibility to Shilts's characterization—that someone facing such trying circumstances and so many unknowns might engage in careless behavior which put others at risk:

> I think it's entirely possible for *a person,* not necessarily for Gaétan but for *a person,* who receives a diagnosis that is in essence a death sentence, and who gets really angry because nobody can really tell them exactly where it came from but they say to them, "Because of who you are, because you are a gay man, because you enjoy sex, because you've been with lots of men, that's why you've got this disease," combine it with a Catholic upbringing which says everything is your fault anyway or God's visiting upon you because of something you *did*, I think it's entirely possible for him to be in a state of denial, anger, whatever emotional turmoil he was in, to go out and have sex with people unprotected, knowing that there was a *chance* that he was doing something that might put them at risk. Not, not maybe deliberately loading the gun and firing it and saying, "I know I'm gonna kill you," but, "I've got it. I didn't do anything to bring this on myself other than be who I am. Why should I be worried about whether or not I'm giving it to you? I'm just bloody pissed off." So I guess in an abstract sense I could understand it if that's what happened, but I . . . didn't know him well enough to understand if that was where he was coming from.[86]

84. Conn, recording C1491/34, tape 1, side A ("a mean bone in his body"); Barbara Dunn, Elaine Watson, and Janice Miller, interview with author, Vancouver, June 10, 2008, recording C1491/26, BLSA (Dunn's defense of Dugas at tape 1, side B).

85. Spencer Macdonell (pseud.), interview with author, Vancouver, June 11, 2008, recording C1491/27, tape 2, side A.

86. Dunn, Watson, and Miller, recording C1491/26 (Watson quoted at tape 1, side B).

The photographic portrait of Dugas in *People* magazine would receive the widest circulation and deployment of any photograph depicting him, appearing as it did in the magazine and weeks earlier on *60 Minutes*. As such, it is illuminating to examine the picture and its wide travels. The image viewers see most clearly shows the flight attendant in a moment of apparently good physical health—tanned, muscled, and lean. Given the emphasis in Shilts's popular history and the surrounding publicity that Dugas had lured hundreds of men into sexual liaisons, it should not be surprising that this photo would be used the most frequently to depict his physical appeal. As it appears in *60 Minutes*, the image has a slightly awkward composition, with the lower edge of frame clipping Dugas's right arm at the elbow, left forearm at the wrist, and most of his lower body at the waist. By contrast, a distant view of the image, held later by the host Harry Reasoner in a medium over-the-shoulder shot as he interviewed one of Dugas's former lovers, one is able to see that this was not its original composition but rather a cropped view, a reduction possibly imposed by producers wary of broadcasting standards and not wanting to engage with complaints about the depiction of Dugas's groin, clad in what appears to be a bodybuilder's posing pouch. It seems likely that the original image was a 5-by-7-inch photograph, probably belonging to one of Dugas's former lovers, a memento sent by the flight attendant while he was out of town. In this sense, Dugas was like many other gay men of the period who sent letters and postcards with enclosed photographs of themselves to distant friends and lovers.[87]

The image was wrenched from this originally private realm, one which acknowledged the physical, sexual relationship connecting two men, and thrust into an overwhelmingly public and disembodied setting—broadcast to millions of North American viewers in their homes. This dislocation is amplified by the cropping the photograph underwent, first by the producers of *60 Minutes* and then in its subsequent incarnations. An even smaller version was printed in *People* magazine. Its appearance now approached that of a standard head-and-shoulders shot, although due to differences of shading and the original angle of the photograph, Dugas's neckless head rather looks as if it has been removed from another body and glued onto a new set of shoulders. The photog-

87. Where they have survived, the correspondence and enclosed photographs in numerous LGBT archives attest to this fact.

rapher's identity was permanently erased, with the caption for the image reattributing the credit: "Photograph by CBS News, 60 Minutes."

People magazine's international circulation facilitated the wide diffusion of this photograph—literally presenting Dugas as "the Face of AIDS," a popular theme in news feature reporting throughout 1987. The owner of one particular copy apparently thought that Dugas personified the group that was responsible for the epidemic. Such was the force of his or her conviction that this person photocopied the magazine page, annotated it, and mailed this palimpsest to the San Francisco AIDS Foundation, in whose archived records it now rests (see fig. 4.5).[88] One can scarcely think of a more different motive for this mailing than the one that may have brought the picture from Dugas to a lover. The original article presents Dugas as a "missing link" to researchers, when in 1987 it was clear that the "links" he represented in the early cluster study were deeply problematic, given the current knowledge of HIV incubation periods. The article likely suggested other "links" to the person mailing the photo, too, given the immediate historical context. In the past year, Lyndon LaRouche had spearheaded a restrictive initiative in California to test and track down PWAs; just weeks before, on October 14, Senator Jesse Helms was fighting in Congress to remove funding from gay-run AIDS prevention services and declared, "Every AIDS case can be traced back to a homosexual act." [89] In this context, the reader who annotated and mailed the image was able to view Dugas/"Patient Zero" as the ultimate embodiment of guilt and the cause of the epidemic. In some instances, then, by delivering to conservatives an exaggerated model of gay male sexuality, *And the Band Played On* and the publicity surrounding it managed to fan the flames of a movement Shilts and Denneny were hoping to counter.

Of the image's many subsequent apparitions, some more public than others, three in particular are worth mentioning. The first, retitled "Proud Lives," appeared in a gay magazine in Vancouver, in an article showing solidarity for fallen community members (fig. 4.6). In contrast

88. San Francisco AIDS Foundation (SFAF) Records, MSS 94–60, carton 2, folder: "Assorted Bizarrities" [mail received] (2 of 2 folders) 1985–91, Archives and Special Collections, UCSF Library and Center for Knowledge Management, University of California–San Francisco (hereafter cited as SFAF Records).

89. For more on the 1987 Helms amendment, see Crimp, "Promiscuity in an Epidemic," 256–66.

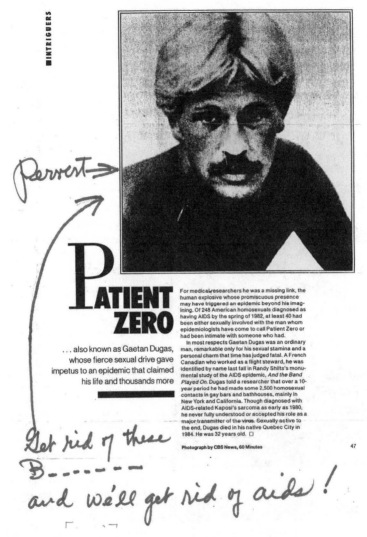

Perverts ⇒

P

ATIENT
ZERO

... also known as Gaetan Dugas,
whose fierce sexual drive gave
impetus to an epidemic that claimed
his life and thousands more

For medical researchers he was a missing link, the
human explosive whose promiscuous presence
may have triggered an epidemic beyond his imagining. Of 248 American homosexuals diagnosed as
having AIDS by the spring of 1982, at least 40 had
been either sexually involved with the man whom
epidemiologists have come to call Patient Zero or
had been intimate with someone who had.
   In most respects Gaetan Dugas was an ordinary
man, remarkable only for his sexual stamina and a
personal charm that time has judged fatal. A French
Canadian who worked as a flight steward, he was
identified by name last fall in Randy Shilts's monumental study of the AIDS epidemic, *And the Band
Played On.* Dugas told a researcher that over a 10-
year period he had made some 2,500 homosexual
contacts in gay bars and bathhouses, mainly in
New York and California. Though diagnosed with
AIDS-related Kaposi's sarcoma as early as 1980,
he never fully understood or accepted his role as a
major transmitter of the virus. Sexually active to
the end, Dugas died in his native Quebec City in
1984. He was 32 years old. □

Photograph by CBS News, 60 Minutes   47

Get rid of these
B------
and we'll get rid of aids!
┌ . ╮

FIGURE 4.5 A palimpsest of hostile views in the archives, ca. 1988. Annotated photocopy of "Patient Zero" page from *People* magazine (December 28, 1987, 47), 21.6 × 35.5 cm (photograph 13.9 × 15.2 cm, excluding frame), annotation in red pen, mailed to the San Francisco AIDS Foundation soon after publication. Courtesy of Archives and Special Collections, Library and Center for Knowledge Management, University of California, San Francisco. Curiously, the anonymous author, one of *People* magazine's 24.5 million readers (according to Donald M. Elliman Jr., "Publisher's Letter," *People*, December 28, 1987), restrains him- or herself from spelling out the apparently intended word *Bastards* in full, despite the general tone of the message and the word *Pervert* being on full display. For the writer of the message, it seems clear that Dugas had become the "face of AIDS."

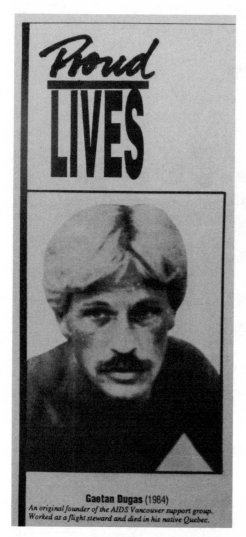

FIGURE 4.6 "*Proud* Lives—Gaetan Dugas (1984)," *Q Magazine,* May 1988, 14; framed photograph measures 6.2 × 8.6 cm. Courtesy of the British Columbia Gay and Lesbian Archives. In the wake of the publicity for *And the Band Played On*, a periodical serving the lesbian and gay community in Vancouver—Dugas's penultimate place of residence before his death in 1984—reappropriated the widely distributed photograph from *60 Minutes* and *People* magazine. Here, noting that he was "an original founder of the AIDS Vancouver support group," the magazine's editor, Rob Joyce, countered the media's depiction of Dugas as a sociopath and included his image in a group photo tribute, alongside those of other local men who had died of AIDS.

to the *People* magazine piece, which focused on Dugas's "fierce sexual drive [which] gave impetus to an epidemic," this defiant entry attempts to reclaim Dugas's reputation, offering him instead as one of the founders of AIDS Vancouver's support group. The second, a rather audacious and self-congratulatory half-page advertisement by *California Magazine* in the *New York Times*, praised its scoop of running the "Patient

Zero" story as an article before any other publication—this, as we have seen, had been one of the earliest sales for any part of Shilts's book. In this version, we see that Dugas's head *has* been removed from its original shoulders and pasted onto a body dressed in a suit and tie to give the semblance of a flight attendant's identity badge, complete with a forged signature and the almost comically ironic phrase (given the frequent recycling of this particular image), "not transferable." If anything, this advertisement only served to amplify the impression that Dugas had single-handedly launched the American AIDS epidemic, which raised the ire of some AIDS activists. Protesters from a San Francisco chapter of ACT UP reproduced the advertisement in a call to action for their members (fig. 4.7). In each of these occurrences, one sees an image that has been seized by certain groups and deployed according to their particular agendas. In each, Dugas's status as a patient and his role as a sick person in a new epidemic was contested, his image used to give force and to personalize each party's claims. As picture and story traveled across the continent and overseas, reaching new publics, they took on new meanings and significance.

While the CDC's cluster study had, in 1982, offered compelling evidence for some readers that AIDS was caused by a sexually transmissible agent, the 1987 "Patient Zero" story provided in its turn a seductive explanation to make sense of the early hidden spread of the epidemic. The fact that an early case subject had been a sexually active flight attendant could explain how AIDS had spread across the country, while the man's resistance to public health officials confirmed age-old apprehensions about the role that willful disease spreading played in an epidemic. Abraham Verghese, an AIDS physician who wrote sensitively of his experiences in a southern American town treating patients afflicted by the disorder, was among those who used the story to map a mental image of sexual connection and viral transmission, one which linked his more remote community to the early urban epicenters of AIDS. "I couldn't help reflecting," Verghese wrote, thinking of the partner of one of his patients who had lived in San Francisco, "that Otis had been in the Castro—1978 to 1985—at the height of the silent spread of the virus through the gay community there. Otis had probably celebrated Gay Pride Week, been on the same dance floor with Gaetan Dugas—*Patient Zero.*" With italic font suggesting a nervous shiver, the doctor ventured an unfinished thought: "It was not beyond the realm of the possible to

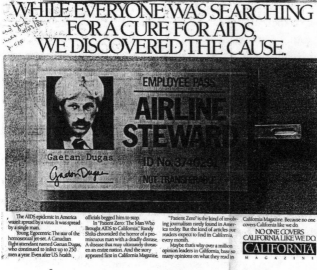

FIGURE 4.7 ACT-UP San Francisco protests *California Magazine*'s claim that it "discovered the cause" of "the AIDS epidemic in America," 1988; photocopied advertisement with typed activist message; 43.9 × 29.7 cm. Courtesy of the Gay, Lesbian, Bisexual, Transgender Historical Society. The original advertisement appeared in the *New York Times* in August 1988 to promote *California Magazine*'s "involving journalism." Declaring that Dugas was "the cause" of AIDS, the advertisement breathlessly notes that he "continued to infect up to 250 men a year. Even after U.S. health officials begged him to stop." Responding to these damaging claims, the San Francisco chapter of ACT UP distributed this photocopied leaflet, urging protesters to demand that the magazine "STOP THE SPREAD OF FEAR AND IGNORANCE!!" Drawing on transnational networks, these AIDS activists are most likely referring to critiques of *And the Band Played On* published by the British journalist Duncan Campbell in the *New Statesman* and *Capital Gay* in March 1988. Campbell interviewed William Darrow, the CDC researcher, who explained that the hypothesis of a short incubation period for HIV infection could no longer be maintained. Darrow told Campbell that he had urged Shilts not to use the names of AIDS patients nor to place reliance on the cluster study's original hypotheses. Tim Kingston, a San Francisco reporter and activist, relayed Campbell's findings to gay San Francisco readers the following month in *Coming Up!* magazine.

imagine that Otis had slept with the Air Canada flight steward, or slept with someone who had slept with Gaetan, or . . ."[90] Other readers, by contrast, focused on Dugas's apparently willful transmission of his infection. Jim Kepner was a gay rights pioneer who had been active in the

90. Abraham Verghese, *My Own Country: A Doctor's Story* (New York: Vintage Books, 1994), 286–87.

Mattachine Society and lived in Los Angeles. In a personal chronology of the AIDS epidemic, he decided that although Dugas was "afflicted with KS in June 80, he did *not* plant the first seeds of AIDS in the U.S." Nonetheless, Kepner continued, "he typified many who felt their sexual freedom must not be limited, & felt that if they'd gotten it, they should pass it on."[91]

And the Band Played On and the media attention accompanying its release drew the ire of people with AIDS and members and allies of lesbian and gay communities. One PWA wrote to *Coming Up!* and the *Bay Area Reporter*, two San Francisco-based gay periodicals, shortly before his death to complain about the repercussions the book had for people living with the disease: "As a PWA (person with AIDS), I myself am infuriated by this book. It makes gay people look like rabid infected disease carriers who can't wait to give AIDS to someone else. [Shilts] himself has admitted that perhaps he got a little carried away with Patient Zero. I encourage everyone in the Gay community to steal this book and burn it."[92] Another San Francisco PWA activist, Dan Turner, would deplore the fact that Shilts was making money from victim blaming: "As a person who has been living with AIDS longer than Mr. Shilts has been writing about it, I found his pot-boiler shots reprehensible. He does not speak for me."[93] Lon Nungesser, a social psychologist with KS whose work had also been published by St. Martin's Press, railed against Shilts as "the most dangerous anti-gay voice in America" and questioned the motives and ethics of his publisher.[94]

A woman, from Orillia, Ontario, wrote to the *Toronto Sun* to complain that the newspaper's recent publication of the "Patient Zero" feature had "undone much of what your more responsible journalists have tried to accomplish in educating your readers about AIDS and the gay

91. Emphasis in original; see "The AIDS Record: A Chronological Account," unpublished typescript, February 1, 1993, s.v. March 30, 1984, Jim Kepner Collection, ONE National Gay and Lesbian Archives at the USC [University of Southern California] Libraries, Los Angeles.

92. Jerry A. Lazier, "Gay Aunt Mary," *Coming Up!* February 1988, 3; Jerry A. Lazier, "Aunt Mary Shilts," *Bay Area Reporter* [San Francisco], January 14, 1988, 8.

93. Dan Turner, letter to the editor, *San Francisco Chronicle*, August 16, 1988, folder: D. Turner Corresp., box 2, Dan Turner Papers, 1990–10, Gay, Lesbian, Bisexual, Transgender Historical Society, San Francisco; *Shilts* written as "Schilts" in original. Turner evidently did not appreciate how Shilts had used his interview; see chapter 3.

94. Lon G. Nungesser, letter to the editor, *Coming Up!* May 1988, 2–3.

community in general." It was bad enough, she asserted, to print the excerpt in full, but "to include the author's declaration that Gaetan Dugas was 'what every man wanted from gay life' is abominable." Dugas was, in her opinion, "criminally irresponsible, as well as perhaps psychotically promiscuous and immature, just the opposite of the overwhelming majority of gay men." To print the segment was, she opined, akin to suggesting "that all heterosexual men seriously want to be murderous Casanovas, homicidal little boys unable to make a real and loving commitment to a long-term partner."[95]

Others agreed with this letter writer's perspective. "Has the AIDS crisis become just another soap opera?" asked one woman writing to the *Seattle Times*, following its printing of the "Patient Zero" feature, which she was disappointed to see had been published without any kind of editorial contextualization. She wrote that she would hate for Dugas's "social irresponsibility," as it was portrayed, to be seen as "indicative of any kind of universal attitude in the gay community. To put it bluntly, gay people are not subversive, immoral and perverted heathens."[96] Stan Persky, a gay Vancouver writer, drew criticism within the alternative press for uncritically repeating Shilts's tale of "Patient Zero" in a magazine article. He used the flight attendant's "reckless sexual conduct" as an introductory example to frame the British Columbia provincial government's controversial 1987 legislative efforts to implement forcible isolation for anyone with an infectious disease deemed likely to expose others.[97] If, as one later critic asked, Gaétan Dugas's example was not representative of gay men as a whole, as Persky had gone on to suggest, then why include it in such a prominent way? The answer, some observers believed, was that any drive to severely restrict the rights of people with AIDS rested on the assumption that some dangerous "carriers" would attempt to infect others.[98] Dramatic examples like the one Shilts had crafted were vital for that project.

In 1989, a *Vancouver Sun* columnist wrote a petulant piece following the death of Kevin Brown, a former acquaintance of Dugas who went on

95. Karen Moore, "Patient Zero Excerpt Showed Bad Judgment," *Toronto Star*, December 29, 1987, A16, ProQuest (435693482).

96. Nora Stern, "'The Band Played On'—Story of First AIDS Victim Was Overly Sensational," *Seattle Times*, November 12, 1987, A19, NewsBank (469938).

97. Stan Persky, "AIDS and the State," *This Magazine* 22, no. 1, March/April (1988): 10–14.

98. Emke, "Speaking of AIDS in Canada," 486–87.

to become an AIDS activist known across North America. In it, he criticized Brown's refusal "to condemn the [homosexual] practices that pass on the HIV virus that leads to AIDS" and also mentioned Dugas as an exemplar of these practices.[99] The columnist's writing provoked an angry letter from a gay reader, who demanded that the journalist apologize for his "smear [of] Kevin Brown just days after his funeral." What the reader found most despicable was the journalist's suggestion that "there were any similarities between Kevin's refusal to condemn the sexual practices of gay men, and Gaetan Dugas who admitted that he was out to infect as many men as possible in vengeance for his own diagnosis. Mr. Lautens makes mention of both of these men as though they were fighting a common cause."[100]

There were thus many people, inside and outside North America's lesbian and gay communities, who accepted the depiction of Dugas in Shilts's book and the wider media coverage and who saw the dead flight attendant's actions as beyond the pale, completely unrepresentative of the behavior of gay men in general. Others, including Jim Kepner, were more mixed in their views, rejecting the notion that Dugas had introduced the virus to North America but seeing him as representative of a widely shared view that rejected any limits to sexual liberation.

"Not Just a Hypothetical Case"

And the Band Played On was published in a year that proved to be pivotal in the emergence of a discourse advocating for the use of criminal law to address HIV transmission. A front-page *New York Times* article from June 1987 noted a number of recent cases, particularly in the military, where individuals stood accused of willfully exposing other persons to the virus. The article emphasized that although several of these cases related to instances of spitting or biting—modes which had not been demonstrated to pose a risk for transmission—these examples still contributed to an effort to rework the public-health statutes in some states, to the opposition of many public health officials and gay rights

99. Trevor Lautens, "As I Like It," *Vancouver Sun*, June 7, 1989, A11, ProQuest (243565235); Kahn, *AIDS, The Winter War*, 77–79.

100. Michael Kalmuk, "An Apology Owed to Brown Family," *Vancouver Sun*, June 22, 1989, A18, ProQuest (243552753).

activists. They feared that politicians had "seized on a handful of peculiar and frivolous cases" to justify action that would lead to a negative effect on public health: it could make those most at risk for HIV infection reluctant to get tested.[101] Attention to this issue continued throughout the summer of 1987, with *Time* magazine and the *Los Angeles Times*, among others, featuring articles and polls on the topic.[102] In a syndicated newspaper column, a professor of public policy noted the sharp contrast with the previous year, which had been, he thought, guided by robust scientific research. In 1987, however, "the Year of the AIDS Politician," "sideshow" efforts intent on scapegoating led to calls for widespread mandatory testing, quarantine of people with HIV, and "new criminal penalties for that almost-mythical character, the deliberate spreader of disease."[103]

These developments played into the Reagan administration's slow-to-develop and socially conservative response to the epidemic. The most important factor shaping the Republican administration's response to AIDS was the lead role taken by members of the Department of Education. The department's secretary, William Bennett, and the under secretary, Gary Bauer, who was also Reagan's advisor on domestic policy issues, developed a response in keeping with the religious support base of the New Right. Their approach took every opportunity to reinforce the supremacy of heterosexual marriage and traditional gender roles.[104] To the notion of the "innocent victim" of AIDS—the HIV-infected blood transfusion recipient, for example—Bennett and Bauer set up a rhetorical counterpoint, the deserving person with AIDS. This idea was articulated in the writing of John Klenk, one of Bauer's former aides: "The most common cause of the spread of AIDS is irresponsible sexual behavior. Anyone who engages in such behavior endangers him (her) self, his (her) partner, his (her) children, and other innocent victims—not to

101. Boorstin, "Criminal and Civil Litigation," A1.

102. Richard Lacayo, "Assault with a Deadly Virus," *Time*, July 20, 1987, 57; Robert Steinbrook, "The *Times* Poll: 42% Would Limit Civil Rights in AIDS Battle," *Los Angeles Times*, July 31, 1987, B1.

103. David L. Kirp, "Politics Is Latest AIDS Sideshow," *Lodi* [CA] *News-Sentinel*, July 9, 1987, 4; https://news.google.com/newspapers?id=BLM0AAAAIBAJ&sjid=YiEGAAAAIB AJ&dq=aids%20kirp&pg=3276%2C926014.

104. Brier, *Infectious Ideas*, 87.

speak of causing enormous medical costs to taxpayers and the public. Society must show its disapproval for such behavior."[105]

It appears that part of Klenk's remit was to assemble documented cases of alleged deliberate transmission. In June 1987, he sent a note to Bauer that listed a compendium of "thirteen 'horror stories'—cases of malicious or irresponsible behavior threatening the spread of AIDS." These included "an Army private who knew he was infected yet had unprotected sex with three soldiers (both sexes), one of them his fiancee"; "a man with full-blown AIDS" who had raped a South Carolina woman; a young bisexual man in San Diego who "boasted he'd infect as many coeds as he could"; several men who had bitten police officers; a "parolee who announced he intended to infect as many prostitutes as possible, 'just to get even'"; and a "civil rights activist who threatened 'blood terrorism' if enough money wasn't provided for AIDS research."[106] Bauer's files grew with other examples, such as of prostitutes returning to work after a diagnosis, and with references to sworn testimony that apparently demonstrated that individuals were transmitting their infection with knowledge and intention. According to one California physician who raised controversy by calling for the quarantine of HIV-infected people, "there exists a population of persons who have been infected and have the misguided opinion that the only means by which this disease will be cured is if it becomes so widespread that the government has to cure it. Their goal," he argued, "is to continue spreading it as fast as individually possible to reach that end."[107]

Also among Gary Bauer's archived files is a copy of the October 1987 cover story of *California* magazine: the serialized "Patient Zero" story sold by St. Martin's Press as part of the book's wildly successful promotional campaign.[108] The timing ensured that the figure of the deliberate, malicious AIDS spreader, which had been forming in a somewhat incho-

105. Quoted in ibid., 92. See also Grover, "AIDS: Keywords," 28–30.

106. John Klenk to Gary Bauer, with attachment, June 10, 1987, folder: AIDS VII (4 of 5), box OA 19222, Gary Bauer Files, Ronald Reagan Presidential Library, Simi Valley, CA (hereafter cited as Bauer Files). It is worth noting that Theresa Crenshaw, a San Diego physician, was the source for the stories about the young man from San Diego and one instance of a man who bit a police officer. She would soon take up a position as a commissioner on the presidential commission investigating the HIV epidemic.

107. William T. O'Connor, "AIDS: The Alarming Reality," report, June 7, 1987, 21, folder: AIDS (2 of 3), box OA 19222, Bauer Files.

108. "Patient Zero: The Man Who Brought AIDS to California," photocopy of Octo-

ate manner earlier in 1987 and which built on previously existing fears of people with AIDS, took root in the public imagination. Perhaps more significantly, this figure now had a name and, following the *60 Minutes* television news special seen by millions of viewers in November 1987, a nationally broadcast face. It became possible to refer to Dugas's example as shorthand for the type of criminally irresponsible person from whom the public needed protection. In addition, this historical case gave lawyers a powerful example of a malicious disease spreader that allowed them to circumvent the difficulties that they would have faced in terms of establishing malice and an intent to infect for a similar case in a court of law.

During the fall of 1987 and in early 1988, both the presidential commission in the United States and the Royal Society in Canada were devising guidelines to deal with the ethical and legal challenges posed by AIDS, in the absence of national-level response frameworks in each country. The background papers to the Canadian Royal Society's report noted, "We have heard anecdotal evidence of a small minority of those infected with HIV who feel doomed and, not caring about the risks to other [*sic*], are concerned primarily with their own pleasure." The authors went on to emphasize, however, that the largest risk of HIV transmission came from voluntary behavior between adults who knew how HIV was transmitted.[109]

In the United States, Dugas's example was adopted in legal texts with remarkable speed. By November 1987, the same month that the book went into wide release, advocates of tough penalties for HIV transmission were mobilizing the "Patient Zero" story. The *State Factor*, a conservative legal publication put out by the American Legislative Exchange Council lobby group, featured Dugas's interaction with Selma Dritz, the San Francisco public health official, in its December issue. The article argued that criminal laws were needed to deal with this "small minority of AIDS victims" who "either are intent on infecting others—or simply do not care enough to change their sexual practices."[110]

---

ber 1987 *California Magazine* cover and article, folder: AIDS VII (2 of 5), box OA 19222, Bauer Files.

109. Martha Mackinnon, Keel Cottrelle, and Horace Krever, "Legal and Social Aspects of AIDS in Canada," *AIDS: A Perspective for Canadians: Background Papers*, ed. Royal Society of Canada (Ottawa: Royal Society of Canada, 1988), 354–55.

110. Douglas J. Besharov, "AIDS and the Criminal Law: Needed Reform," *State Factor* 13, no. 8 (1987): 1.

In this period, legal scholars arguing for tougher sanctions often used the "Patient Zero" story to strengthen their case. In 1989, one author, an associate law professor at the Catholic University of America, cited Shilts's work repeatedly and focused on the journalist's description of Dugas. There was some doubt, the author admitted, following Shilts, about whether Dugas was the first person to bring HIV to the United States. "But there is no debate as to Gaetan's conduct right up to the moment of his death. He continued to have multiple and random sexual partners, living a code of conduct that held: 'It's my right to do what I want to do with my own body.'" The author continued that it was "this type of intentional and reckless activity" that led to the presidential commission's recommendation that states adopt criminal laws to regulate the reckless behavior of individuals.[111]

Even those who opposed the criminalization of HIV transmission felt it necessary to engage with Dugas's example. Two Harvard law professors, who in early 1988 argued against the implementation of criminal penalties, conceded:

The AIDS victim who deliberately exposes others in order to gain revenge, for example, is no less culpable than a person who deliberately injects a victim with a lethal poison in the hope of causing death. Nor is culpability doubtful in other instances that are likely to count as murder under the Model Penal Code: for example, the prostitute who knows he or she is contagious and nonetheless plies his or her trade without precautions, indifferent to the number of persons thus fatally infected, or the person who, knowing he has AIDS, rapes another and so eventually causes his or her death.[112]

In a footnote to document the existence of those attempting to spread the virus out of revenge, the authors noted, "The example of Gaetan Dugas . . . suggests this is not just a hypothetical case."[113]

111. Raymond C. O'Brien, "AIDS: Perspective on the American Family," *Villanova Law Review* 34 (1989): 256–57.

112. Kathleen M. Sullivan and Martha A. Field, "AIDS and the Coercive Power of the State," *Harvard Civil Rights–Civil Liberties Law Review* 23 (1988): 164.

113. Ibid. The authors also use "the now notorious 'Patient Zero,'" on p. 153, as an example of "the HIV-infected person who tells his doctors, despite their warnings, that he will not give up unprotected sexual intercourse." The authors had published an earlier version of this article before Shilts's book was released; see Sullivan and Field, "AIDS and the Criminal Law," *Law, Medicine and Health Care* 15 (1987): 46–60.

And the Band Played On and the "Patient Zero" story influenced the work of the Presidential Commission on the Human Immunodeficiency Virus Epidemic that President Reagan had assembled in the summer of 1987. The commission held its first hearings in September, just as the prerelease publicity for Shilts's book began to take hold in the national media, and continued its deliberations until June 1988. During the intervening time, the book became a nonfiction best seller. One legal scholar has intimated, albeit on scant evidence, that the temporal overlap of *Band*'s release and the commission's hearings demonstrates that the book had an impact on the commission's recommendations, which proved influential in legitimizing the subsequent use of criminalization as an appropriate response to the epidemic.[114] This assertion is valid, but it requires a more careful consideration of the evidence.

There were several instances where the story had the potential to influence the commission's work. First, commissioners were mindful of anecdotes that they heard outside of the documented hearings. For example, in their discussion of the legal implications of HIV transmission in April 1988, Admiral James Watkins, the commission's chair, emphasized the importance of "answering the question that's so often asked me after many of these hearings."[115] In this instance he was contemplating the need for mandatory HIV testing for rapists in criminal cases, providing recommendations that might do "a lot to allay public fears, even though those circumstances in which the HIV may be transmitted by that means may be small."[116] Thus, although it was apparently uncommon, the *possible* threat posed by a small group of individuals was emphasized and, unsurprisingly, the undocumented concerns of citizens from outside of the commission were imported into its deliberations.

Second, witness testimony and the commissioners' discussions reveal a sense of urgency in dealing with the possibility of dangerous disease spreaders. One witness before the commission, a prosecutor from Genesee County, Michigan, had attempted unsuccessfully to prosecute an individual with HIV for attempted murder for spitting at a police offi-

114. James B. McArthur, "As the Tide Turns: The Changing HIV/AIDS Epidemic and the Criminalization of HIV Exposure," *Cornell Law Review* 94 (2009): 712–14.

115. Transcript, "Hearing on Societal and Legal Issues," Presidential Commission on the Human Immunodeficiency Virus Epidemic, April 5 and 6, 1988, 136, NCAIDS Records.

116. Ibid., 137.

cer. This prosecutor urged the commission not to be deterred from making strong recommendations in favor of criminalizing the transmission of HIV, in spite of a perhaps inconvenient lack of evidence. "It should be stressed," he acknowledged, "that the percentage of AIDS carriers who will maliciously or irresponsibly place others at risk is largely speculative." Nonetheless, he continued immediately, "This fact should not deter us from developing a legislative framework to control such conduct."[117]

Most compellingly, the language used by one commissioner demonstrated the way in which the term *patient zero*, originally coined as an epidemiological term to denote the Los Angeles cluster study's nonresident case of KS, had evolved over only a few months of widespread public discussion to become synonymous with Shilts's portrayal of Dugas as a dangerous disease spreader. Theresa Crenshaw, a sex therapist and one of the commission's more socially conservative members, presented a justification for focusing on a small number of dangerous individuals. She had recently read that 5 percent of the "carriers," for sexually transmitted diseases other than AIDS, were responsible for 80 percent of the cases. This meant, she reasoned, "that a very sexually active small group has an enormous impact on our society." She continued, employing a telling choice of words, that "we're hearing such emphasis on the rarity of the patient zero or some of the individuals that you've alluded to, that have been prosecuted, whether they're rare or whether they're not rare we really must act promptly and effectively to prevent many others from becoming infected as a result of antisocial behavior."[118]

The commissioners were evidently concerned with the potential risk posed by individuals like Shilts's "Patient Zero." Their final report contained a separate section on criminalization in which the commission encouraged "continued state efforts to explore the use of the criminal law in the face of this epidemic."[119] Source material from the commission's support staff indicates that this section was based "almost verbatim" on Sullivan and Field's article.[120] Notably, however, the final report's

117. Testimony of Robert E. Weiss, Presidential Commission on the Human Immunodeficiency Virus Epidemic, April 6, 1988, 4, NCAIDS Records.

118. Transcript, "Hearing," 253, NCAIDS Records.

119. Presidential Commission on the Human Immunodeficiency Virus Epidemic, *Report of the Presidential Commission on the Human Immunodeficiency Virus Epidemic* (Washington, DC: US Government Printing Office, 1988), 130.

120. Barry Gaspard [staff assistant to Commissioner Frank Lilly] to Members of

criminalization section disregarded Sullivan and Field's conclusion that "any deterrence that criminal enactments might add to incentives that already exist is not worth the disadvantages of using the criminal law as a tool to contain the AIDS epidemic."[121] Though the final report cautioned that "the use of criminal sanctions should not substitute for use of public health measures to prevent transmission," it seems likely that its recommendations for increased use of criminal law and the powerful stories of deliberate disease spreading typified by the example of Dugas may have contributed to just this type of trend.[122] Between 1987 and 1989, twenty states enacted statutes that sought to criminalize the knowing transmission of HIV.[123]

In 1990, the US Congress passed the Ryan White Comprehensive AIDS Resources Emergency Act, which incorporated many of the presidential commission's recommendations, to direct relief to the areas of the country most affected by HIV. Among its many provisions, the act required that, as a condition of federal funding, states have in place "adequate" criminal laws to prosecute HIV-infected individuals who, knowing their infection status, intentionally exposed others to HIV without their consent.[124] By the end of the 1990s most states had in their statutes some form of legislation that addressed the deliberate transmission of HIV—an often feared though seldom demonstrated phenomenon. This controversial approach was subsequently transferred internationally to several western African countries, through the process of "model HIV law," where ready-made legal frameworks were exported abroad as part of US-funded development aid. This process has, in turn, been cited as an important factor in more recent efforts to further criminalize the transmission of HIV.[125] Thus, not far below the surface of current global

the AIDS Consortium, memo [June 1988], folder 4, box 390, Gay Men's Health Crisis (GMHC) Records, Manuscripts and Archives Division, New York Public Library, Astor, Lenox, and Tilden Foundations.

121. Sullivan and Field, "AIDS and Coercive Power," 196.

122. Presidential Commission, *Report*, 130.

123. Bayer, *Private Acts*, 254.

124. Ryan White CARE Act of 1990, Pub. L. No. 101–381, 104 Stat. 576 (1990), https://history.nih.gov/research/downloads/PL101-381.pdf; Raymond C. O'Brien, "A Legislative Initiative: The Ryan White Comprehensive AIDS Resource Emergency Act of 1990," *Journal of Contemporary Health Law and Policy* 7 (1991): 183–206. White was a young HIV-positive hemophiliac who rose to national prominence when he was subjected to intense discrimination at school based on fears surrounding his disease. He died in 1990.

125. Richard Pearhouse, "Legislation Contagion: The Spread of Problematic New HIV

HIV politics lurks the legacy of *And the Band Played On*'s depiction of Gaétan Dugas.

Resistance from North American Lesbian and Gay Communities

Resistance and suspicion were exhibited in several segments of the lesbian and gay communities across North America in response to the mainstream praise and media attention devoted to Shilts's book. In New York, Michael Denneny's business partner, Charles Ortleb, skewered the book in an editorial note in the *New York Native* for what he saw as its display of the author's "agenda of self-hate." He was scornful of the fact that when Shilts had arranged to interview him for the book, "he told me what role he wanted me to play in the book. I then told him what role I had played in reality, which he ignored, because he knows better." Ortleb had grown increasingly dismissive of the direct link between HIV and AIDS and suggested that instead of buying Shilts's book, readers should purchase two copies of a new book by Harris L. Coulter that explored the links between AIDS and syphilis. In a swipe at both Shilts and Denneny, Ortleb ended his editorial with the dig, "'Patient Zero' is the biggest crock since Hitler's diaries.'"[126]

The year 1987 saw the formation of ACT UP, signaling a resurgence of activist outrage at injustices for PWAs, not simply in terms of their access to treatment but also in terms of their representation in the media. Emerging first in New York, the organization quickly developed chap-

---

Laws in Africa" (paper presented at the Seventeenth International AIDS Conference, Mexico City, August 6, 2008); Lucy Stackpool-Moore, *Verdict on a Virus: Public Health, Human Rights and Criminal Law* (London: International Planned Parenthood Federation, 2008), 13, http://www.ippf.org/resource/Verdict-Virus-Public-health-human-rights -and-criminal-law.

126. Charles L. Ortleb, "Randy Shilts's Agenda," *NYN*, October 19, 1987. Ortleb would later lampoon *Band* in his and Denneny's other joint publication, *Christopher Street*, in an article entitled "Scientist Zero," a piece that criticized the work of the CDC scientist Donald Francis and advanced Ortleb's view that HIV did not cause AIDS. "Millions of people," the magazine's cover read ironically, "believe that HIV is the cause of AIDS. Thanks to Randy Shilts, that idea has been traced back first to a cluster group of scientists, and then to one single scientist who spread the idea from coast to coast. This is the story of Dr. Donald Francis: SCIENTIST ZERO." See Charles L. Ortleb, "Scientist Zero," *Christopher Street*, March 1989, cover.

ters across the country. As mentioned earlier in the chapter and shown
in figure 4.7 there, one of ACT-UP San Francisco's "zaps" involved its
organization of a protest against *California Magazine*, which in August 1988 ran a lurid advertisement, complete with a doctored version of
the *60 Minutes* Dugas photograph, promoting the "kind of investigative
journalism rarely found in America today." A flyer urged members to
contact *California Magazine* and "tell them what you think about their
'kind of involving journalism.'"[127] The flyer noted that the theory "was
dismissed in May by the same doctor who began it. Was there a story in
California Magazine about that?" Word had begun to spread in activist circles about Bill Darrow's alleged repudiation of the cluster study,
which British activists had reported in the gay press in April 1988, in
London.[128]

Jon-Henri Damski, a prominent gay journalist and activist from Chicago, was particularly condemnatory of an article combining an interview with Shilts and a description of the "Patient Zero" story, which
appeared on the Chicago *Sun-Times*'s front page on October 11, 1987.
He found the title, "Victim Zero," which the *Sun-Times* journalist had
coined, to be particularly galling, given years of efforts by those living
with AIDS not to be labeled "victims." Damski deemed it "a total disaster" that while one of the largest gay and lesbian protest marches in history was taking place that weekend in Washington, DC, news of it was
eclipsed by the mass-marketed "Patient Zero" story. "On the very Sunday we were making history in Washington," he wrote bitterly, "the Chicago *Sun-Times*' front-page lead story headlined 'Victim Zero,' made
myth of us and people with AIDS." This statement is suggestive of the
silences generated by the unequal access to the means of cultural and
historical production or, in this case, to contributing content to mass-
circulating newspapers. "It was a book review that wasn't a book review," Damski continued. "It was an opinion piece that wasn't an opinion piece; it was soft news, almost porn, placed where a reader expects
hard news and real fact. It was urban myth replacing journalism." With
a faith in scientific order that, in retrospect, appears optimistic, Dam-

---

127. Shown earlier in the chapter in fig 4.7; ACT-UP San Francisco, "Stop the spread
of fear and ignorance!" photocopied flyer, circa August 1988, folder: AIDS-Related, box:
Legal Size Ephemera, AIDS Ephemera Collection, Gay, Lesbian, Bisexual, Transgender
Historical Society, San Francisco.
128. Crimp, "Miserable Failure," 120–27.

ski believed that "if science knew the first person who had AIDS, they would have called that person Number 1, Patient 1. He or she would have a definite number and place in scientific history. The 'Victim Zero' story is pure urban myth." The reporter also considered the racial consequences of such a numbering system, noting that the flight attendant had, according to the report, acquired HIV from an African in France: "That makes Africans and blacks less than zero."[129]

Theresa Dobko, a counselor working for the AIDS Committee of Toronto from 1984 onward, echoed this perspective in an interview in 2008. She recalled having to address the issues raised by the "Patient Zero" story in the education sessions she gave to various groups:

> So I remember it coming up and I remember that then our work became very difficult because we were trying to balance people's homophobia in saying, "No, this is *not* a gay disease, and no, it's not spread by people who are intentionally trying to infect other people." And then we've got all this cluster research where they're trying to *find the one source of entry* for this, which made me quite insane, because I knew it wasn't going to end up being one person, this was far too complex. So I was very frustrated at this sort of attempt to pin down to the very first person who brought it into North America. I found it also really racist, to be honest, too, because why are you focusing so much on one person who brought it from one country to another, as if that's somehow more meaningful than all the people in Africa who may have had it before the white man who brought it over?[130]

Bernard Courte (who would later join the Toronto-based AIDS Action Now!) wrote to French- and English-language news media to protest against the story. He emphasized in a letter to the mainstream *Maclean's* magazine that Shilts had distorted the chronology of Dugas's case and that at that time, "no one knew exactly what caused the then so-called 'gay cancer.'" He continued, "Furthermore, even if he is connected to nine of the first 19 AIDS patients in Los Angeles, how can that make him 'Patient Zero'? What about the other 10 cases? In the

129. Jon-Henri Damski, "The Victim Zero Story," *Windy City Times*, October 22, 1987, 12. A copy of this story appears in Shilts's files, stapled to Damski's business card; folder 8: Clippings "Scrapbook," 1987, September–October, box 1, Shilts Papers.

130. Theresa Dobko, interview with author, Toronto, September 15, 2008, recording C1491/49, tape 1, side A, BLSA; emphasis on recording.

same line as some Japanese who blame AIDS on Filipino prostitutes, or North Americans who try to pin it on Haitians or Central Africans, it seems that Shilts wants a foreigner as scapegoat for the 42,000 U.S. AIDS cases."[131] In a similar letter he sent to the French Canadian gay magazine *Sortie*, published under the heading "A Scapegoat," Courte faulted Shilts's speculative construction of the flight attendant's behavior. He asked why "would Dugas not also have frequented the baths in Montreal and Quebec City? Does this mean that he was anglophobic (wanting to kill the Anglos)? Or francophobic (not wanting to have relations with his French-speaking brothers)?" Any hypothesis was possible, he explained, yet remained strictly in the realm of the hypothetical.[132] When *La Presse*, Montreal's respectable broadsheet newspaper, published a front-page article on the story, a Montreal man wrote a letter to its editor, which he copied to *Sortie*. He likened this "latest media scoop" to the tale of Adam and Eve and condemned the media for having spread an "ignoble, anti-scientific, and profoundly ridiculous" story. He concluded, "I congratulate the journalists who knew to keep silent in the face of this foolishness, and I wish all the necessary courage to the family of 'this Montrealer' (his identity was reported!) to confront the author of this ignominy."[133]

The mainstream media coverage dismayed Bob Tivey, the former representative of AIDS Vancouver and friend of Dugas whom Shilts had interviewed during his Vancouver visit in 1986. He told a reporter from *Q Magazine*, a Vancouver-based gay periodical, that Shilts had lied to him about not using the flight attendant's name in his book. "I don't want to let him get away with this," he stated, seeing the journalist as having exploited the information he gathered to create a sensationalized story to sell *Band*. "I feel he is sort of cashing in, and as a gay man I resent that." Given the success of recent campaigns to raise gay men's

131. Bernard Courte, "The Spread of AIDS," *Maclean's*, November 30, 1987, 6.

132. B[ernard] Courte, "Un bouc émissaire," *Sortie*, February 1988, 7; my translation of "pourquoi Dugas n'aurait-il pas aussi fréquenté les bains sauna de Montréal et Québec? Aurait-il été anglophobe (voulant tuer les Anglais)? Ou francophobe (ne voulant pas baiser avec ses concitoyens francophones)?"

133. André L. Roy, "Un montréalais contamine les USA!' *Sortie* [Montreal], November 1987, 6; my translation of "dernier scoop des medias," "elle est ignoble, anti-scientifique et profondément ridicule," and "Je félicite les journalists qui ont su garder le silence face à la bêtise, et je souhaite le courage nécessaire à la famille de 'ce montréalais' (son identité fût rapportée!) afin de poursuivre l'auteur de cette ignominie."

awareness of risk factors for AIDS, Tivey highlighted how different the situation was from just a few years previously. He urged others not to "look back and judge somebody's actions, because if Gaetan were here today he would certainly be behaving a lot differently too." He also lamented the "wasted energy" of attempting to identify who was "responsible for AIDS"; as he explained, "There are too many other things that need to be done to stop this epidemic."[134]

To counterbalance Shilts's actions, Tivey took advantage of another form of naming as a form of protesting Dugas's having been singled out as separate from his gay brothers. First in Toronto and then later in Vancouver, gay activists organized AIDS memorials as a means of honoring the dead. The Toronto memorial grew out of the profound impact the AIDS Quilt and the Vietnam Memorial had made on Toronto activist Michael Lynch when he took part in the March on Washington in October 1987. In June 1988, Lynch coordinated the first incarnation of the Toronto AIDS Memorial, which appeared as a temporary display during the city's Pride festivities.[135] Tivey submitted Dugas's name for inclusion for the memorial in Toronto.[136] This would have been in the first collection of names, since an early promotional brochure for the memorial, requesting additions for 1989, lists Dugas's name alongside nearly three hundred others from the memorial's first display.[137] Eventually, the names would be ordered by year of death, accompanied by a year of birth, when known, and engraved on metal plaques mounted to a semicircular row of concrete pillars in Cawtha Square Park. Each plaque could hold about twenty-five names; with one death each recorded for 1981 and 1982, these years shared one plaque. For 1983 there were twelve deaths recorded on one plaque, and Dugas's name was one of eighteen to be listed on a separate metal sheet for 1984. This would also be the final year of the era before highly active antiretroviral therapy that twelve months of deaths would fit on a single plaque.[138]

134. Ross, "Media Finds Easy Target," 5.

135. Michael Lynch, "The Power of Names," *Xtra!* [Toronto], February 26, 1988; Silversides, *AIDS Activist*, 161.

136. Robert (Bob) Tivey, interview with author, Toronto, September 9, 2008, recording C1491/44, tape 2, side A, BLSA.

137. "The AIDS Memorial: A Celebration of Life," folded leaflet, ca. 1988, folder: AIDS Memorial Committee (Toronto), Vertical Files: Canada, Canadian Lesbian and Gay Archives, Toronto.

138. I base my count on a visit to the memorial on August 30, 2008. It is possible that

Tivey would do the same for the Vancouver memorial in the late 1990s, a project whose organizers included one of his former boyfriends. This memorial would eventually assemble nearly one thousand names in random order on several gently curving red steel sheets, located a few hundred meters from where Dugas lived in 1983, overlooking the beach at English Bay in Vancouver. Reflecting on the act of remembering and the memorials' significance in 2008, Tivey explained their importance to him:

> As we move along and things change and time goes by, there's not a lot of things to remind us, and that's why we need to have one place to go. Which I did when I was out in Vancouver recently. I just sat there, on one of those stones in front of the Memorial, and read a couple of plaques, and then had to stop and then read some more. I pick out all the people that I knew, but it is very important. It's not to live there all the time, but the need to go back and to remember, and, I don't want those people to ever be forgotten. [*Pause*] Even though I know *eventually* [*chuckling*], as we all leave this earth, things will change but we have to do as much as we can, I think, to keep their spirits alive and their names alive.[139]

Thus, among their many other commemorative functions, these two Canadian AIDS memorials served as a symbolic yet durably physical means for Tivey and other individuals to mark their silent protest of the scapegoating of Gaétan Dugas, which occurred during 1987 and 1988.[140] Bringing in the scapegoat from the desert, washing the communal sins from his head, and resolutely giving him a place of remembrance, sur-

---

more names have been added since then. To accommodate the large increase in deaths later in the epidemic, the plaques for the years from 1993 onward use a smaller font, which allows up to eighty names to be included on each plaque.

139. Tivey, September 9, 2008, recording C1491/44, tape 2, side A; emphasis on record-ing. Tivey died in March 2011.

140. More information on these two memorials can be found online at http://www.aidsmemorial.info. Archived captures of a defunct website for the Vancouver AIDS memorial can be viewed at http://web.archive.org/web/20070818223015/http://www.aidsmemorial.ca/Home/Home-1.htm. Readers are also invited to visit the websites of the NAMES Project AIDS Memorial Quilt (http://www.aidsquilt.org) and the Canadian AIDS Memorial Quilt (http://www.quilt.ca) to view quilt panels submitted to commemo-rate Gaétan Dugas.

rounded by the names of fellow community members—these actions speak to a quiet, reflective, yet powerful rejection of the centuries-old practice of exclusion which often accompanies times of crisis.

* * *

The idea of "Patient Zero" was marketed around North America over a short and sustained period in the fall of 1987 and winter and spring of 1988. The choice of this story was a deliberate attempt by Shilts's publisher to take advantage of the media's propensity for exaggeration in order to promote *And the Band Played On*, and in that sense the "yellow journalism" strategy was successful. The book became a best seller, providing a detailed and passionately written account of the first years of the American epidemic and raising awareness about AIDS. Less successful, though, were efforts to downplay the significance of the flight attendant's role after the publicity had begun. Shilts learned this to his continued frustration as he struggled to reorient discussions toward his critique of the Reagan administration. Throughout this process, Dugas's name and image were widely circulated, adapted, and reappropriated by groups and individuals around the continent for various purposes.

As soon as *Band* was released, the idea of "Patient Zero" was mobilized by social conservatives who saw in it a powerful image of an irresponsible PWA, a rhetorical figure for whom they had been searching for some time. When Shilts provided them with Dugas, the flight attendant and his alleged sociopathic behavior were used to argue for the need of stronger criminal punishments for the sexual transmission of HIV. This mobilization was nonetheless contested on several fronts, albeit with limited success. Compared to the resources, connections, and coordinated strategy of St. Martin's Press, as well as those marshaled by the political forces that adopted the "Patient Zero" idea, Dugas's family and members of North American lesbian and gay communities had diminished access to the means of cultural production. Nonetheless, they attempted, through a range of strategies, to dispute the dominant depiction of Dugas as "Patient Zero." These attempts would continue into the 1990s, as the next chapter will show.

This chapter closes with a final example of the traveling idea of "Patient Zero," to give a further sense of its ongoing, global peregrinations. On October 31, 1992, the president of the American Medical Association (AMA), the largest and most influential organization of American physicians, stood before an audience assembled for the Third Japan/US Health Care Symposium in Kobe, Japan, to deliver a speech about the global threat of HIV/AIDS. His oration offered an occasionally rambling mix of familiar statements intended to highlight the medical community's need to fight several battles: against HIV, against the fear of the disease, and against the costs that it presented to health-care systems globally. To explain to Japanese health-care workers how history had shaped the American experience, the AMA president plagiarized Shilts's history, embellishing where necessary. His comments emphasized the porousness of national boundaries, which permitted the easy flow of bodies, viruses, and scapegoats: "Many today believe the real story started with an international airline steward who came to be known as—Patient Zero. His story bears lessons for all nations—not the least because it shows the terrible damage just one infected person can inflict on others. Patient Zero was a familiar figure in homosexual communities on three continents. Highly mobile, crisscrossing the Atlantic. Collecting partners with abandon—he carried a deadly virus that was ticking away just like a time bomb."[141]

In case his audience was in doubt, the AMA president offered his moral assessment: "An innocent he was not. He eventually told health investigators that during the 1970s he'd had some 2,500 sexual contacts with men in Europe, Canada, South America—and in the large centers of gay lifestyle in New York and California. In the later years, he knew he had what he called the 'gay cancer.' And knew he was passing it on to others. Criminal? Demented? No one knows. But we do know he never changed his own behavior." He continued, repeating a by now familiar refrain: "The full extent of the damage caused by Patient Zero was never determined. He was lost to any CDC follow-up because he was Canadian and lived in Quebec City. He was only 31 years old when he died, but he'd already earned his own sad brand of medical immortality. Because he was such a lethal agent of infection, Patient Zero is to AIDS in America what Typhoid Mary was to an earlier epidemic."[142] This concluding scenario offers a compelling example of a powerful narrative stripped of its contextual features and exported to a new international

141. John Lee Clowe, "The Changing World of AIDS: We Are All At Risk," *Vital Speeches of the Day* 59, no. 5 (1992): 136.
142. Ibid., 136.

audience. The speaker took for granted the widespread applicability and appeal of the story, even while further wrenching it from its original settings of time and place. The science supporting the accusations contained in the statement had long ceased to be persuasive, but the moral framing and storytelling power of the idea remained strong. Such ideas can travel well.

CHAPTER FIVE

Ghosts and Blood

I'm not the first, but I'm still the best,
Make me true, make me clear,
Make me disappear.
—The character of Zero, a ghost, in *Zero Patience*, 1993[1]

The focus was not on 'Gaétan's a bad guy,' but . . . about Gaétan as a missed opportunity for Canadian public health. — *Douglas Elliott*, counsel for the Canadian AIDS Society, Commission of Inquiry on the Blood System in Canada, 1993–97[2]

For lawyer Douglas Elliott and the other participants in the Commission of Inquiry on the Blood System of Canada, the work was difficult, and it soon became emotionally draining. In autumn 1993, Canada's federal government, facing a mounting barrage of criticism in the press, had called for a commission of inquiry into the safety of the Canadian blood system. The inquiry, led by Mr. Justice Horace Krever, an Ontario Court of Appeal judge, was to "review and report on the mandate, organization, management, operations, financing and regulation of all activities of the blood system." Under particular scrutiny were "the events surrounding the contamination of the blood system in Canada

1. *Zero Patience*, made in 1993 by the Toronto-based Zero Productions, was later released on DVD; see *Zero Patience*, directed by John Greyson (New York: Strand Releasing Home Video, 2005), DVD.
2. Douglas Elliott, interview with author, Toronto, August 27, 2008, recording C1491/39, tape 2, side B, BLSA. The deposited recording includes the additional interviews the author conducted with Elliott on August 30 and September 6, 2008.

in the early 1980s," when more than a thousand Canadians had been infected with HIV as a result of receiving blood products and transfusions—a breakdown in safety which contemporaries labeled as "the country's worst ever heath-care disaster." It would later be recognized that more than two thousand Canadians had become infected with HIV and an additional sixty thousand with the hepatitis C virus through their unsuspecting use of the dysfunctional system.[3]

Two days of preliminary hearings in November 1993 established which groups could be granted standing as *interveners*—parties with an interest in the proceedings who might offer the inquiry a useful perspective through their participation. Elliott, whose experiences as a young gay man had led him into AIDS activist work in the early 1980s, sought and received standing on behalf of the Canadian AIDS Society, an umbrella organization of regional AIDS support groups made up predominantly of gays and lesbians. After these initial sessions, the intervening parties assembled their witnesses and developed their strategies, and the commission's staff commenced the arduous process of requisitioning the many thousands of documents that would bear on its work.

The public hearings commenced in earnest on Valentine's Day 1994, their home base a large room on the twentieth floor of the Maclean Hunter Building on downtown Toronto's Bay Street. After a week of introductory witnesses, who provided an overview of the complicated network of actors making up the Canadian blood system—national institutions, governments (federal, provincial, and territorial), regulators, pharmaceutical corporations, hospitals, donors, and individual consumers—the

3. Horace Krever, "Appendix A," in Krever, *Commission of Inquiry*, 3:1081; André Picard, "Hearings to Mix Blood, Politics and Drama," *Globe and Mail* [Toronto], February 14, 1994, A5. Picard's sustained reporting, along with that of his *Globe and Mail* colleague Rod Mickleburgh, undoubtedly contributed to the government's decision to call an inquiry. Alongside the final report produced by Krever and his commission counsel, Picard's book, first published in 1995, is considered the authoritative account of the blood disaster: see André Picard, *The Gift of Death: Confronting Canada's Tainted-Blood Tragedy*, rev. ed. (Toronto: HarperPerennial, 1998); I have relied on his estimates for the numbers of infected Canadians. In his book's acknowledgments, Picard cited the "debt of gratitude" that "any journalist" writing on the AIDS epidemic owed to Randy Shilts, whose book "set a standard of quality and dedication that is a model for all journalists writing about disease in modern society." This may explain why one of Picard's book's chapters, "Death Touches Down: AIDS in Canada," begins and ends with a Shilts-like depiction of Gaétan Dugas. See Picard, *Gift of Death*, vii, 51–67.

commission began to hear testimony from those the system had failed: some of the thousands of Canadians who had become sick after receiving HIV- and hepatitis C–infected blood. Fears that some of these individuals might not live for long factored into the commission counsel's decision to hear from these witnesses—including infected health-care workers, transfusion recipients, and hemophiliacs—as soon as possible.

At the end of the first week of grueling testimony from blood and blood product recipients and their family members, *Zero Patience*, an off-beat feature film challenging the myth of "Patient Zero" by Toronto-based filmmaker John Greyson, began its exclusive hometown engagement at the small Carlton Cinema.[4] The theater was located in the city's gay district near the intersection of Church and Wellesley, a short walk from the hearings in the Maclean Hunter building—a high-rise that some lawyers participating in the inquiry had darkly christened the "Vampire State Building."[5] Soon after the film's opening, and no doubt in need of respite from the hearings' intensity, Elliott took part in an evening outing to see *Zero Patience*, attending with a journalist covering the inquiry and Bob Tivey, one of Gaétan Dugas's friends from Vancouver who had since returned to his native Toronto and who would occasionally attend the hearings. The lawyer recollected that the film gave them pause for thought: "we went out for a beer afterwards and talked about what we thought of the movie and about the real Gaétan, and about the Shilts book."[6] It seems that this evening was influential. Although I am not suggesting that *Zero Patience* inspired Elliott's strategy at the Krever inquiry, it certainly informed it.

These two attempts to invert the widely accepted depiction of "Patient Zero" that had been presented in *And the Band Played On* form the subject of this chapter. Sharply contrasting in form yet thematically, culturally, and geographically overlapping, both efforts emerged in the 1990s from Toronto, Dugas's onetime home. At first glance, it may appear unusual—indeed, bizarre—to hold Greyson's film *Zero Patience* in the same analytical frame as the national commission of inquiry on the Canadian blood system. The first was a quirky, independent feature film musical about AIDS made by a small cast and crew on a shoestring bud-

---

4. Based on a search of advertisements in Toronto's *Globe and Mail* newspaper, the film's nine-week run at the Carlton reached from February 25 to April 28, 1994.

5. Elliott, August 27, 2008, recording C1491/39, tape 2, side B.

6. Elliott, September 6, 2008, recording C1491/39, tape 1, side B.

get of just over $1 million.[7] The second was a large-scale state apparatus, involving dozens of counsel and support staff, hundreds of witnesses, hundreds of thousands of pages of documentation, and costs stretching between an estimated $17.5 and $57 million.[8] Yet, as I will demonstrate, these two arenas were the sites of the two most significant and wide-reaching attempts that decade by AIDS workers to challenge the history contained in *And the Band Played On*. By examining their more subtle similarities and contrasting their divergent approaches, we can gain a more nuanced appreciation for the continued use and significance of the idea of "Patient Zero" during the last years of the North American HIV/AIDS epidemic's first phase, preceding the rollout of highly active antiretroviral therapy (HAART). The chapter's main questions are as follows: In what types of AIDS work did the idea of "Patient Zero" re-surface in the 1990s, what new forms did it take, and why? What did such an idea illuminate? And to what extent were these challenges to the dominant narrative successful?

This chapter follows historian Jennifer Brier's approach in grouping activities often described separately as AIDS activism and AIDS service provision as "AIDS work" and those involved as "AIDS workers." Doing so recognizes the extent to which the various activities existed on a spectrum of politicization, with no straightforward points of division.[9] It also allows for the inclusion of the work carried out by a lawyer such as Elliott, who was a board member for the AIDS Committee of Toronto (ACT) and who represented AIDS organizations and people living with the syndrome, alongside Greyson and individuals like him, who might more typically be viewed as activists. Furthermore, testimony from activists including Ed Jackson and Tim McCaskell suggests that the situation in Toronto had managed to avoid the dichotomous split between activism and service provision that has been observed in other places, most notably New York City.[10]

And why Toronto? Intrusive raids by the city's police force—first on

7. John Greyson, interview with author, Toronto, September 2, 2008, recording C1491/41, tape 1, side A, BLSA.

8. Michael J. Trebilcock and Lisa Austin, "The Limits of the Full Court Press: Of Blood and Mergers," *University of Toronto Law Journal* 48, no. 1 (Winter 1998): 29–30.

9. Brier, *Infectious Ideas*, 4.

10. Jackson, recording C1491/48, tape 1, side B; Tim McCaskell, "A Brief History of AIDS activism in Canada," *Socialist Worker*, November 24, 2012, http://www.socialist.ca/node/1453.

the offices of the collective that produced the *Body Politic* newspaper in 1977 and later as part of a massive series of arrests in the city's bath-houses in early 1981—formed a historic backdrop that galvanized large sections of the city's gay population, the largest in the country, to re-sist authorities seen as overstepping their jurisdiction. Susan Knabe and Wendy Gay Pearson, the authors of a book-length critical analysis which situates *Zero Patience* and Greyson's activism within a wider political context, suggest that the 1981 police raids on the bathhouses in that city helped focus the community's activism around explicit sexuality and the right to share sexual spaces. Thus, in their words, "AIDS emerged into a politicized community that had a particular ideological investment in the defence of sexual practice and was sensitized to the various ways sex-uality was being policed."[11] This high sensitivity, together with skepti-cism toward mainstream media reporting on sexuality and relatively easy travel links to such influential US cities as New York and Washing-ton, DC, also help account for the emergence of a vibrant platform of left-leaning protest which underpinned the two revisionist approaches to the idea of "Patient Zero" from Toronto in the 1990s.[12]

In their analysis of the film, Knabe and Pearson drily note that "*Zero Patience* is a difficult film to summarize."[13] Heeding their counsel, and given the extensive analysis the film has received elsewhere, particularly in Knabe and Pearson's excellent book, this chapter's concern is with the film's production, distribution and reception, with only a brief outline of its contents. The Krever inquiry, on the other hand, has received much less historical attention. Thus, more space will be allotted to describing the inquiry's genesis, internal workings, and proceedings, before the final section of the chapter evaluates the relative efficacy of these two Toronto-based interventions in refuting the dominant "Patient Zero" story.

AIDS Theatricality and Transnationalism

John Greyson's film has received a significant amount of attention from other authors who have critiqued Randy Shilts's vision of "Patient

---

11. Susan Knabe and Wendy Gay Pearson, *Zero Patience: A Queer Film Classic* (Van-couver: Arsenal Pulp Press, 2011), 144.

12. Ibid. See also Silversides, *AIDS Activist*, 12–14.

13. Knabe and Pearson, *Zero Patience*, 27.

Zero."[14] Writers have praised its wit, its creativity, and its energetic expression of the spirit of protest generated through the treatment activism of groups including the AIDS Coalition to Unleash Power (ACT UP) and AIDS Action Now! Little argument is required, on the one hand, to demonstrate that a film—and particularly one which appropriates the most self-consciously aware of cinematic genres: the musical—is *theatrical*, a term which can suggest the knowing adoption of roles, following a predetermined "script," and illuminating particular moral messages. On the other hand, a commission of inquiry could benefit from a few words of explanation to tease out the ways in which it could be viewed as a theatrical performance.

Like many other official commissions before it, the Krever inquiry was set up by government to investigate a matter of concern to the state. These official processes have been described by some commentators as "symbolic rituals within modern States" and, more boldly, "theatres of power." Their work can be usefully divided into three stages: the investigative, the persuasive, and the archival.[15] It is during the investigative phase, when witnesses are called to deliver testimony, that an inquiry is at its most evidently theatrical. In many ways similar to a traditional courtroom, the commissioner sits at the head of the hearing room, facing a room full of interested parties, their representatives (typically lawyers), members of the press, and the general public. The Krever inquiry was similar to others in that its proceedings were televised, with key exchanges frequently excerpted for the evening news. With an eye to the evidentiary power of the second two phases of the inquiry, lawyers acting as counsel and representing interveners assembled panels of witnesses to give testimony and submit documents. This evidence would, they hoped, influence the writing of the commissioner's report (which many would also hope to be persuasive) and inhabit the official inquiry's archive and thus serve as the articulation of an official historical truth. Frequent interviews by counsel to journalists covering the inquiry also served as parallel attempts to shape the emergent historical truth.

Both the Krever inquiry and *Zero Patience* were, in different ways,

14. For critical responses to the film, see Crimp, "Miserable Failure," 124–28; Treichler, *Theory in an Epidemic*, 312–14; Wald, *Contagious*, 254–56; and most recently Tiemeyer, *Plane Queer*, 191–93.

15. Adam Ashforth, "Reckoning Schemes of Legitimation: On Commissions of Inquiry as Power/Knowledge Forms," *Journal of Historical Sociology* 3, no. 1 (1990): 1–22.

concerned with HIV/AIDS as a transnational phenomenon. Both were in dialogue with developments in other countries, such as public health measures and activist responses, and were attentive to the ways in which flows of bodies, ideas, and products, ranging from expertise to artistic works to blood products, crossed into and out of Canada. The Krever inquiry had as its task to investigate the ways in which the Canadian blood system had caused the infections of thousands of Canadians with HIV and hepatitis during the 1980s. This complex industry was at its heart a transnational one, with a dizzying overlap of players, regulators, donors, and recipients, dispelling any notion of clearly articulated and carefully monitored national borders and health systems. The inquiry invited experts from the United States to give testimony, and a substantial section of its report examined the response to HIV/AIDS in other resource-rich countries based on an extensive review of the international literature.

Greyson's film drew on more than a decade of his experiences of gay activism and experimental art and video work in Canada, the United States, and Europe, work which would anchor him within the networks of activists who were involved in the treatment activism of the late 1980s and early 1990s. This activism, though drawing its initial impetus from New York, spread widely and vigorously to cities in both the United States and Canada, as well as overseas.[16] It dealt with a disease that did not recognize borders, in the context of states increasingly attempting to do so, particularly in terms of erecting travel restrictions on people living with HIV.[17] The film's chances of success were from the outset based on the prospect of reaching international audiences at film festivals, and its funding would involve backers in Canada and the United Kingdom.[18] It is to the genesis of this project that we now turn.

16. See Brier, *Infectious Ideas*, 156–200; Mandisa Mbali, *South African AIDS Activism and Global Health Politics* (Basingstoke, UK: Palgrave Macmillan, 2013), particularly 107–35.

17. Crimp, "Miserable Failure," 118.

18. Anna Stratton, John Greyson, and Louise Garfield, "Release & Marketing Proposal," draft, January 18, 1992, 1, file: Zero Patience—Marketing, Acc. 2003–007–05.486, John Greyson Collection, Film Reference Library, Toronto (hereafter cited as Greyson Collection). Canadian financiers included Telefilm Canada, the Ontario Film Development Corporation, the Canadian Film Centre, the Canada Council, the Ontario Arts Council, and Cineplex Odeon Films; Channel 4 Television U.K. also provided funding; *Zero Tabloid* [tabloid-style promotional material] (Toronto: Cineplex-Odeon Films, 1993), 5, folder 240, box 9, Michael Callen Papers, LGBT Community Center National History Archive, New York City (hereafter cited as Callen Papers).

Zero Patience for Accusations

Between 1986 and 1990, John Greyson divided his time between Toronto and Los Angeles, where he spent half of the year teaching at a local arts college. In October 1987, a friend showed him the "Patient Zero" article featured on the cover of that month's edition of *California* magazine. "Wait a sec, I thought. By 1987, they'd already identified North American cases of AIDS dating back to the late sixties, so this story was clearly suspect. Yet in the weeks and months that followed, Patient Zero was taken up by the mainstream media to such a degree that today it's accepted by many as a proven 'fact.' I decided to do a film about the politics of such dubious 'facts,' and *Zero Patience* is the result."[19] Greyson had not met Dugas while the flight attendant was still alive, despite their perigrinations bringing them to Toronto and New York concurrently during the early 1980s. He was, however, only one step removed, since two of his friends had had sex with him.[20] Greyson explained, "In our film, we never deny that Patient Zero was promiscuous. . . . We don't really think it's that important. Lots of people, gay and straight, are promiscuous. We're much more interested in why society needs a Patient Zero, a scapegoat that they can distance themselves from. The film refuses to treat Patient Zero as a pariah—it tries to reclaim him, warts and all, as one of us."[21]

In 1990, John Greyson took up a directing residency at the Canada Film Centre in Toronto. As part of his program application, he had developed an outline for an AIDS musical, and in 1991 he wrote the script's first draft, researching information about the flight attendant's life, international AIDS activist issues, and current theories and controversies regarding the disease's "causes, cures and treatment."[22] A de-

19. "The Whole Truth: Patient Zero Myth Debunked," in *Zero Tabloid*, 3 Callen Papers; emphasis in original. See Christine Gorman, "Strange Trip Back to the Future: The Case of Robert R. Spurs New Questions About AIDS." *Time*, November 9, 1987, 75.

20. Greyson mentions a friend named Michael; Greyson, recording C1491/41, tape 1, side A. The director was also friends with Ed Jackson, whose sexual contact with the flight attendant was discussed in the previous chapter.

21. "Culture of Certainty? We Don't Buy It!" in *Zero Tabloid*, 8, Callen Papers.

22. "ZERO PATIENCE—Development Summary," 23 October 1991, file: Zero Patience—Current, acc. 2003–007–05.0481, Greyson Collection. Among the critiques of the "Patient Zero" story that influenced Greyson was an extended book review of *And the Band Played*

velopment outline for the film hinted strongly at the direction it would take (and anticipated a point of resonance with the blood recipients who would later testify in the Krever inquiry): "Scientists, the media and governments all seemed more concerned with identifying and isolating the 'cause' of the plague than they were with finding and treating the millions who are now infected."[23] Over the course of writing four subsequent drafts, Greyson's film project received funding support from several Canadian arts councils, attracted colleagues from the film center's producing program as coproducers, and gathered interest from domestic and foreign distributors.[24]

Drawing its inspiration from the efforts of groups such as ACT UP and video artists including Stuart Marshall, Greyson's film set out to challenge the orthodoxies of science and the media's claims to represent truth. Embodying its aim of critiquing simplistic narratives spun by the media, the film's complicated story line and songs brim with witty references to AIDS activism of the 1980s and deliberately blend cinematic realist and surrealist touches. As cultural critics have noted, Greyson deliberately calls attention to the constructedness of the story he tells, in contrast with Shilts, whose journalistic history attempts to erase such scaffolding.[25] In the film, Sir Richard Burton—the eminent Victorian explorer famous for searching for the source of the Nile and for his fascination with cross-cultural sexualities—is still alive, following "an unfortunate encounter with the Fountain of Youth." He works as a taxidermist and curator at Toronto's Natural History Museum, his character representing an overconfident culture of scientific certainty. Responsible for developing a new exhibit for the museum's Hall of Contagion, Burton decides to focus his work on "Patient Zero," the French Canadian flight attendant blamed for bringing AIDS to North America. Meanwhile, Zero, the ghost of this otherwise unnamed flight attendant, is trapped in

---

On by Duncan Campbell which accompanied the book's British release: "An End to the Silence," New Statesman, March 4, 1988, 22–23. A clipping of this review accompanies other press materials in a funding application submitted by the producers in July 1992; file: Zero Patience Funding Application, acc. 2003–007–05.0485, Greyson Collection.

23. John Greyson, "Zero Patience: Outline for a Musical," 1, file: Zero Patience—Current, Acc. 2003–007–05.0481, Greyson Collection.

24. The Producers [John Greyson, Louise Garfield, Anna Stratton], "Details of Production," 2 July 1992, file: Zero Patience Funding Application, Acc. 2003–007–05.0485, Greyson Collection.

25. Crimp, "Miserable Failure," 127–28.

a watery, limbo-like existence. Zero wishes for his story to be told and his life to be saved; mysteriously, his wish is partly granted. His ghost returns to the present day, arising in the middle of a gay bathhouse hot tub. To his sadness, however, Zero is invisible to everyone he encounters—the men in the bathhouse, his former lover, and his mother—to everyone, that is, except for Burton.

The film's labyrinthine plot moves between several sites which would hold symbolic significance for many North American people living with AIDS and their family members: a doctor's office, where Zero observes his former lover receiving treatment for an AIDS-related infection that threatens his eyesight; a gay bathhouse; and an ACT UP meeting at a community center, where Burton attempts to gather video evidence for his research. Much of the action also unfolds at the Natural History Museum, where multiple struggles over the meanings and causes of AIDS take place. Burton interviews a doctor involved in the 1982 cluster study, and Zero's mother as well. Initially convinced of Zero's guilt, Burton edits his video footage into a montage that wrenches witness statements out of context and frames Zero as a deliberate disease disseminator. Burton even manages to manipulate Zero's mother's recorded testimony to make her appear to exclaim that "Zero was the Devil."

Zero confronts Burton on his duplicity and decides eventually to collaborate with him, determined to become visible and have his voice heard. As the two draw closer and eventually begin a romantic relationship, Burton gradually comes to doubt the certainties of his science and the story he is telling. He becomes particularly swayed when he and Zero come face-to-face—through a microscope view of a slide of Zero's blood—with Miss HIV, a microscopic drag queen virus floating in a bloodstream swimming pool, played by longtime AIDS activist Michael Callen. Miss HIV clarifies what the 1982 cluster study had set out to establish and that Zero had not been identified as the first AIDS patient in North America. Although Burton wishes to have Zero proclaim his innocence on video, they are unable to catch Zero on tape for longer than a few seconds. At this point fate intervenes: the museum's director, Dr. Placebo, insists on broadcasting Burton's original slanted video montage, saying that, in any case, he preferred that version of the story. The distorted myth of Patient Zero is subsequently disseminated wholesale via the media. Riled by the museum's willful misinformation, and singing that "We've got zero patience for accusations, zero patience for blame," ACT UP members stage a protest; they rearrange Burton's

Hall of Contagion exhibit to evoke a more patient-centered health-care history. Ultimately, to Burton's sadness and dismay, Zero wishes to be allowed to disappear. Reluctant to let his otherworldly lover depart, Burton finally acquiesces and helps Zero short-circuit the museum's "Patient Zero" display. Zero is at last able to return to his limbo-like existence, freed from the never-ending attempts to frame his existence within straitjacket-like AIDS narratives.[26]

Greyson later expressed his fondness for the film's lyrics and the ideas and spirit of the time it captured. At the same time, despite being produced on a much greater budget than his previous experimental video work, the production's resources were roughly a third of what he needed to realize his vision and thus constrained the production quality.[27] Reviews were mixed. A Quebecois reviewer in Montreal defined the film as "impossible to classify" and "a unique experience."[28] An Anglophone critic noted that despite it being "a movie that you really *want* to like," *Zero Patience* was "disappointing" and "often appear[ed] amateurish." At the same time he acknowledged that the film was laudable for its political message and "admirably uncompromising" in its depiction of gay life—with "such in-your-face segments as a duet performed by two animated singing anuses"—and could not, like Jonathan Demme's film *Philadelphia*, be accused of sanitization.[29] The timing of the film's release and its originality compelled audiences and critics to pay attention. As Greyson recalled:

It was released the same week as *Philadelphia* in theatres and so it *immediately* had . . . the most brilliant juxtaposition imaginable because the critics had a great hook, you know, on the one hand *Philadelphia*, four-hanky weepie, on the other *Zero Patience*, and so . . . it almost forced the critics to take a stand in terms of politics, as opposed to simply around film. And so while most critics were pretty hard on the film in terms of its craft, there was an acknowledgment that it was stirring the pot, intervening, saying something that hadn't been said before in a semi-mainstream context.[30]

26. On this point, see Knabe and Pearson, *Zero Patience*, 11, 150.

27. Greyson, recording C1491/41, tape 1, side A.

28. Éric Fourlanty, "Zero Patience," *Voir*, March 10, 1994. My translation from the French original: "inclassable" and "une expérience unique."

29. Scott Steele, "AIDS, the Musical: Zero Patience," *Maclean's*, March 7, 1994, 60.

30. Greyson, recording C1491/41, tape 1, side A; emphasis on recording. Interestingly, Douglas Elliott recalled the cathartic and emotional response he had each time he

Though less accessible to many mainstream audience members by virtue of its intellectually challenging approach and niche cinema distribution, *Zero Patience* benefited from the near simultaneous release of two Hollywood contributions: the movie *Philadelphia* and the HBO television miniseries of *And the Band Played On*. *Zero Patience* held its main premiere in Toronto during the Festival of Festivals (precursor to the Toronto International Film Festival) on September 11, 1993. By coincidence, this was the same day the TV miniseries of Shilts's book was broadcast on cable television, an adaptation in which the figure of "Patient Zero" played only a small role.[31] Shilts, possibly having been stung by criticism from AIDS activists, had insisted that the TV miniseries minimize the role of the flight attendant.[32]

In addition to showing the film at various North American gay film festivals, Greyson sought to make use of a network of AIDS organizations to promote the film. In a letter to the film's marketing coordinator, he noted that "the range and scale of AIDS groups across the country is breath-taking" and that there would be a symbiosis to the relationship between the film distributor and these groups: "They'll want to work with us as much as we'll want to work with them."[33] In discussing the possibility of gala fund-raising evenings, he distinguished, however, between AIDS service organizations and his preferred activist organizations. Given the relative success of the former in raising financial contributions, "Groups like ACT [the AIDS Committee of Toronto] and Casey House [an organization providing palliative care for people living with AIDS] don't need Zero Patience," he wrote.[34] Greyson wished to preserve a space for dissident voices—for people living with AIDS, for critics of the health-care system, for activists in general—amid what

---

viewed *Philadelphia*, identifying strongly with Denzel Washington's character of a lawyer who knew that his client with AIDS would soon die; Elliott, September 6, 2008, recording C1491/39, tape 2, side A.

31. *Philadelphia*, directed by Jonathan Demme (TriStar Pictures, 1993; Burbank, CA: Columbia TriStar Home Video, 1997), DVD; *And the Band Played On*, directed by Roger Spottiswoode (HBO Pictures, 1993; Warner Home Video, 2004), DVD.

32. Deborah Hastings, "Shilts Says Film Version of His Book Still Alive," *Indiana Gazette*, October 30, 1991, 31.

33. John Greyson to Virginia Kelly, 4 May 1992, file: Zero Patience—Distribution, Acc. 2003–007–05.0483, Greyson Collection.

34. John Greyson to Virginia Kelly, undated, file: Zero Patience—Distribution, Acc. 2003–007–05.0483, Greyson Collection.

he and others saw as the institutionalization and professionalization of AIDS. "AIDS runs the risk," he wrote in a November 1991 outline for the film, "of becoming as respectable as cancer: an acceptable tragedy, and a multi-billion dollar industry that doesn't really cure anyone. Alternative theories, therapies, and treatments are being suppressed because they threaten not just the profit margins of the pharmaceuticals, but the very authority of the medical establishment."[35] The resulting marketing plan would enthusiastically describe "the support and communications network spawned by the AIDS crisis" as "formidable and wide reaching," and it highlighted the need to work through the Canadian AIDS Society "to reach primary and secondary audiences."[36] Also, the opening gala held in advance of the film's general release was a benefit screening for the activist group AIDS Action Now! and Inside Out, a collective which organized an annual gay and lesbian film festival (see fig. 5.1).[37]

By the 1990s, AIDS service organizations had become relatively mainstream, no longer considered by many as activist in a political sense. A decade earlier, however, the fledgling efforts of these organizations would have been considered essential foundational work, given their active campaigning against the status quo, amid a widespread lack of institutional response to AIDS, and the media's often discriminatory depiction of those with the disease. It is to this earlier group of AIDS workers that the discussion now turns.

The Krever Inquiry

The Krever inquiry's primary investigative phase stretched from early 1994 until the end of the following year. During this initial stage, the commissioner, his counsel, and teams of lawyers traveled across the country to hold regional hearings from Vancouver to St. John's.[38] They listened to many of the Canadians who had been infected with HIV and

35. "*Zero Patience*," outline, 12 November 1991, 1, file: Zero Patience OAC—Canada Council, Acc. 2003–007–05.0487, Greyson Collection.

36. VK & Associates, "Positioning of Project and General Marketing Approach," June 30, 1992, 3, file: Zero Patience—Funding Application, Acc. 2003–007–05.0485, Greyson Collection.

37. See the promotional advertisement for the film "Zero Patience [/] A John Greyson Movie Musical," *Xtra!* [Toronto], February 18, 1994, 2.

38. For a comprehensive summary of the inquiry's schedule, see Horace Krever, "Ap-

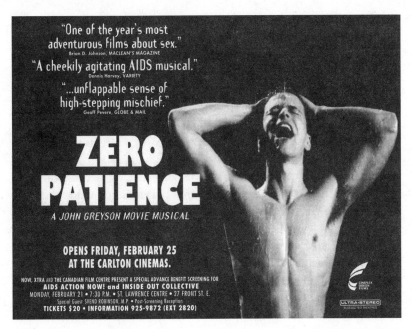

FIGURE 5.1 Promotional advertisement for *Zero Patience*, 24.8 × 18.9 cm, reprinted from *Xtra!* February 18, 1994, 2. Courtesy of the Canadian Lesbian and Gay Archives, Toronto. © Zero Patience Productions. Used with permission from John Greyson, and from Ken Popert on behalf of Pink Triangle Press. This poster, depicting the actor Norman Fauteux in the role of the ghost Zero, also illuminates the connections Greyson had with AIDS activism work in Toronto, for which this advance gala was to be a fund-raiser. The film's producers relied on such activist networks as a way of finding audiences and promoting the film.

hepatitis C through infected blood and blood products, as well as the regional representatives of the organizations whose safety and regulatory measures were under investigation. The inquiry's second investigative phase began in early 1995 at the commission's Toronto headquarters. There, national experts testified about their roles in Canada's blood system during the 1980s, and roundtables of experts discussed current issues facing the blood system.

While the Krever inquiry was chiefly concerned with the events and (in)actions leading to an HIV- and hepatitis C–infected blood system, the motives of the different parties granted standing varied consider-

pendix I," in Krever, *Commission of Inquiry*, 3:1136–38; and Trebilcock and Austin, "Limits," 25–28.

ably. Having been permitted to represent the Canadian AIDS Society, Douglas Elliott believed that the inquiry offered Canadian gay communities their only opportunity to document officially their early responses to AIDS in the face of governmental inertia and widespread homophobia. During the hearings he advanced several arguments contesting the widely held view that these communities had perpetuated the epidemic's spread. Among the accepted truths that Elliott challenged was the by then often-told story of "Patient Zero," part of his wider strategy to challenge the history of the lesbian and gay community's response put forward by Randy Shilts. This widely read perspective clashed with his own personal recollection of the early response to AIDS in Canada.

In July 1983, a twenty-six-year-old Douglas Elliott was articling for Bassel, Sullivan and Leake, a Toronto law firm, having recently graduated from the University of Toronto Law School. One day, his lover passed on news of a disturbing phone call he had received from a friend and former sexual partner, who had been working in New York City as a model: "'Darrell just called and you know this AIDS thing, he's got it, and he doesn't have any health insurance, so he's coming back to Canada to die.' And that was one thing we knew for sure about AIDS at that time was the average time from diagnosis to death was six months. Everybody who got it was dying."[39] Elliott had been following news of the disease ever since initial reports of a "gay cancer" had left him and others deeply skeptical. Over time, though, this skepticism gave way to uncertainty, then apprehension, about "a real medical threat."[40]

Having a friend diagnosed with the condition made the threat even more apparent. Elliott, realizing he needed more detailed information to assist Darrell, sought guidance from the newly formed ACT, which had recently held a press conference to inform the public that it was organizing a response to the condition.[41] Elliott was disconcerted by what he saw: "I'm looking around, and they had these crappy offices over top of the Kentucky Fried Chicken, dirty and grimy and a few sticks of furniture, and I'm thinking, 'This is the frontline of defence against this terrible epidemic? You've got to be joking.'" Elliott and his partner became involved with ACT while they juggled looking after their dying friend and Elliott's studying for his upcoming bar exam. Darrell died in 1984;

39. Elliott, August 27, 2008, recording C1491/39, tape 1, side B.
40. Ibid.
41. Silversides, *AIDS Activist*, 54.

soon after, Elliott was elected to ACT's first board of directors and continued his work with the group, becoming one of the earliest lawyers in
the country to be involved with AIDS issues. He recalled that his professional background made him stand out from other members of the
board: "It was a pretty laid-back, kind of lefty grassroots organisation
and meeting in a big, open, grimy room . . . with the smell of Kentucky
Fried Chicken permeating the air, and I'm the only guy in a suit, and
they say, 'Well, you should be on the executive, we need guys in suits for
when we meet politicians.'"[42]

In the first months after its foundation in mid-1983, ACT worked hard
to address what its members viewed as the media's propensity for "blaming the victim for the illness," monitoring and responding to media reports displaying strong bias.[43] Members of the organization also protested vigorously against the gay community's lack of representation on
the nascent National Advisory Committee on AIDS (NAC-AIDS). This
expert committee had been appointed to advise the federal minister of
health, Monique Bégin, and was initially coordinated by the director
general of the Laboratory Centre for Disease Control (LCDC), Alastair
Clayton.[44] Elliott recalled the "strained" relationship between the two
organizations early in their history and that "one of our big bones of
contention in those years was that the NAC-AIDS would not have an
openly gay community representative on their board." He remembered
the derision with which his fellow ACT members viewed this situation:

All you have is a bunch of public health officials, all of the people who are doing *nothing* about AIDS [*laughing wryly*], all of the people in white lab coats
that are sitting around reading CDC reports and things like that and thinking great thoughts—they're the people that are sitting around the table. The
people that are actually *doing* something about AIDS, who are on the front-
lines and experiencing AIDS and making a difference with respect to education and stuff like that—they're the people in the community organizations

42. Elliott, August 27, 2008, recording C1491/39, tape 1, side B.

43. ACT's early activities are outlined in its meeting minutes and *AIDS Activities Bulletins*, printed from August 16, 1983, onward: "Minutes of the General Meeting," October 18, 1983, 1, attached to *AIDS Activities Bulletin*, no. 6, October 31, 1983. The ACT Library closed in the spring of 2010, though as of July 2014 the minutes and bulletins were
still held at the organization's head office in Toronto.

44. Charlotte Montgomery, "Begin Appoints Advisers to Study AIDS," *Globe and
Mail* [Toronto], August 16, 1983.

that you're shunning. . . . We have expertise to share. You want to communicate with the gay community and you wouldn't know a gay person if they bit
you in the ass.[45]

Elliott remained involved with ACT's board through 1986, the year
when the second national AIDS conference was held in Toronto. At this
meeting, representatives from AIDS service organizations from across
the country finalized plans to found the Canadian AIDS Society (CAS).
The society developed as a national organization to help overcome the
geographic distance separating the largely gay-run community AIDS organizations in various far-flung Canadian cities, to share information,
and to engage with the federal government as a national body representing these disparate local groups. Between 1986 and the beginning of the
Krever inquiry, Elliott took on AIDS-related briefs for the fledgling
CAS in addition to his developing specialty in AIDS-transfusion civil
cases. As the AIDS epidemic grew in Canada and spread beyond the
large cities where the syndrome was first noticed, the CAS grew as well.
By the mid-1990s, the coalition represented roughly one hundred community AIDS organizations across the country.[46]

In mid-September 1993, the federal government announced its commitment to a blood inquiry. Simultaneously, the country's provincial
and territorial governments announced that time-limited compensation
packages would be made available to recipients of infected blood.[47] Elliott was in Ottawa for a previously arranged meeting with the Red Cross
regarding his own cases involving recipients of infected blood. The meeting was very brief; the Red Cross was not interested in any further nego-
tiations in the wake of the recent compensation announcement. With a
few hours to spend in the country's capital before returning to Toronto,

45. Elliott, August 27, 2008, recording C1491/39, tape 1, side B.
46. D. Steele, "Evolution of Canadian AIDS Society," 39–61.
47. All provincial and territorial governments took part in this announcement apart
from Nova Scotia, which had already developed its own program. To receive compensation, those who had received infected blood and blood products would be required to sign
waivers promising not to pursue any future lawsuits against the compensating parties,
which included not only the regional governments but also the Canadian Red Cross Society and a number of insurance and pharmaceutical companies; see Picard, *Gift of Death*,
157–94. It has been suggested that the inquiry was called to deflect criticism during a general election; see Nicholas d'Ombrain, "Public Inquiries in Canada," *Canadian Public Administration* 40, no. 1 (1997): 94.

Elliott visited the CAS office and spoke with the organization's Director of Programmes, Russell Armstrong, who was an old friend:

So we had a little chat, and I explained what was going on . . . and he had read the Shilts book. When I talked about the Gaétan Dugas thing, he just sort of rolled his eyes and said, "Yeah, I know, but what can we do?" And I said, "Well, I think you need to be at this Inquiry." He said, 'Well, it's really about [the] Canadian Hemophilia Society—it's their ballgame." I said, "Well, do you really want them presenting the role of the gay community in responding to AIDS?" He said, "Absolutely not" [Elliott laughing].[48]

Elliott received Armstrong's blessing to represent his organization. At the inquiry's organizational hearings in November 1993, the CAS was granted intervener standing and funding, an important point since the CAS had no discretionary funds to allocate to such an undertaking.

A newsletter article distributed during the inquiry summed up the approach Elliott would follow, stating the importance of "the social underpinnings of the spread of HIV." It suggested that homophobia and racism had influenced the spread of HIV infection through the blood system and that the "indifference with which AIDS was treated in the early 1980s was justified by the institutional parties by the identity of the first groups affected by AIDS and their marginalized place in society." The article listed several examples of the effect of homophobia: an unwillingness of medical directors in the Red Cross to contact gay organizations, reluctance to use the word *gay* in health brochures, a lack of will on the part of provincial governments to fund AIDS service organizations before the mid-1980s—given the prevailing view that these were political rights groups—and ignoring the work these organizations were doing, some of which may directly have served to protect the blood supply.[49]

The participation of CAS in the inquiry was controversial in some quarters, as a 1994 article in the conservative *Alberta Report* indicates. Subtitled "Gays turn their tainted-blood culpability into an asset," the article lamented the "farce" of the "homosexual lobbying" and its "gay

48. Recounted in Elliott, August 27, 2008, C1491/39, tape 2, side B. Elliott recalled there being a "very bad relationship" between ACT and the Canadian Hemophilia Society.
49. Patricia A. LeFebour and Douglas Elliott, "Inquiry into the Blood System in Canada: The Krever Commission," *Canadian HIV/AIDS Policy and Law Newsletter* 1, no. 3 (1995), http://www.aidslaw.ca/site/download/9189/.

disinformation" at the inquiry's hearings in the province of Alberta and put forth exactly the views that Elliott had feared might be in the majority. It argued that "gays should themselves accept much of the blame for their determined effort to subvert public discussion of the true nature of the disease's transmission" and that "successful lobbying against implementing . . . standard public health measures was led by militant gays." The article ended with a quote from an epidemiologist in Ontario, who offered a condemnatory assessment of the gay community's guilt: "'Gays gave blood even once they knew they were high-risk. . . . And a lot of them were scared they'd get quarantined if it remained strictly a homosexual disease.'"[50] Once again, the centuries-old specter of a group determined to spread a disease to others had been raised.

Inquiries as Arenas of Historical Production

In the absence of an established historiography for the Canadian epidemic, it is not surprising that there were fears that another historical explanation might fill the void. This alternate version, Elliott feared, was likely to be the story portrayed in Shilts's book, where the author dismissed civil rights concerns as "public relations" and offered examples of gay community members urging each other to lie about their sexuality or to engage in "blood terrorism" if the government did not fund AIDS research.[51] Elliott's efforts to seek a place at the inquiry for the CAS is significant, as it demonstrates the potential power of popular narratives to shape high-level interpretations of the "official" history of an epidemic. Elliott was concerned that the influence of *And the Band Played On* would dominate the consciousness of the parties represented in the Krever inquiry and that, as in Shilts's book, many would try to blame the gay community for the contamination of the blood supply.[52]

---

50. Joe Woodard, "Bad Blood and Bad Medicine," *Alberta Report* 21, no. 21 (1994): 26, Academic Search Complete, EBSCOhost (9406077701). Ivan Emke criticizes the tone of the AIDS coverage in the *Alberta Report* during the 1980s, notes the conspiratorial overtones the journal implied in its use of the phrase AIDS "carrier," and suggests that the blood supply is the modern version of the poisoned well; see Ivan Emke, "Around the Bush Yet Again: Reflection on Reckless Vectors, Past and Present," *Sexuality Research and Social Policy* 2, no. 2 (2005): 95–98.

51. Shilts, *Band*, 170–71, 238, 309.

52. In his thesis, Steele notes the broad influence of Shilts's book; one of his inter-

What I read in his book troubled me on a number of levels, not least of which it was describing the American experience and I knew that the Canadian experience had been quite a bit different than what it had been in the United States. For example, it was very clear when you read Randy Shilts's book that he felt that the leadership in the lesbian and gay community in San Francisco had been irresponsible, especially in their opposition to closing the bathhouses. And whether that's true or not, I knew that in Toronto . . . ACT had always opposed closing the bathhouses but for very legitimate reasons . . . . And I thought, "Oh no, here we go again. Now we got somebody in the *in-*side of the gay community saying that *we're* responsible for the AIDS epidemic, after we've worked so hard to try and get away from that 'gay plague' stuff." [53]

This scapegoating of the lesbian and gay community he felt to be particularly likely given the absence of any nationally recognized coalition of gay rights organizations seeking standing in the inquiry. The history of AIDS in Canada, not covered in any popular accounts, would, he feared, be covered by and subsumed within the Krever inquiry's investigations and final report. It would, he believed, be a disaster to leave the creation of this history to the Canadian Hemophilia Society, a group with which ACT had not enjoyed a good relationship.[54] For Elliott, "one of the key issues was to highlight the positive role that the gay community had played in responding to AIDS, and to dispel this notion that somehow *we* poisoned the well, the Shilts thesis, that between irresponsible community leaders who refused to close the bathhouses, and Typhoid Marys, like Gaétan Dugas, that *we're* the ones who are responsible for the AIDS epidemic. I was very concerned that we were going to be scapegoated, that gay people in general were going to be scapegoated and that some individuals like Gaétan were going to be in particular scapegoated."[55]

Elliott was not alone in this view. A longtime gay activist, Ed Jackson, who was one of Dugas's former sexual partners and also a friend

---

viewees mentioned that it made a distinct impression on Perrin Beatty, the Minister of National Health and Welfare from 1989 to 1991; D. Steele, "Evolution of Canadian AIDS Society," 21.

53. Elliott, August 27, 2008, C1491/39, tape 2, side A; emphasis on recording.

54. Hemophiliacs were also often portrayed in the media as "innocent victims" of HIV infection; Patton, *Sex and Germs*, 23; Emke, "Speaking of AIDS in Canada," 543–44.

55. Elliott, August 27, 2008, C1491/39, tape 2, side B; emphasis on recording.

of Greyson, later recalled his partipation in the hearings, where "every document" was carefully interpreted:

> There were many vested interests represented there. The room was *littered* with lawyers, all representing some organisation or other whose reputation or legal culpability was going to be called into question so they were protecting each other. You certainly had a sense of the adversarial nature of this. The important thing from our perspective was to ensure that the role of the gay community was not maligned, was not misrepresented, [and] was made as visible as possible in that situation. Because there wasn't a lot of visible documentation before that that people could rely on to counter what might be misrepresentations or accusations of failure to respond appropriately. You felt the ominousness of that. This was important to get it right because it could have repercussions later.[56]

Gary Kinsman, an activist and academic, voiced similar concerns in 1997, writing before the release of the commission's final report later that year. Along with the media coverage it generated, Kinsman believed that the Krever commission "could establish an official history of AIDS that marginalizes the stories of gay men and community activists. This is especially the case given that some officials in the Red Cross have argued—in contrast to the actual safe sex and blood-donation responsibility efforts of early AIDS groups—that they could not properly screen the blood supply because of supposed 'resistance' from the gay community; and that they could not implement HIV testing because they feared gay men would flood the testing with the possibility of infection because of the period between infection and the appearance of HIV antibodies."[57] In addition to sharing these men's concerns about blame, Elliott believed, like Kinsman, that the inquiry would produce the authoritative version of the epidemic's history in Canada. "And I just knew that [gay community resistance] wasn't a true picture of what happened. We had been fighting AIDS at a time when governments didn't give a shit, or were *glad* to see AIDS cleaning out the riffraff from the populace. And

---

56. Jackson, recording C1491/48, tape 2, side A; emphasis on recording.

57. Gary Kinsman, "Managing AIDS Organizing: 'Consultation,' 'Partnership' and 'Responsibility' as Strategies of Regulation," in *Organizing Dissent: Contemporary Social Movements in Theory and Practice*, 2nd ed., ed. William K. Carroll, 219–20 (Toronto: Garamond Press, 1997).

I, having my history background, I wanted the historical truth on the record. And I also realized that this story would never be told again. That this was going be the one time that you were going to get the official history of Canada's response to the AIDS epidemic." Elliott also believed that Krever, as commissioner, would "be receptive to this, but that he just might not know. So I thought we should be there."[58] Thus Elliott sought to challenge "the Shilts hypothesis," as he put it,[59] by attempting to insert into the public record the efforts that members of the gay community had undertaken in the early 1980s, at a time of sluggish, antipathetic, or nonexistent institutional responses. One pillar of this strategy was to present a reconfigured view of "Patient Zero," the most sensationalized character of Shilts's history and the media response which publicized it.

"A Missed Opportunity for Canadian Public Health"

In the questions he posed during the inquiry's hearings, Elliott demonstrated a novel take on Gaétan Dugas's role as "Patient Zero." Like Greyson in Zero Patience, he portrayed Dugas not as a recalcitrant disease carrier but as a reasonably concerned gay man, willing to assist authorities with contact tracing in order to offer more information about the new disease. In addition, Elliott showed that an AIDS patient, identified at an early stage by the CDC as a person of extreme interest, was living in communities across Canada unbeknownst to local health authorities. In this way, Elliott was able to add to the impression of a country with very weak public health surveillance abilities. In the popular version of the "Patient Zero" myth, Dugas's listing of his sex partners' names in an address book represented the narcissistic excesses of unrestrained gay sexuality. In Elliott's reformulated version, this address book contained key epidemiologic information: names and contact information of his sexual partners, all potential blood donors and all potentially infected with the agent that caused AIDS. In this new version, each recorded name represented a chance for officials to trace a contact,

58. Elliott, August 27, 2008, recording C1491/39, tape 2, side B; emphasis on recording. Elliott had pursued an undergraduate degree in history at the University of Western Ontario; Elliott, August 27, 2008, recording C1491/39, tape 1, side A.

59. Elliott, August 27, 2008, recording C1491/39, tape 2, side A.

identify a potential AIDS patient, and prevent him from donating blood. In Elliott's words, "the focus was not on 'Gaétan's a bad guy,' but . . . about Gaétan as a missed opportunity for Canadian public health."[60]

The number of times the concept was raised in the hearings suggests the importance of the flight attendant to Elliott's strategy. A search of the inquiry's transcripts indicates that the phrases "Patient 0," "Patient Zero," "Gaetan Dugas," or similar references to the flight attendant were raised in at least twenty separate instances during seventeen days of the inquiry (see table 5.1).[61] This finding alone suggests that, more than seven years after the publicity surrounding Shilts's book and more than ten years after the flight attendant's death, the "Patient Zero" narrative retained some important presence in the imagined history of AIDS in Canada. Nine mentions occurred during the regional hearings held across the country; the remainder took place during the national hearings, current issues presentations, and final oral submissions in Toronto. Since the lawyers representing the intervening groups often pooled their cross-examination questions to save time, other participants touched on the subject as well; nonetheless, counsel for the Canadian AIDS Society revisited the idea nine separate times, the most of any group, of which Elliott led eight.

Time restrictions also affected the examination strategies adopted by the commission of inquiry and the intervening parties. Initially faced with an impossibly short period of less than twelve months in which to conduct his hearings and write a report, Krever protested and was granted more than one extension. Even so, with more than twenty parties granted standing and nearly forty lawyers directly involved in the proceedings, the inquiry was constantly wrestling with time constraints.

60. Elliott, August 27, 2008, recording C1491/39, tape 2, side B. Elliott nonetheless believed that Dugas had likely been careless in his sexual behavior: "Doubtless he caused some infections, and doubtless some of that was done in an irresponsible way, but he didn't single-handedly cause the epidemic" (ibid.).

61. I have not included in this count a fascinating metaphorical reference by one participant, Alan Powell, who employed the term *patient zero* to suggest that the lack of a primary case among recipients of hepatitis C–infected blood hindered the commission's ability to establish an official history for their infections: "Since we didn't have a patient zero we couldn't do the backtracking involved to find out when and where it first became prevalent in North America or anywhere else in the world"; quoted in *Verbatim Transcripts of Commission of Inquiry on the Blood System in Canada*, 247 vols. (Gloucester, ON: International Rose Reporting, 1997), CD-ROM, 199:42196.

TABLE 5.1. **Instances in which participants employed the words "Patient Zero," "Patient 0," "Gaetan Dugas," "Gaétan Dugas," and similar references to the flight attendant during the Commission of Inquiry on the Blood System in Canada, 1994–1996**

Date	Inquiry Phase	Location	Transcript (Volume:page)	Counsel (& Affiliation)	Person(s) Appearing (& Affiliation)	Words Recorded in Transcript
March 28, 1994	Regional hearings	Vancouver, BC	23:4272–73	Céline Lacerte-Lamontagne (Commission Counsel)	Dr. Timothy Johnstone (Director, Division of Epidemiology, British Columbia Ministry of Health, 1982–1986)	Patient 0
July 27, 1994	Regional hearings	Halifax, NS	60:12605–8	Douglas Elliott (Canadian AIDS Society)	Dr. Pierre Lavigne (Provincial Epidemiologist, Nova Scotia Department of Health, 1980–1988) Dr. Wayne Sullivan (Administrator, Community Health Services, Nova Scotia Department of Health, 1980–1991)	Gaetan Dugas; Patient Zero
July 29, 1994	Regional hearings	Halifax, NS	62:13174–75	Douglas Elliott	Robin Metcalfe (Chair, Gay Alliance for Equality, 1983)	Gaétan Dugas; Patient 0
September 23, 1994	Regional hearings	Montreal, QC	77:16534–42	Céline Lacerte-Lamontagne	Dr. Richard Morisset (President, Comité SIDA-Québec, 1982–1987; Member, NAC-AIDS Committee, 1983–1984) Dr. Jean Robert (Chief, Département de Santé communautaire, Hôpital Saint-Luc, 1977–83; Secretary, Comité SIDA-Québec, 1982–1987)	*un Montréalais; cas initial; patient zéro*
September 23, 1994	Regional hearings	Montreal, QC	77:16718–21	Dawna Ring (Janet Conners*)	Dr. Richard Morisset Dr. Jean Robert	Patient Zero
September 26, 1994	Regional hearings	Montreal, QC	78:16980–81	Dawna Ring	Dr. Antony Alcindor (President, Association des médecins haïtiens à l'étranger, chapitre Montréal, 1982–1989; Coordinator, Comité haïtien sur le SIDA, 1983–1985) Dr. Alix Adrien (Montreal-based physician) Marlène Rateau (Teacher, Ministère du Service de Santé, la Commission des écoles catholiques de Montréal, 1974–1988)	patient zero

(continued)

TABLE 5.1. **(Continued)**

Date	Inquiry Phase	Location	Transcript (Volume:page)	Counsel (& Affiliation)	Person(s) Appearing (& Affiliation)	Words Recorded in Transcript
September 28, 1994	Regional hearings	Montreal, QC	80:17404–5	Patricia LeFebour (Canadian AIDS Society)	Dr. Michel Pelletier (Director, Planning and Programs, Health and Social Services Council, Bas Saint-Laurent, Gaspésie, Îles-de-la-Madeleine region, 1979–1986) Dr. Marc Dionne (Director, Beauceville Public Health Department, 1979–1983)	Patient Zero
September 30, 1994	Regional hearings	Montreal, QC	82:17906–7	Douglas Elliott	Reynald Gagnon (Chief, Short-term Care Programmes, Ministère de la Santé et des Services sociaux, 1980–1983)	Gaetan Dugas; Patient Zéro
October 11, 1994	Regional hearings	Toronto, ON	83:18010–11	Douglas Elliott	Dr. Philip Berger (Toronto-based physician treating patients with HIV)	Gaétan Dugas
March 7, 1995	National hearings	Toronto, ON	100:21590–98	Marlys Edwardh (Commission Counsel)	Dr. Donald Francis (Assistant Director for Medical Science, Hepatitis and Viral Enteritis Division, US CDC, 1978–1983)	Patient Zero
March 9, 1995	National hearings	Toronto, ON	102:21926–33	Douglas Elliott	Dr. Donald Francis	Gaeten Dugas [sic]; Patient Zero
March 14, 1995	National hearings	Toronto, ON	104:22339–40	Roy Stephenson (Commission Counsel)	Dr. Thomas Zuck (Chief, Department of Pathology, Walter Reed Army Medical Center, Washington, D.C., 1977–1980; Deputy Director, Armed Forces Institute of Pathology, and Consultant in Pathology to the Surgeon General, United States Army, 1980–1982)	"case 'zero'"; "the Air Canada steward"

Date	Event	Location	Citation	Witness	Officials	Term
April 17, 1995	National hearings	Toronto, ON	115:24510–18	Marlys Edwardh	Dr. Norbert Gilmore (Chair, NAC-AIDS Committee, 1983–1989) Dr. Richard Mathias (Member, NAC-AIDS Committee, 1983–1986) Dr. Frances Shepherd (Member, NAC-AIDS Committee, 1984–1986) Dr. Colin Soskolne (Member, NAC-AIDS Committee, 1983–1985)	Gaetan Dugas
April 20, 1995	National hearings	Toronto, ON	117:25108–17	Douglas Elliott	Dr. Norbert Gilmore, Dr. Richard Mathias, Dr. Frances Shepherd, Dr. Colin Soskolne	Gaetan Dugas
April 20, 1995	National hearings	Toronto, ON	117:25138–40	Dawna Ring	Dr. Norbert Gilmore, Dr. Richard Mathias, Dr. Frances Shepherd, Dr. Colin Soskolne	Gaetan Dugas
October 13, 1995	National hearings	Toronto, ON	198:41786–93	Douglas Elliott	Dr. Alastair Clayton (Director General, LCDC, 1979–1987)	Gaetan Dugas; patient zero
October 23, 1995	National hearings	Toronto, ON	199:42196	Dr. Alan Powell (Canadian Hepatitis C Survivors Society†)	Dr. Peter Gill (Director, Bureau of Microbiology, LCDC, 1979–1988)	patient zero
November 22, 1995	Current issues presentations	Toronto, ON	216:45476–77	William Selnes (Canadian Hemophiliacs Infected with HIV)	Dr. Joseph Losos (Director, Bureau of Infection Control, LCDC, 1979–1986; Director General, LCDC, 1988–1996) and four other health officials (Dr. Richard Mathias, Dr. Donald Wigle, Dr. Donald Sutherland, Dr. Paul Gully)	"a cluster of cases of homosexuals in Southern California"; "a Canadian"

(continued)

TABLE 5.1. *(continued)*

Date	Inquiry Phase	Location	Transcript (Volume:page)	Counsel (& Affiliation)	Person(s) Appearing (& Affiliation)	Words Recorded in Transcript
November 22, 1995	Current issues presentations	Toronto, ON	216:45512–13	Douglas Elliott	Dr. Joseph Losos, Dr. Richard Mathias, Dr. Donald Wigle, Dr. Donald Sutherland, Dr. Paul Gully	"a Canadian was at the centre of the original cluster study on AIDS"
December 9, 1996	Final oral submissions	Toronto, ON	241:49460–61	Paul Nesseth (Gignac, Sutts Group†)	None	patient zero
December 10, 1996	Final oral submissions	Toronto, ON	242:49486–87	Dawna Ring	None	"patient zero, the most noteworthy person with AIDS in North America"

Source. Electronic word search of *Verbatim Transcripts of Hearings of Commission of Inquiry on the Blood System in Canada*, 247 vols. (Gloucester, ON: International Rose Reporting, 1997), CD-ROM.

*Conners was an HIV-infected woman granted intervener standing at the inquiry.

†Dr. Powell was the national president of the Canadian Hepatitis C Survivors Society.

‡Nesseth represented a group of infected hemophiliacs from Ontario.

This demanding schedule in turn limited the questions which different lawyers were able to ask of those giving testimony and forced them to prioritize their lines of interrogation, often at the last minute. Given this shortage of time, it is suggestive that some lawyers repeatedly prioritized the idea of "Patient Zero" as a question point for a number of witnesses throughout the inquiry.

Border Guards or UN Observers?

Elliott summarized his general line of attack—into which Dugas's story would fit—during his April 1995 examination of Dr. Richard Mathias, a provincial epidemiologist based in British Columbia who had also been a member of NAC-AIDS. Although Krever's main task was to determine what had gone wrong with the blood system, the commissioner and his counsel clearly realized that to fulfill this mandate, they would need to gather information about the state of the provincial and national public health systems for the period in question. A safe blood supply depended in part on a strong public health system that efficiently gathered and distributed information regarding health risks to Canadians.

Only partially addressing his witness, Elliott ended his questioning of the epidemiologist with a rhetorical flourish, drawing a comparison between interprovincial cooperation and international affairs. He asking the hearing room, "Do we have the right—do Canadians have a right to expect that provincial epidemiologists are going to act like border guards, and defend us from epidemics, rather than UN [United Nations] observers who merely report on the damage after the fact?"[62] Elliott's line of questioning posited public health as a space delimited by boundaries of region and nation. In this geographically and politically defined environment, interregional communication and cooperation would prove essential in preventing the spread of infectious disease across a continent whose borders were decidedly porous in terms of travel and trade. Elliott later recalled the transnational dimensions of the inquiry's subject matter:

62. Statement of Douglas Elliott, April 20, 1995, *Verbatim Transcripts of Commission*, 117:25117.

The AIDS epidemic, the blood business, the pharmaceutical business, it's all international. It's an international problem, so it points out the frailties of national systems coping with international problems. Armour Pharmaceutical can come in and sell their product in Canada, and then when something goes wrong with it, they can say, "Hey, we're in the USA. You can't get us here." When the patient zero cluster study is being done, a Canadian goes down to the United States, gives the information, but then the information doesn't flow back north. I mean it goes to anyone who needs it in the United States but it ain't goin' north of the border. This is one of the things that was highlighted for me by this whole tragedy.[63]

In the early 1980s there existed very little in terms of an official framework to allow cooperation and swift information flow, either between regions in Canada or between Canada and the United States, particularly in a response to a new disease. As the commission would learn throughout the hearings, the Canadian public health system's capabilities to respond to new infections were substantially less than that of their American neighbors. Dr. Alastair Clayton, LCDC's director general from 1979 to 1987, explained the difference to the commission: "Whilst we did the same sort of things in Canada as they did in the U.S., they were much, much larger. We were about 150 people and they were 2,000 or more I believe. And their budget I once worked out was 300 times larger than ours. So we were never able to do all the things we would like to do, and they were so often extremely helpful to us."[64] While the CDC had the staffing to redirect a team of nearly a dozen dedicated to the new disease (though admittedly on a low budget), the LCDC had only Clayton and Dr. Gordon Jessamine, the chief of the Field Epidemiology Division, as staff members with any sort of epidemiological training. According to their colleague, Dr. Richard Mathias, neither of them had any expertise, however, in "the aggressive management of communicable diseases," nor the resources to devote large amounts of time to following up what appeared at the time to be a small problem.[65]

Other sources would support the view that LCDC was not proactive

63. Elliott, September 6, 2008, recording C1491/39, tape 1, side B.

64. Testimony of Dr. Alastair Clayton, October 11, 1995, *Verbatim Transcripts of Commission*, 196:41381.

65. Additional information about the state of the Canadian public health system is drawn from Mathias, recording C1491/16, tape 1, sides A and B.

in tracking early cases. In early 1982, when asked by Nathan Fain, a health writer for the *Advocate,* to confirm CDC reports that a young man from Montreal had been diagnosed with Kaposi's sarcoma in New York City, Jessamine could only reply that no such case had been reported to him.[66] Fain wrote again in May to gain an update on the Canadian situation. Jessamine responded that, in addition to the first reported case in Canada, which was featured in the March 1982 *Canada Diseases Weekly Report,* "other information reaching us indicates that a young man with immunodeficiency (I believe) from Montreal was diagnosed in New York. I have no further details on this patient." Jessamine further noted that "lack of resources have not permitted us to follow up more intensively listings of Kaposi's sarcomata, provided to us by the Provincial Tumour Registries. This was to be undertaken, but the epidemiologist involved left us for a position with Environmental Health." With only one confirmed case and three possible ones, Jessamine wrote that "observations and conjectures volunteered on the basis of the above information, especially with regard to the transmissibility of the syndrome, would be somewhat out of line and rather unscientific." Further underlining the scarcity of funding, Jessamine concluded by assessing that "the problem in Canada is rather small (as yet identified) and it would be difficult to dissipate our rather meagre epidemiological resources when other major problems confront us continually."[67]

As it would turn out, the province of Quebec had sent the reports of its first cases directly to the US Centers for Disease Control (CDC) in Atlanta, which in time passed the information back to its Canadian counterparts at the LCDC. On this early list of Canadian patients, case number 8 was initialed "GD," though on being questioned, Alastair Clayton admitted that he did not become aware that this identification

66. Nathan Fain, "Is Our 'Lifestyle' Hazardous to Our Health? Part II," *Advocate,* April 1, 1982, 19.

67. Gordon Jessamine to Nathan Fain, 1 June 1982, folder: Fain, Nathan Correspondence, box 1, Lawrence Mass Papers, Manuscripts and Archives Division, New York Public Library. The first reported case in Canada to which Jessamine referred was a gay man in Windsor, Ontario. Reports of earlier cases surfaced in later years, including a Canadian bush pilot who worked in Zaire and died from an AIDS-like condition in 1979, and a young Haitian man visiting relatives in Canada in 1976 and 1977 who received treatment for a devastating combination of infections at a Montreal hospital; see "AIDS Killed Cdn. in '79," *Medical Post,* October 4, 1988, 59; and Richard Morisset, interview with author, Montreal, July 9, 2008, recording C1491/29, tape 1, side A, BLSA.

might signify Gaétan Dugas until reading Shilts's book many years later. Clayton explained that "we did not know who [GD] was or where he was from."[68] LCDC was hampered by its reliance on passive surveillance information sent by each of Canada's ten provinces and two territories, whose regional governments were almost wholly responsible for the provision of the country's health-care services. Physicians who diagnosed a case of a notifiable illness would send a detailed report to the local public health authority, which would then forward the information to the provincial or territorial department or ministry of health.[69] Detailed information such as name, age, sex, and relevant clinical data would be held at the regional level, but only a consolidated report that listed numbers of cases would be sent to LCDC.

Three additional complications further aggravated the ability of LCDC to coordinate reports and verify cases. First, physicians chronically underreported cases. Second, each province or territory had its own list of notifiable diseases—and in some cases, most notably that of Quebec, provinces might not send notices through the appropriate channels. Finally, although there were field epidemiologists to assist the national office, in a system patterned on the CDC Atlanta's Epidemic Intelligence Service (EIS), funding difficulties meant that there were far fewer epidemiologists to cover the country than originally envisaged. When questioned during the hearings about LCDC's minimal use of active surveillance, particularly in the period following the report of the first Canadian case in March 1982, Jessamine responded that "it is the norm in Canada. This is the way that all cases of communicable disease are notified. If we had persisted in getting direct supervision or direct notification from physicians or if we—I think the provinces would have disagreed that we were—with us, that we were invading their territory."[70]

At one stage in 1982, it appears that respect for regional autonomy, as well as a recognition of its fiscal limitations, led LCDC to abandon its national attempts to coordinate surveillance, with a request that provincial epidemiologists report any cases directly to the US CDC in Atlanta,

68. Testimony of Dr. Alastair Clayton, October 13, 1995, *Verbatim Transcripts of Commission*, 196:41787.

69. For more about the agencies involved in public health in Canada during the 1980s, see Horace Krever, "The Public Health Environment," in Krever, *Commission of Inquiry*, 1:148–62.

70. Testimony of Dr. Gordon Jessamine, October 11, 1995, *Verbatim Transcripts of Commission*, 196:41521.

copying LCDC in on the message.[71] In addition, during his testimony, Jessamine lamented the lack of seriousness with which some provincial epidemiologists were approaching the situation, as some were resisting requests to make AIDS notifiable. He claimed that one even responded, "Ah, this will be over in six weeks, we will forget about it."[72] With these aforementioned problems impeding its surveillance system, LCDC was not in a position to be a guardian of the public health system and certainly not, to return to Elliott's image, a border guard. Indeed, in the hearings, the former director general renounced the idea that his organization could be a "guardian," settling instead for a role as "monitor" of the nation's health.[73]

Regional Divisions, Professional Networks

Regional efforts show differing levels of awareness of the perceived significance of "Patient Zero" and were similarly characterized by a lack of coordination. In Toronto, public health authorities were not aware that Dugas had spent any time living within their jurisdiction. According to Clayton, a field epidemiologist affiliated with LCDC was sent to follow up with an individual with the initials "GD" reported in Toronto, but "unfortunately, she missed him by a short time and we understand that he went—because he was a flight attendant—he went off."[74] In Montreal, two infectious disease specialists who were affiliated with the city's hospitals had been alerted by Dr. Paul Wiesner, the chief of CDC Atlanta's sexually transmitted disease section, whom they knew from academic conferences, that "Patient Zero" had listed Montreal as a base. These two doctors were subsequently able to verify that Dugas had in fact been treated locally; they decided, however, that they should not pass on this information to LCDC since Wiesner had shared it in confidence.[75] This informal network might explain, however, the communica-

71. Krever, *Commission of Inquiry*, 1:197.

72. Jessamine testimony, October 11, 1995, *Verbatim Transcripts of Commission*, 196:41431.

73. Ibid., 196:41382.

74. Testimony of Dr. Alastair Clayton, October 13, 1995, *Verbatim Transcripts of Commission*, 198:41787.

75. Testimonies of Dr. Richard Morisset and Dr. Jean Robert, September 23, 1994, *Verbatim Transcripts of Commission*, 77:16534–41; refer also to the recorded interviews the

tion of early Quebec cases directly to the US CDC in Atlanta, bypassing regional authorities and Ottawa. Two regional health officials in Quebec at that time testified before the inquiry that they had not been aware that "Patient Zero" had been treated in Montreal.[76] Officials in Halifax, one of Dugas's bases while he was with Air Canada, had attempted unsuccessfully to follow up with Dugas after the flight attendant had tested positive for syphilis; they testified to the Krever commission that no one from the US CDC had contacted them regarding Dugas's status as an AIDS patient.[77] Finally, the chief epidemiologist of British Columbia testified that he had become aware "anecdotally" around January 1983 that the man "subsequently called Patient 0" was residing in British Columbia, and that "CDC Atlanta had a great deal of interest in him."[78] Although he did not specify in his testimony from which source he received the information, a journalist present at the hearings reported that a senior member of the CDC had contacted this epidemiologist, urging him to take action against the man.[79]

A chance social encounter between a US CDC official and a Vancouver doctor at an infectious disease conference held in early 1983 in Waikiki may have prompted this call. As Brian Willoughby, the Vancouver physician who cared for Dugas, later related in an interview, "And, at the meeting in Hawaii that I went to, Harold Jaffe from the CDC had been invited to speak and this was after our day of meeting we were having a cocktail party. And for what it's worth, on the twenty-seventh floor of the Hyatt Regency Waikiki, at a cocktail party, Harold Jaffe said to me: 'Oh, we have found Patient 0. He's an Air Canada steward who lives

---

author conducted with each in July 2008: Morrisset, recording C1491/29; Jean Robert, interview with the author, July 14, 2008, recording C1491/33, BLSA.

76. Testimonies of Dr. Michel Y. Pelletier and Dr. Marc Dionne, September 28, 1994, *Verbatim Transcripts of Commission*, 80:17404.

77. Testimony of Dr. Wayne Sullivan, July 27, 1994, *Verbatim Transcripts of Commission*, 60:12605–8. While testifying, this witness hesitated before divulging Dugas's sexual health information. The commissioner verified that the patient was dead before urging him to continue, with the implication that the duty of confidentiality no longer applied. See also the commissioner's earlier statement in which he opined, "It's an old problem, whether the obligation of confidentiality that is owed to a patient survives the death of the patient. That is not answered the same way in all jurisdictions, but it's an old problem"; July 14, 1994, *Verbatim Transcripts of Commission*, 56:11735.

78. Testimony of Dr. Timothy Johnstone, March 28, 1994, *Verbatim Transcripts of Commission*, 23:4272.

79. Picard, *Gift of Death,* 67.

in Montreal.' And I said 'No, no. He moved to Vancouver.' And Harold Jaffe said, 'Oh, lucky you.'"

Willoughby took from this interaction that the CDC was confident "that you could trace backwards to him, and not very well beyond him."[80] This anecdote reinforces the impression of the cluster study's significance and the role of "Patient 0" communicated by KS/OI Task Force members through 1982 and into the beginning of 1983. Taken together, the aforementioned examples illustrate the limitations of the passive surveillance system in responding to a newly emerging disease. More important, they demonstrate how informal conversations across personal and professional networks would supplement, and sometimes circumvent, the official systems in place.[81]

Although some readers might question the US CDC's decision not to share Dugas's details with its national counterparts in Ottawa, if it in fact was in communication with health workers in Montreal and Vancouver, the legislative framework for such information sharing at this time was quite limited. International conventions of the time had developed around marine shipping and travel in the late nineteenth and early twentieth centuries and not yet adapted to the speed of air travel. These conventions required reports of only cholera, plague, and yellow fever to the World Health Organization. In the context of a perceived decline of infectious disease in resource-rich nations during the mid-twentieth century, mechanisms for rapidly sharing personal health information between countries did not exist.[82] Thus, when it did move, the information often flowed through more expedient unofficial channels instead.

80. Willoughby, recording C1491/18, tape 1, side A, BLSA. Jaffe, for his part, recalled attending the meeting but not this conversation; Harold Jaffe, e-mail to author, June 9, 2016.

81. On this point, see Bayer and Oppenheimer, *AIDS Doctors*, 109–12. These examples also demonstrate the extent to which practices of sharing information relating to individuals with AIDS among health professionals has changed considerably in the intervening period; on this point see Carol Levine, "Ethics and Epidemiology in the Age of AIDS," in *Ethics and Epidemiology*, ed. Steven S. Coughlin and Tom L. Beauchamp (Oxford: Oxford University Press, 1996), 241–44. Indeed, amid concerns by persons with AIDS about their information, and in line with the codification of guidelines for AIDS research, in November 1984 Jaffe would instruct employees within the Epidemiology Section of the CDC's AIDS Branch on the importance of keeping identifiable records in locked filing cabinets and allowing only authorized CDC employees to have access to them. See Jaffe, "Records Security Procedures [/] AIDS Epidemiology Records," memo, November 19, 1984, folder: AIDS Task Force 1983–85, Darrow Papers.

82. Lorna Weir and Eric Mykhalovskiy, "The Geopolitics of Global Public Health

The emergence of HIV had shattered any perceptions of declining infectious disease risk, and many observers viewed the existing slow-moving communications channels as inadequate. Dawna Ring, a lawyer representing an HIV-infected Nova Scotia woman, advanced the view of a global "infectious disease crisis." "We are no more than 16 hours away from any part of the world," Ring noted in her final oral submissions to the inquiry. Highlighting the risks of global travel, she reminded those assembled "that patient zero, the most noteworthy person with AIDS in North America," lived in Nova Scotia "between 1978 and 1982, at the beginning of AIDS entering into our blood systems." His importance, she suggested, in an argument based more on correlation that causation, was "to show to us that we truly are a global community, and that we cannot look at the epicentres of where a disease is currently occurring and thinking that that is the only place where the disease is present." In her warning that "every small and rural community is at risk of exposure," the flight attendant's example was emblematic of the dangers of a more closely and quickly interconnected world.[83]

Defining the Importance of "Patient Zero"

During his testimony as an expert witness at the national hearings in Toronto in March 1995, Dr. Donald Francis of the US CDC was called on by the commissioner to offer a definition of the term "Patient Zero." Krever asked, "Is that simply the person who is common to a lot of peo-

---

Surveillance in the Twenty-First Century," in *Medicine at the Border: Disease, Globalization and Security, 1850 to the Present*, ed. Alison Bashford (Basingstoke, UK: Palgrave Macmillan, 2006), 240–63; David P. Fidler, "From International Sanitary Conventions to Global Health Security: The New International Health Regulations," *Chinese Journal of International Law* 4, no. 2 (2005): 325–92. These World Health Organization regulations, first named the "International Sanitary Regulations" in 1951 and later "International Health Regulations" in 1969, originally included the three aforementioned diseases, as well as smallpox, typhus, and relapsing fever. The latter two were removed from the regulations in 1969, and smallpox was removed in 1981, following its global eradication; see Gian Luca Burci and Claude-Henri Vignes, *World Health Organization* (The Hague: Kluwer Law International, 2004), 135.

83. Oral submission of Dawna Ring, December 10, 1996, *Verbatim Transcripts of Commission*, 242:49486–87; see also Tomes, "Germ Panic," 195. Ring's client, Janet Conners, had contracted the virus through sexual contact with her husband, a hemophiliac who had received HIV-infected blood products.

ple or is it the first identifiable case?" Not having been directly involved in the cluster study carried out by his colleagues, Francis ventured his own definition: "This was the individual who really served as the—at least presumed movement in this cluster of cases, and only—they were numbering cases 1, 2, 3, 4, 5, and then finally, there was this one person who was the first case in all of this that joined it together."[84] Francis smoothed over the process by which the flight attendant received his eventual designation: "Not having any number, I think they just called him Patient Zero."

The scientist later attempted to coin a back-formation for the term, relating it to the earliest spread of HIV and taking it even further from its original use as a referent for the "Out-of-California Patient":

> As far as I know, Patient Zero had no—presumably, the first case had sexual activity in Africa, and I do not know that this individual did. I—we also know that AIDS was introduced into these countries periodically and so there were other Patient Zeros that never had Patient One come from them. It was just— and we've never known the individual that brought it into—presumably into the gay bath houses in this part of the world that really allowed for the amplification of it. Then I would presume that this Patient Zero picked it up from Patient Zero Zero, and then moved it on to the subsequent ones.[85]

It seems doubtful that Francis's attempt—to link the CDC's 1982 term "Patient 0" to what had in the years since become the consensus view on the spread of HIV—clarified matters for the commission. The scientist did, however, offer a clear corrective to the media's focus on Dugas, which helped support Greyson's and Elliott's reformulated portrayals of the flight attendant: "You should make it very clear, by the way, for the Canadians, that it was his cooperation and his notebook and the cooperation with the investigators that allowed us to do the investigation. It wasn't that one Canadian spread AIDS all the way across the United States. There were lots of people doing this, a lot of them Americans.

84. Testimony of Dr. Donald Francis, March 7, 1995, *Verbatim Transcripts of Commission*, 100:21597. In a later interview, another epidemiologist ventured a more succinct definition, which indicated how the term's meaning had evolved since the 1980s: "the first person who was infected from an animal source who then transmitted it to another human." Mathias, recording C1491/16, tape 1, side A.

85. Testimony of Dr. Donald Francis, March 7, 1995, *Verbatim Transcripts of Commission*, 100:21598.

This guy just happened to be cooperative and kept a date book, and so he had people's names and so a—the investigation was possible thanks to him, not that he started AIDS in the world or the United States."[86] Francis also told the inquiry that he believed that the CDC would have complied if Canadian authorities at LCDC had requested specific information about Canadian cases of AIDS.[87]

This disclosure set the scene for Elliott's encounter with Alastair Clayton, the former head of LCDC, seven months later. Elliott had declared in a newspaper interview that "the key to unlocking the tragedy was a Canadian," who had shared his information with American authorities. "Yet Canada got no advantage in having that advance information." Clayton, Elliott later explained, was his "most important target," and he would interrogate him as to why there had not been closer communication with the Americans about Dugas and the cluster study.[88]

On October 13, 1995, on the twentieth floor of the Maclean Hunter Building, Dr. Alastair Clayton sat before a microphone at the witness stand at the front of the large room, near the desk of stoic-faced Commissioner Krever. Clayton faced five rows of lawyers and a small audience in the public seating area, as well as a TV camera capturing the proceedings for live broadcast.[89] Elliott, his inquisitor, sat at the table closest to the witness. As it turned out, Clayton proved to be a self-assured witness, seemingly thriving on the adversarial position in which—after a decade—he once again found himself with Elliott. "It would have been very difficult without a name to identify this person and to institute contact tracing unless he had come forward or unless he had been treated in Canada by a physician who would be doing these things," he explained to Elliott. "But we would not at the federal level, or even at the provincial ministerial level, know his name, nor should we have done. Your

86. Ibid.

87. Ibid., 102:21928.

88. See two articles by Ellie Tesher, "Blood Inquiry a Sorry Litany of Errors," *Toronto Star*, September 8, 1995, A2, ProQuest (1355573880); and "Blood Drama Unmasks Bland 'Stars,'" *Toronto Star*, October 13, 1995, A2, ProQuest (1357140608).

89. Timothy M. Paterson provides a rich ethnographic description of the national hearings and their physical location in the first chapter of his thesis: "Tainted Blood, Tainted Knowledge: Contesting Scientific Evidence at the Krever Inquiry" (PhD thesis, University of British Columbia, 1999), 36–37, doi: 10.14288/1.0089863. Elliott's interviews are also a useful source for the inquiry's inner workings.

organization, Mr. Elliott," he added—in a baiting manner, perhaps—
referring to ACT's early activities, "was instrumental in making sure
that confidentiality was paramount in this situation, a movement which I
applaud greatly."[90]

Presented with a witness who was skillfully deflecting his questions,
Elliott continued nonetheless: "And I am not suggesting that confidentiality ought to have been breached, Dr. Clayton, but the evidence
of Dr. Francis and I think it is borne out by the evidence from Randy
Shilts' book and from others who have known Mr. Dugas is that he was
very cooperative with public health authorities, that he was quite prepared to open up his extensive records of sexual contacts to scientific investigators in an effort to assist them in understanding this disease and
helping control its spread."[91] Clayton, meanwhile, stated that he had assumed that confidentiality reasons would have precluded such a request
and as a result did not place one.[92] As we have seen, information was difficult enough to share between provinces within a nation in the absence
of a legal framework, so the prospect of sharing specific details internationally would have appeared even more daunting and unlikely. As Clayton testified, "Those circumstances could easily be repeated again, because of the lack of names, as I have mentioned, the importance of lack
of names. Whether or not CDC should have come to us and said, 'We
have this person, this is his name, this is what he is doing[,]' I think could
be very difficult for us—for them to do and us to accept." He concluded,
"Had we been informed, we would have been very happy to try to coordinate, but it is difficult to imagine how the U.S. government would
have come to us and said, 'You have one patient whose name is so and
so, he is a flight attendant who is doing this that and the next thing.'"[93]
With his time running down, and his "most important target" maintaining his ground, Elliott relinquished his focus on "Patient Zero" and
switched to another line of questioning.

90. Testimony of Dr. Alastair Clayton, October 13, 1995, *Verbatim Transcripts of Commission*, 198:41790.

91. Elliott's cross-examination of Dr. Alastair Clayton, October 13, 1995, *Verbatim
Transcripts of Commission*, 198:41790.

92. Ibid., 41787–89.

93. Ibid., 41793.

The Efficacy of Ghosts and Blood

The Krever commission's 1,138-page final report was tabled in Canada's House of Commons on November 26, 1997. The report was deeply critical of the dysfunctional system, or, as Krever himself articulated in an interview, "the so-called 'system,' which I found was not a system at all."[94] Described by journalists as an "exhaustive chronicling of the 'unprecedented disaster,'" the report's initial section represented the first concerted effort to construct a comprehensive outline of the history of the AIDS epidemic in Canada.[95]

Chapter 10 of the *Final Report* outlined key events in the early response to AIDS in Canada. At one point it noted that Jessamine, the chief of LCDC's Field Epidemiology Division, stated in a February 1982 interview that it was "only a matter of time" before AIDS would appear in Canada. The report immediately went on to remark that Jessamine, in saying this, was unaware that "the Centers for Disease Control had recently linked a Canadian flight attendant to several cases of AIDS in New York and California. The flight attendant had travelled extensively to the gay urban centres of Canada and the United States between 1979 and 1983."[96]

Ultimately, this passage was the sole oblique reference to Dugas and the idea of "Patient Zero" in the entire report, apart from a discussion of the perceived significance of the cluster study in the United States.[97] Yet this brief mention masked a series of encounters that took place in the inquiry's hearings across the country, during which the powerful image of "Patient Zero" was brought back into public debate. More than ten years after his death, the flight attendant, dressed first by John Greyson

94. Horace Krever, interview with author, Toronto, September 10, 2008, recording C1491/46, tape 1, side A, BLSA.

95. André Picard and Anne McIlroy, "Tainted Blood Tragedy: Never Again," *Globe and Mail* [Toronto], November 27, 1997, A1.

96. Krever, *Commission of Inquiry*, 1:196. This statement, however, is inaccurate; as outlined in chapter 2, the CDC's Darrow and Auerbach did not link Dugas with other AIDS cases until later in spring 1982.

97. The *Final Report* presented the 1982 cluster study as an "important milestone" to support the theory that an infectious agent caused AIDS: Krever, *Commission of Inquiry*, 1:xxi, 185; 2:592.

and then by Douglas Elliott in a different uniform, had touched down once more in cities across Canada.

Later, when asked about Elliott's general strategy, Justice Krever suggested that "I don't think there's any question that I heard a lot about the background of gay 'communities' in Canada, Toronto and Montreal, some of which was relevant for contextual reasons, but as I said anybody with standing had a particular—I don't like the word—*agenda* that wasn't necessarily mine. That's inevitable. And the task is to see that it doesn't interfere with the Commissioner's agenda."[98] Regarding the report's brief mention of "a Canadian flight attendant," the commissioner reflected:

> It was put in because that was part of the background. That was part of the context, but it was *never significant*. In my mind, it *didn't matter*. The nature of the problem that I was inquiring didn't in any way turn on who the first person was. It was just something that was in the material, in the literature, but of no great significance. So I don't think I said, "I'm going to reduce this because of it," it was just in passing, "This is a bit of information." . . . And even if that was wrong, it didn't affect anything in the Inquiry. And the fact that even if it was right it didn't affect anything—it was just *there*.[99]

Though Krever's *Final Report* contained scarcely a reference to Dugas, Elliott's broader strategy—of gaining a foothold in the "official history" of AIDS in Canada—was more visibly successful. Krever devoted several pages of the *Final Report* to outline the history of gay activism in Canada, with accounts of discrimination and the community's fears of being scapegoated. He also provided a detailed description of community-based efforts to protect the blood system, "despite the lack of communication with, direction from, or assistance by the Red Cross."[100]

Taken together, John Greyson's *Zero Patience* and Douglas Elliott's work at the Krever inquiry demonstrate the continuing influence of Randy Shilts's construction of Gaétan Dugas as "Patient Zero" in Canada through the final pre-HAART years of the HIV/AIDS epidemic. In highly contrasting ways that point to the diversity of AIDS work dur-

98. Krever, recording C1491/46, tape 1, side B.
99. Ibid.; emphasis on recording.
100. Krever, *Commission of Inquiry*, 1:234–37 and 252–57.

ing this period, these two theatrical productions from Toronto investigated the transnational history of the epidemic, the production of historical truth, and the creation of scientific "facts." One defied classification and standardization; its postmodern delight in building then deconstructing stories and mashing ideas and genres served to challenge tidy media narratives about the disease and what a film about AIDS could and should be. It existed on the edge of establishment yet, considering its sheer inventiveness and originality, made remarkable strides into the mainstream. The other took place resolutely within the system, part of a long-established mechanism for resolving state crises and generating standardized histories. While it yielded, in the final official history, a foothold for a group that had for years been excluded to the fringes, it consigned to the briefest of mentions an individual deemed, in the end, to be "of no great significance."

Both productions bore witness: the film to the style, intelligence, and sophistication of activist groups such as ACT UP and to the very sexually active and loving gay men who had died; the inquiry, through the CAS's presence and the witnesses it brought forward, to those infected and to the efforts of the first responders to the epidemic. Both viewed the involvement of the CAS as crucial to their success in advancing a gay-friendly history of AIDS. And both mounted a sustained challenge to a singular notion of "Patient Zero" as an individual representing disease origins and deserving of blame.

One need look no further than a book published in the same year as Krever's *Final Report*, and several years in the wake of *Zero Patience*, to demonstrate the challenges faced by any attempt to rehabilitate Dugas's role as "Patient Zero." Despite displaying an apparent awareness of the blood inquiry's investigations, the authors of *The Canadian 100: The 100 Most Influential Canadians of the 20th Century* would nominate Dugas for inclusion in their book. As they explained, in Shiltsian tones, "This Canadian, in a tragic, bizarre way, had an impact on the lives of untold thousands around the world"—namely, "the thousands he directly or indirectly infected with the killer virus."[101] With a similar degree of misrepresentation, the entry for *patient zero* in *Mosby's Medical Dictionary*,

---

101. H. Graham Rawlinson and J. L. Granatstein, "79: Gaétan Dugas," *The Canadian 100: The 100 Most Influential Canadians of the 20th Century* (Toronto: Little, Brown Canada, 1997), 305, 307. The authors also misstate the year of Dugas's birth as 1953, not 1952.

the definition used as a departure point for this book, was published for the first time the following year.

In both the film and the inquiry, Gaétan Dugas featured significantly—and yet at the same time did not. Greyson's film was directly inspired by the ways in which Dugas was represented in the media as part of the production of Shilts's history; it aimed to deconstruct the misunderstandings that created this myth. Yet at the same time, the director chose to rename the ghost of the flight attendant "Zero." In the Krever inquiry, Douglas Elliott and his colleagues repeatedly questioned public officials about their knowledge of and interactions with Gaétan Dugas. However, apart from a cursory mention, this strategy did not garner the flight attendant's name a place in the commission's final report. The commissioner's silence on the issue and on the flight attendant's name—after deciding that the matter was of no great importance to the history of AIDS in Canada—demonstrated the idea's inconsequence; but it also allowed widespread allegations to smoulder away undisturbed.

Douglas Elliott deployed Dugas and the "Patient Zero" story as an index case, literally *to point* to weaknesses in the Canadian public health response to AIDS and a blood crisis, and to undermine any wholesale attempts to import and impose an American-imagined history onto Canada's past. John Greyson reimagined a fictionalized ghost of the flight attendant to critique the historical fictions put forward by Shilts and the news media. In his film, however, it was not possible for Gaétan Dugas to become visible in the limited schemes of representation available for people with HIV/AIDS in the early 1990s; in response, the flight attendant's ghost chose to disappear.

As Krever was writing the commission's final report, a revolution in treatment was transforming the HIV/AIDS landscape in North America. Exciting results presented in Vancouver at the 1996 World AIDS Conference demonstrated that HAART was proving astonishingly successful in keeping the virus under control in the bodies of those infected with it. On this treatment regimen, many patients who had previously been close to death were restored to nearly full health. With many HIV-positive individuals in North America subsequently able to live well on medication, it would appear, from one perspective, that matters had clearly moved on since the early 1990s. At that time, Greyson's ghost Zero wished to be allowed to disappear rather than be trapped within the limiting discourses about AIDS available then. Perhaps, then—at a distance of more than thirty years from the flight attendant's death in 1984—it is possible to retell a story about Gaétan Dugas that does not fall into the same traps of old?

On the other hand, critics have complained that the successes of HAART have led to the collapse of community-based organizing around HIV, in favor of same-sex marriage and family rights. This decrease in activism has, they maintain, diminished support and increased pressure on people living with HIV diagnoses: these individuals are now viewed as bearing chief responsibility for the continued existence of the epidemic. Such a focus on the visible, "irresponsible," and more easily regulated threats, as opposed to the inherently cocreated nature of sexual risk behavior and the importance of sexual health education, suggests that, in some ways, matters may not have changed significantly from the pre-HAART era.[102] Perhaps, then, it is as important as ever to revisit, by name, Gaétan Dugas's historical experience of the early AIDS epidemic. It may be true that Greyson's film demonstrates the risks in examining Dugas's experience with AIDS—any attempt to do so will be trapped by preexisting narratives surrounding the disease.[103] Yet, as the persistent misunderstandings about Dugas's role as "Patient Zero" can attest, doing nothing poses its own risks as well.

102. Whitaker, "Thirty Years of AIDS,"; Gary Kinsman, "Vectors of Hope and Possibility: Commentary on Reckless Vectors," *Sexuality Research and Social Policy* 2, no. 2 (2005): 99–105.

103. Knabe and Pearson, *Zero Patience*, 11.

CHAPTER SIX

Locating Gaétan Dugas's Views

"I am trapped in a dungeon where the guards wear white coats," he pleaded. "Please rescue me." — The character of Gaetan Dugas in *And the Band Played On*, 1987[1]

I feel like an <u>allien</u>. — *Gaétan Dugas*, 1982[2]

On a sunny but bitterly cold winter's day in late January 1982, Gaétan Dugas left his apartment in downtown Montreal to post a letter to Ray Redford, a former lover in Vancouver with whom he remained friends. As he hurried through the snow-filled streets near the city's emerging eastern gay village, Dugas may have pondered the contents of the message he was sending, in which he had reflected on his recently troubled state of health.

---

1. Shilts, *Band*, 412. Portions of the material presented in this chapter first appeared in Richard A. McKay, "Sex and Skin Cancer: Kaposi's Sarcoma Becomes the 'Stigmata of AIDS,' 1979–83," in *A Medical History of Skin: Scratching the Surface*, edited by Jonathan Reinarz and Kevin Siena, 113–27 (London: Pickering and Chatto, 2013); Richard A. McKay, "'Patient Zero': The Absence of a Patient's View of the Early North American AIDS Epidemic," *Bulletin of the History of Medicine* 88, no. 1 (Spring 2014): 161–94, published by The Johns Hopkins University Press, doi:10.1353/bhm.2014.0005.

2. Gaétan Dugas to Ray Redford, 22 January 1982, Personal Papers of Ray Redford, Vancouver (hereafter cited as Redford Papers); underline in original. For ease of reading I have quoted exactly from Dugas's letter and reproduced the original spelling and grammatical errors without marking each one with *sic*. Dugas wrote his message in an elegant cursive on the backs of three postcards (each measuring 12.8 by 19.8 cm, or about 5 by 7 inches), explaining at one point, "Ray, today is so cold again that I dear not go outside—to get some paper to write. Sorry about these little cards but you would understand if you be here."

Dugas began his letter by complimenting Redford on his attractive new partner. "Obviously all the hot men are on the West Coast. [He] Has beautiful eyes & an inviting moustache. Really Handsome!!" He continued—with words and spelling that hinted at his acquisition of English as a second language—by providing his friend with an update on his health and thanking him for his concern. "Well, my mind is finding peace again. Thank you for your encouraging letter—it is the best medicine so far.—You are right I must upgrade my attitude towards a full recoverage—but you know, there is always the storm that strike you when at least less expected."[3]

Evidently Redford had asked, in a previous letter, some questions about "gay cancer" based on an article he had read. Dugas noted that he could only have "gathered very few informations off that article," but he attributed this lack of knowledge to the generally poor level of research about the disorder: "it was writing by the only sources they had!" He added that he found taking vitamin A to be "very good, so I overdose myself everyday."[4]

Dugas thanked his friend for an invitation to visit him in Vancouver, adding, "I will hurry to grow my hair—even if you think a look better." Having shaved his head in anticipation of chemotherapy, Dugas felt self-conscious without his usually immaculately styled blond locks, a fact which compounded his altered sense of self from being sick with cancer. "I feel nude," he wrote, "& too many people turn around when I walk in the city." He added, "I feel like an allien," underlining this thought with a single stroke of his pen.[5]

Evidently, he drew a warm comfort from their correspondence. "It is always a great please to read you," Dugas confided, "and look forward to your letter." He ended the message by noting that he was waiting for the weather to improve so that he could visit his family who lived in a small community on the outskirts of Quebec City; "but as I speak to them regularly, my parents send you all their Best Wishes for this New Year! Love & Affection [/] Gaétan oxo."[6]

3. Ibid.

4. Ibid.

5. Ibid., emphasis in original.

6. Ibid. The photographs of Dugas and the quotations from his letter appear with the generous permission of his two surviving sisters. Dugas's sisters and Ray Redford have expressly asked for their privacy to be respected and for no media representatives of any kind to contact them.

"Patient Zero": The Absence of a "Patient's View"

As the previous chapters have established, much has been written about Gaétan Dugas, his sexual exploits, and his controversial refusal to obey the recommendations of public health officials in the early 1980s. Dugas, the man at the center of the "Patient Zero" story, was described by journalist Randy Shilts—and later echoed by newspapers around the world—as "the Quebeçois [sic] version of Typhoid Mary." The early date of his infection has been invoked repeatedly by his critics, who allege that, as the sexually active "Patient Zero," he must have infected a significant number of people. More than one physician accused him of being a "sociopath," and his reported refusal to give up sex—in the face of allegedly strong evidence suggesting the sexual transmissibility of an AIDS-causing agent—is still cited as proof of a profound disregard for social responsibility.[7]

In assessing the appropriateness of this judgment, however, it is worth considering how difficult it would have been to be diagnosed with a disease whose origins and mode of transmission were unclear, whose sufferers drew heavy moral condemnation, and which—as it became ominously evident—carried a high mortality rate. Furthermore, the accusations have been based on testimony that is increasingly viewed as suspect or, at the very least, one-sided. As we have seen, *And the Band Played On,* the main source for virtually all subsequent discussions of Dugas, has drawn criticism for its reliance on rumor and hearsay and for its overimaginative reconstruction of the thoughts of the people it portrays, particularly those of Dugas. Cultural theorists, including Douglas Crimp and more recently Priscilla Wald, have criticized the way by which Dugas came to be categorized as "Patient 0" by the US Centers for Disease Control (CDC) and "Patient Zero" by Shilts.[8] Crimp focused on Shilts's construction of Dugas as "the book's arch-villain," while Wald questioned the scientific validity of the evidence underlying Dugas's

7. At the 2008 Annual Meeting of the American Association for the History of Medicine, for example, the author met a psychiatrist who reported using Dugas's case in teaching as a "classic" example of sociopathic behavior, following the views of Friedman-Kien, Conant, etc.

8. Crimp, "Promiscuity," 237–71; Crimp, "Miserable Failure," 117–28; Wald, *Contagious,* 213–63.

transformation into "Patient Zero." They agreed that Shilts's portrayal of Dugas was highly problematic; both also gave favorable mention to *Zero Patience* (1993), John Greyson's agitprop musical film, discussed in chapter 5. It is worth noting that uncovering new evidence about the flight attendant's lived experience, as one of the first diagnosed cases of AIDS-related Kaposi's sarcoma (KS), was not central to Greyson's argument (nor was it a priority for Crimp or Wald). Thus, although these critics were influential in complicating the flight attendant's status as "Patient Zero," they did not add any substantially new information to the details about Dugas initially provided by Shilts in his book.

The historian Roy Porter, writing in 1984 as fears of the newly recognized epidemic took hold, acknowledged the difficulty of accessing "the patient's view" in a history of medicine focused on physicians. Nonetheless, he challenged historians to rediscover how "ordinary people in the past have actually regarded health and sickness."[9] He noted that critics of patient-focused histories would point out the methodological obstacles—namely, that it was predominantly physicians who left records, effectively rendering the patients mute.[10] Furthermore, because access to medical records is so often restricted to protect patient privacy, modern patients' voices are, in a sense, doubly muted.

Medical accounts of the AIDS epidemic have made it clear that, after several decades of growing confidence about their ability to treat infectious diseases, physicians experienced the appearance of the first recognized cases of AIDS in the late 1970s and early 1980s as a significant paradigm shift.[11] Fierce, interconnected debates ensued at both the expert and lay levels about the causes of the syndrome. These debates would characterize a period of tense uncertainty and fear that lasted until the ascendance and eventual consolidation of a new paradigm in the spring of 1984, one which held that a previously unknown retrovirus was the cause of AIDS."[12] The uncertainty that such discussions raised for members of the lay public recalls the historical example of "Typhoid Mary" Mallon, though for different reasons than Shilts's comparison im-

9. Porter, "Patient's View," 176. Porter's call has more recently been extended by the literary scholar John Wiltshire, "A Patients' History of Medicine," *Clinical Medicine* 7 (2007): 370–73.

10. Porter, "Patient's View," 182.

11. Bayer and Oppenheimer, *AIDS Doctors*, 63–64.

12. Epstein, *Impure Science*, 45–78; Brier, *Infectious Ideas*, 26–44.

plied. In her sensitive examination of the Irish American cook's life in the late nineteenth and early twentieth centuries, the historian Judith Walzer Leavitt explored the coping difficulties experienced by an individual when the terrain of scientific and medical knowledge dramatically shifted around her vantage point. Mallon faced repeated and lengthy incarcerations when the scientific and medical authorities of her day modified their way of imagining disease transmission in response to novel observations. Their new paradigm allowed for the existence of healthy carriers, capable of transmitting infections while displaying no signs of disease. This shift did not translate into Mallon's worldview, and her reluctance to concede to new public health demands left her vulnerable to demonization in subsequent historical accounts. Not surprisingly, Leavitt specifically compared the experiences of Mallon and Dugas, both being vulnerable to public health scrutiny following their identification as disease "carriers" by experts.[13] This chapter extends this comparison as it investigates a key difficulty presented by such paradigm shifts: the challenges faced by individuals whose behavior comes to be judged by a new paradigm's standards.

In this chapter I oppose the assertion that Dugas ignored incontrovertible information about AIDS and was intent on spreading his infection. The information available to him and to others between April 1982 and June 1983—the period during which his actions have faced the most scrutiny—and on which they based their decisions and actions, was far less stable, coherent, and self-evident than it was often later portrayed to be. The chapter combines interview and documentary evidence to interpret how members of several North American gay communities made sense of the threat of the condition that would become known as AIDS. Throughout, readers might ask themselves: To which sources would a gay man turn to obtain what he perceived to be reliable information about a growing risk to his health? How would he have perceived the advice of doctors and public health officials? At what stage did the threat of AIDS move from the realm of distant to present danger? And, crucially, in what theories of causation and cure might he have believed? Keeping these questions in mind is essential if we are to position Gaétan Dugas's responses to AIDS in a historically sensitive manner. A revised view emerges of Dugas's experience as a KS patient, and later as a person with AIDS, based in part on reading Shilts's research mate-

13. Leavitt, *Typhoid Mary*, 14–38, 162–201, 234–38.

rials against the grain.[14] Drawing from these notes, Shilts would suggest in his book that from March 1983 onward, Dugas's "sexual prowling had reached near-legendary proportions." He believed that the man attempted to infect others on the basis of internalized homophobia. The journalist also wrote, dismissively, "At one time, Gaetan had been what every man wanted from gay life; by the time he died, he had become what every man feared."[15] Challenging Shilts's perspective, this chapter demonstrates that, while Dugas did indeed struggle with his diagnosis and with some physicians' interventions, he also made attempts to change his behavior, was able to offer assistance to others, and maintained close contact with friends and family whom he loved. In the process, he shared much in common with other early KS patients and would, shortly after his death, be eulogized for symbolizing strength and determination in the face of adversity.

Gaétan Dugas's Early Life

Dugas was born on February 19, 1952, and adopted into a large Quebecois family living in the small town of Ancienne-Lorette, a parish roughly thirteen kilometers (about eight miles) west of Quebec City which could trace its roots to the seventeenth century. His adoptive parents hailed from farming families in the more remote Gaspé Peninsula and had moved to their new community by the mid-twentieth century.[16]

14. Porter suggested several works as exemplars to guide efforts at patient-centered histories of medicine, including Carlo Ginzburg, *The Cheese and the Worms*, trans. John Tedeschi and Anne Tedeschi (Baltimore: Johns Hopkins University Press, 1980). This "microhistory" provides an excellent example of reading evidence—in this case the inquisitorial trial records of a sixteenth-century miller accused of heresy—"against the grain" to reconstruct the worldviews of a man who would typically have been left out of the historical record. This tactic has been widely employed by postcolonial scholars as well, following a provocative and widely discussed lecture by Gayatri Chakravorty Spivak in the 1980s; see Rosalind C. Morris, ed., *Can the Subaltern Speak? Reflections on the History of an Idea* (New York: Columbia University Press, 2010), 1–7.

15. Shilts, *Band*, 251–52, 439.

16. Dugas's adoptive parents were married in 1935 in Ste-Anne-des-Monts, Quebec, and worked at the time as a day laborer ("journalier") and a domestic worker ("travaux domestiques"); Bulletin statistique de mariage no. 104443, formulaire de mariages, 1935, Bibliothèque et Archives nationales du Québec, Montreal. The 1911 Census of Canada lists several families with their surnames in the surrounding area.

In the 1950s, like today, two landmarks dominated Ancienne-Lorette: at its heart, the towering twin spires of the Notre-Dame de l'Annonciation church, and, to the southwest, an expansive airfield. Farming land and a small glove factory offered ready employment for its residents, while improving transportation links to Quebec City and gradual expansions to the airfield strengthened the town's connections to the wider world and held the prospect of growth. Following its use as an air force base and air observer school during the Second World War, the community's airfield was inaugurated as a commercial airport in late 1957.[17] The airport's increasing size helped drive the small town's development, and it seems likely that Dugas's dreams of flying, and of the wider world beyond Ancienne-Lorette, would have been stirred at a young age. By training as a hairdresser he initially followed in the footsteps of several female family members who worked in the hair and beauty profession, though the young Dugas may also have been influenced by an older brother-in-law who worked as an airman.[18] A friend later recalled him praising his family members for their steadfast acceptance of his nonconforming expressions of gender and sexuality.[19] Given his nurturing upbringing, it seems likely that Dugas would feel confident in eventually choosing a profession that married the glamour of hair and makeup with the horizon-breaking excitement of air travel.

These youthful stirrings were quite possibly further encouraged by the 1967 world's fair in Montreal, an event of international significance marking Canada's centennial year and the host city's 325th anniversary. Held between April and October, and with participation from more than sixty countries, Expo '67 set attendance records and drew more than fifty million visitors, a number more than double the host country's

17. Lionel Allard, *L'Ancienne-Lorette* (Ottawa: Éditions Leméac, 1979), 361–62. It seems that the townspeople enjoyed good relations with the international airmen who trained at the base during the war and who were remembered as "congenial and courteous young men." A record kept at the airport, possibly written by the local chaplain, pointed out the "providential" fact that the town's namesake, Notre-Dame de Lorette, was also the recognized patron saint of fliers; see "Village Founded in 1667," clipping, ca. 1945, institutional records, l'Aéroport international Jean-Lesage de Québec. The author is indebted to Claude Savard, the airport's director of safety and security, for taking the time to locate this material during a visit in December 2007.

18. I have derived this employment information from a review of marriage records compiled by Institut généalogique Drouin and accessible with a paid subscription to Genealogy Quebec, https://www.genealogiequebec.com/en/.

19. Conn, recording C1491/34, tape 1, side B, BLSA.

population.[20] Whether Dugas attended remains in the realm of speculation. However, it would seem strange if the fifteen-year-old had *not* visited the fair—one of the most significant events to take place in North
America that year—which took place less than a three-hour car journey
from his quiet hometown. Air Canada's pavilion—a distinctive structure
topped by a helix of cantilevered triangular blades rising into the sky—
was a crowd favorite, drawing regular queues and an average of nine
thousand visitors each day.[21] Visitors were guided along an artfully designed journey of darkness and light, projected slides and sixteen milli-
meter film, through a history of flight culminating in "the airplane's conquest of time and geography." The finale was a projected film sequence,
depicting Montreal as a gateway to the world and climaxing in a mosaic
of exciting travel destinations—"a colourful spectrum of simultaneous
worlds, not just to be talked or read about, but *experienced*." At a bud-
geted cost of $1.5 million, the pavilion's interior was carefully planned
to avoid any explicit advertising message for Air Canada. Yet the promotional benefits to the company were clear and even extended beyond
the aim of inspiring among visitors the desire to travel by air at a cost
within their reach.[22] As the draft for a company speech noted optimistically, "Such personal contact with compressed knowledge on air transportation may even invite visitors in seeking a career in aviation."[23] If, in
1967, the teenaged Dugas was one of the several hundred thousand visitors to pass through this celebration of the glamour, opportunity, and
adventure of mid-twentieth-century aviation, the experience could indeed have been a formative one.

Certainly, Dugas decided in his teenage years that he would become
a flight attendant, and in 1972, he took advantage of a recent federal gov-

20. Bureau International des Expositions, "1967 Montreal," accessed February 2, 2017,
http://www.bie-paris.org/site/en/component/k2/item/102–1967-montreal.

21. J. M. Jackson to P. S. Turner, 12 July 1967, folder 9000–4-1c, vol. 264, RG70–10-b,
Air Canada Expo 67 Pavilion, Air Canada fonds, Library and Archives Canada, Ottawa
(hereafter cited as Air Canada fonds).

22. Meeting minutes and attached summary of design objectives and comments of the
Air Canada Expo Committee, September 6 and 7, 1966, folder 500–3, vol. 260, RG-70–
10-b, emphasis in original document, "Comments on Pod 3"; budget outlook figures from
Expo 67 Operating Plan, folder 9000–4-1c, vol. 264, RG-70–10-b, Air Canada fonds.

23. Lillian Lancaster to Chris de Lavison, 17 February 1966; Chris de Lavison, "Notes
on Air Canada's Participation to Expo 67," p. 4, 25 February 1966; both in folder 500–8,
vol. 260, RG-70–10-b, Air Canada fonds.

ernment initiative to encourage bilingualism. This program subsidized the cost of immersion language training for Canadians wishing to learn either French or English as a second language in areas where this was the primary language spoken.[24] Because Air Canada required flight attendants working in Quebec to be able to speak both languages, Dugas traveled with a friend to Vancouver to learn English in the spring of 1972 (see fig. 6.1). Staying in dormitory residences at the University of British Columbia, he met Ray Redford, and by the end of that summer the two young men had begun an intense love affair. Redford recalled a visit to stay with Dugas's family in December of that year, which demonstrated to him how well integrated his lover was within his adopted family. Dugas tried to find work in British Columbia as a hairdresser; their relationship lasted for a couple of years until the strains of Dugas's frequent traveling and parallel romances overwhelmed it.

Following some help from Redford in the application process, Dugas was hired as a flight attendant with Air Canada in 1974. The airline had recently opened up the former "stewardess" position to male applicants, and Dugas began to travel widely. Although this appears to have doomed their relationship as lovers, Redford and Dugas would remain in touch as friends. Dugas moved frequently between bases in Canada and spent periods living in Toronto (1976–1979), Halifax (1977, 1980), Ancienne-Lorette (1980), Montreal (1981–1983), and Vancouver (1983–1984).[25] Work with Air Canada permitted him to fly to Europe, the Caribbean, and extensively across the United States. He even married a California woman in 1977, a friendly and convenient exchange which, he explained to a friend and coworker, allowed him and his wife to move with greater ease between each other's countries.[26] As another flight attendant friend

24. Matthew Hayday, "Confusing and Conflicting Agendas: Federalism, Official Languages and the Development of the Bilingualism in Education Program in Ontario, 1970–1983," *Journal of Canadian Studies* 36, no. 1 (2001): 50–79.

25. In addition to details Shilts provides in *Band*, this reconstruction is based on a review of telephone directories for these Canadian cities for the years spanning 1972–1984; Library and Archives Canada, Ottawa. No record of the flight attendant was found in the directories covering the city of Halifax and the neighboring town of Dartmouth, Nova Scotia. Nonetheless, Shilts's notes indicate that Dugas was based in Halifax in 1977 (interview with "Simon," p. 1, folder 23, box 34, Shilts Papers), and his colleague Desiree Conn recalled his presence there in 1980; Conn, recording C1491/34, tape 1, side A, BLSA.

26. Jacques Menard, interview with author, Vancouver, August 19, 2008, recording C1491/37, tape 1, side A, BLSA; marriage registry certificate, June 27, 1977, County of Los Angeles, California.

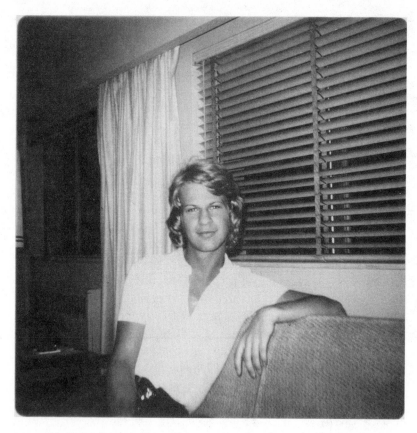

FIGURE 6.1 Gaétan Dugas in Vancouver, summer 1972; 7.7 × 7.7 cm. Scan of a photograph, which was printed from a slide original. Reproduced with permission from Ray Redford and from Richard A. McKay, who holds rights to the digital image. This candid photograph of a relaxed and confident-looking Dugas, at the age of twenty, was taken by Ray Redford at his downtown Vancouver apartment, near the beginning of their relationship.

recalled in 1986 when he was interviewed by Randy Shilts, it was "hard to keep track" of Dugas's movements, a difficulty which remains as true for later historians as it was for Shilts, and for William Darrow tracing Patient 57's travels in 1982.[27] The flight attendant thrived amid the social networking afforded by his position, and he was also able to treat family members, particularly his adoptive mother with whom he was very close, to travels beyond their regular means. Furthermore, Dugas was able to

27. "Simon," interview notes, p. 3, Shilts Papers.

take part in a gradually more visible gay culture in cities across North America. Canada's urban gay communities began to be more open and active following the 1969 decriminalization of consensual sexual acts between two adults of the same sex in private. This cultural enlivening paralleled developments south of the border, as the gay liberation movement gathered momentum.[28]

Dugas's coworkers at Air Canada fondly recalled that he had unfailing optimism, was an exceptionally hard worker, and had a delightful and mischievous sense of humor, which made him popular with passengers, to whom he delivered outstanding service. They recalled the care and attention he took to looking his best—he would joke that he was "the queen of the queens"—with perfectly applied makeup, carefully styled "Marilyn Monroe" blond hair, and a tailor-adjusted uniform that "fit him like a glove."[29] A female colleague remembered, with good-natured exasperation, that it was impossible to keep up with his insuperable energy:

I can remember doing a flight to London with him out of Toronto. And those flights went at night and you flew all night and you hauled your butt into London and got on the bus for an hour and went downtown, and usually ended up feeling like you'd been dragged through a knothole backwards, went upstairs to my room, put stuff away and got changed, came down and there was Gaétan, dressed *to the nines* [*laughing*], looking like he'd had ten hours of sleep, much better than *any of us*, his makeup was nicer [*laughing together with colleagues*] his hair was better, his clothes were nicer. We're all kind of standing there looking at each other [*colleagues laughing*] and Gaétan was on his way out on the town. And I will never forget that feeling of inferiority [*laughing together with colleagues*]. He was somebody I could never aspire to match [*colleagues laughing*]. And we'd laugh about it, like we'd say to him, "God—I can't *ever* look *that* good." [*Imitating Dugas's response:*] "Of course not, darling [*laughing*]. Why would you even try?" [*All laughing together*][30]

28. Warner, *Never Going Back*, 61–95.

29. Menard, recording C1491/37, tape 1, side B (quotations "the queen of the queens" and "fit him like a glove"); Dunn, Watson, and Miller, recording C1491/26 (discussing makeup, Dunn at tape 1, side B; Watson at tape 1, side A); Pedro Levaque, interview with author, Toronto, September 8, 2008, recording C1491/47, tape 1, side A, BLSA (describing "Marilyn Monroe" blond hair).

30. Dunn, Watson, and Miller, recording C1491/26 (Watson at tape 1, side A); emphasis on recording.

Dugas's confident, and sometimes defiant, flamboyance occasionally resulted in confrontations with conservative male pilots, for whom—in a point made by several flight attendants—non-standard displays of gender behavior were sometimes perceived as threats to their own masculinity.[31] Pedro Levaque, a roommate and fellow Air Canada flight attendant, recollected that "he was shocking in a way because he was so outrageously gay and so bluntly gay to your face." With his head-turning style and makeup, "Gaétan was flamboyant number one, you know."[32] Richard Bisson, another flight attendant, echoed this view, describing his friend as "outrageous" and "lit up from the inside."[33] Redford agreed, emphasizing that Dugas was "completely imbued with the spirit of Stonewall."[34] At work, there were complaints about Dugas wearing makeup: he borrowed mascara from female coworkers and occasionally used foundation and blush, "depend[ing] on his mood."[35] He protested to the union, however, and the company ultimately decided that, in an era of lawsuits surrounding sexual inequalities, both men and women could wear makeup if it was done well—which Dugas's always was.[36] It was not unknown for him to confront a passenger for homophobic behavior too. A colleague recalled witnessing a fiery exchange between Dugas and a businessman on one flight. When the passenger reacted to the flight attendant's "flamboyant" finger wagging with a hostile and homophobic retort, Dugas spun around, declaring, "I'm not a queer, I'm a queen."[37]

Levaque and Dugas met and became fast friends while working aboard Air Canada's Rapid Air service, which provided frequent flights linking Toronto with Montreal and Ottawa. Levaque recalled that at one point in the 1970s the two lived next to each other in an apartment building located midway between the downtown core and Toronto International Airport. During these years, Dugas also moved between apartments in Toronto's City Park complex, which was set in a burgeoning gay

31. On this point, see Phil Tiemeyer, *Plane Queer*, 68.

32. Levaque, recording C1491/47, tape 1, side B ("he was shocking . . ."); tape 2, side A ("Gaétan was flamboyant . . .").

33. Richard Bisson, interview with author, Vancouver, August 21, 2008, recording C1491/38, tape 1, side B, BLSA.

34. Redford, "Reminiscences," Epilogue.

35. Conn, recording C1491/34, tape 1, side A.

36. Dunn, Watson, and Miller, recording C1491/26 (Dunn recollection at tape 1, side B).

37. Conn, recording C1491/34, tape 1, side A.

village near the intersecting streets of Church and Wellesley. The city afforded gay men like them many locations to cruise one another for sex: at Buddy's bar, for example, in the Barracks or Club Baths, or on the lakeshore beaches of Toronto's harbor islands—in fact, as one of Dugas's acquaintances later reflected, "any place was potentially a cruising area."[38] Levaque recalled that both he and Dugas were at one point meeting up to three new partners a day. Dugas had a large sexual appetite—"more than anybody I ever met"—and was able to capitalize on his urges by being so perfectly coiffed, with a buoyant personality to match.[39] One man who had sex with the flight attendant on a number of occasions recalled Dugas's forthright nature and confidence at their first meeting. This man, a health-care professional, remembered getting dressed one day, around 1978, in the changing rooms of the downtown YMCA, situated at that time on College Street near Bay Street.[40] A young man entered, wearing a pair of minuscule shorts that were "flamboyant, even for the 1970s." He noticed the shirtless professional, walked straight up, and said, "My name is Gaétan Dugas. That's *Gay*, *Gay*-tan Dugas."[41]

As a gay male flight attendant, Dugas joined a fraternity of young, physically attractive, and fun-loving professionals whose ranks stretched around the globe. Proud of their jobs, their uniforms, and their social cachet, they often spent time together at layovers and after work.[42] One of Dugas's acquaintances remembered attending a raucous "stews' party" and seeing him in uniform, standing side by side with stewards from other airlines:

38. Levaque, recording C1491/47, tape 1, side A (discussion of Rapid Air); Macdonell, recording C1491/27, tape 2, side A (discussion of Buddy's, Barracks, Club Baths); Tivey, September 7, 2008, recording C1491/44 tape 1, side A (discussion of lakeshore beaches); Elliott, August 27, 2008, recording C1491/39, tape 1, side A (discussion of Buddy's); Elliott, August 30, 2008, recording C1491/39, tape 1, side A (discussion of lakeshore beaches), tape 1, side B (discussion of Club Baths); Jackson, recording C1491/48, tape 1, side A (quotation "any place was potentially a cruising area").

39. Levaque, recording C1491/47, tape 1, side B.

40. The YMCA building, undoubtedly the site of many instances of gay cruising like the one described here, was eventually demolished and replaced, in 1988, by the headquarters of the Toronto Police Service.

41. Health-care professional, telephone interview with author, May 18, 2011. This man made initial contact by e-mail after learning of this research project following a public lecture by the author in Toronto in April 2011.

42. Tiemeyer, *Plane Queer*, 120–21.

Oh Goddess, that was hilarious. There was like stews from every airline . . .
and it was huge—oh, booze everywhere, drugs everywhere, sex everywhere—
but the party piece was . . . more than ten stews in . . . their various different uniforms . . . all from different airlines, all doing the Boeing 747–400
safety drill in different languages choreographed all together . . . and it's
this *cacophony*, 'cause it's like Finnish, French, English, German, Spanish,
Russian—everything you can imagine, and it's all with a little bit of a *lisp*
[*laughing*].[43]

Like many other gay male flight attendants, Dugas could and did take
advantage of his occupation to meet and make closer connections with
male passengers.[44] On occasion, he might buy a customer a drink, chat
with him, and then slip him a business card on which he had written his
home phone number.[45] Some of his closer colleagues and acquaintances
recalled him speaking of sex constantly—"way too much information,
Gaétan," his friend and colleague Desiree Conn remembered joking—
and that he would refer to himself good-humoredly as "a slut."[46] One
friend explained, in an interview with Shilts, that for Dugas, "sex was a

---

43. Macdonell, recording C1491/27, tape 2, side A; emphasis on recording. Similar to
Macdonell's recollection of the flight attendant as a "party boy," Jacques Menard recalled
of Dugas, his friend and colleague, "This guy used to party *big time*." He also remembered, with a laugh, how Dugas would make light of his later hospital visits. "He would say
to us, 'I tried to get more drugs out of there but they won't give me any more.'" Menard,
C1491/37, tape 1, side A; emphasis on recording.

44. See Tiemeyer, *Plane Queer*, 120. According to their recollections, it seems that the
flight attendants who spoke with Tiemeyer recalled that they would wait for the passengers
to present *their* business cards. Dugas was, perhaps, bolder in his behavior, though Rink
Foto, a San Francisco photographer who had covered events in the lesbian and gay community since the late 1960s, also recalled occasions when flight crew members—a pilot and
a flight attendant—gave him their cards; Rink Foto, interview with author, San Francisco,
July 19, 2007, recording C1491/06, tape 1, side A, BLSA.

45. Thirty years after the flight attendant's death, a former passenger donated to Toronto's Canadian Lesbian and Gay Archives the business card that Dugas had shared with
him on a flight from Toronto to Ottawa in April 1979 (accession 2014–054). The passenger
recalled that Dugas interacted with him in just this way but that, for reasons unstated, he
never tried to telephone Dugas.

46. For example, Conn, recording C1491/34, tape 1, side A; Menard, recording C1491/
37, tape 1, side A; Rand Gaynor and Robin Metcalfe, interview with author, Halifax,
July 31, 2008, recording C1491/35, BLSA (Gaynor at tape 1, side A).

way of expressing himself. Everything was sexual—the way he looked, talked + dressed."[47]

Some physicians would later suggest that Dugas's high sexual activity was suggestive of a compulsive behavior.[48] It was not, however, outside the norms of a young urban gay male culture that was centered around commercial sex establishments in the years following gay liberation. Also, some medical practitioners took a more nuanced view of this behavior, evaluating whether it disrupted the individual's life. For example, in a book published in 1986, a New York–based psychiatrist gave an example that was strikingly similar to Dugas's case as a demonstration of well-adjusted sexual behavior: "A 31-year-old gay man has frequent, anonymous sex with other men that he meets in a park near his home, or in bars in other cities. He works as an airline steward. He enjoys living alone, traveling, and not having the responsibilities of a lover relationship. He finds that these encounters satisfy his need for sex, and his sexual style fits nicely into the overall pattern of his life."[49] While the author acknowledged that a behavior becomes compulsive when it is repeated to deal with stress in other areas of a person's life, the distinction serves as a useful reminder for the way in which a sexual compulsion was not straightforwardly indicated by a high number of sexual partners.

In summary, from the evidence emerges an image of Dugas as an attractive and charismatic young man who was sexually confident and active—and defiantly proud of being gay. He deployed a keen sense of humor to strike up friendships easily and maintained strong family ties. An eager learner, he brought a strong will to his personal and professional interests, worked hard to enjoy life's pleasures, and displayed a fierce resistance to actions he perceived to be unfair or homophobic.

47. "Simon," interview notes, p. 8, Shilts Papers.

48. For example, Conant, "Founding the KS Clinic," 166–67; Lawrence Mass, interview with author, New York, April 28, 2008, recording C1491/25, tape 2, side A, BLSA; David Ostrow, interview with author, Vienna, July 21, 2010. Said Mass: "He was a sex addict. And we didn't have those terms or concept, we had no programs, nothing in those days." Some critics, meanwhile, have maintained that depictions of people with HIV and/or AIDS often rely on a trope of "hypersexual[ity]"; see, for example, Worth, Patton and Goldstein, "Introduction to Special Issue," 7–8.

49. Ronald E. Hellman, "Facing Up to Compulsive Lifestyles," in *Gay Life: Leisure, Love, and Living for the Contemporary Gay Male*, ed. Eric E. Rofes (Garden City, NY: Doubleday, 1986), 34.

Facing "Gay Cancer"

Dugas received a KS diagnosis in May 1980 at the age of twenty-eight. The difficulty he had with this news was evident to Desiree Conn, a new coworker and friend. In the spring of 1980, immediately after her initial training course, she received her first posting to Halifax, the easternmost and smallest operations base for Air Canada. Dugas was stationed there as a purser, and the two soon flew together and became friends. While the city's small size contrasted with his usual habit of big-city living, there was a lively and well-organized gay and lesbian community, which drew men and women from across Canada's maritime provinces, and the city provided a well-located base for transatlantic flights to London.[50]

Conn recalled that one day Dugas asked her over to the house with a harbor view that he shared with a friend in nearby Dartmouth. He was scared and upset, and he smoked a large joint to calm his nerves. He confided to her that he had been diagnosed with cancer and was very frightened about dying. He had just begun to live, Dugas told her, in tears. There were so many more people in the world he wanted to meet, places he wanted to see, and he had dreams of starting his own gay airline, catering to lesbian and gay passengers hoping for grievance-free travel. Dugas had heard from colleagues that Conn had spent time caring for her father before he had died of cancer, and he wanted to learn about the types of medication that her father had received. Conn tried to reassure her friend, telling him that although her father had succumbed to his illness, there were now powerful new drugs that gave cancer patients a much greater chance of survival. She also remembered Dugas lightening the mood somewhat by repeatedly encouraging her to share his joint, which she, in turn, repeatedly declined. Soon after, Conn learned that Dugas had left Halifax and switched to another base; she recalled him mentioning during their bittersweet conversation a wish to move closer to his family and to pursue cancer treatment elsewhere.[51]

---

50. Gaynor and Metcalfe, recording C1491/35, tape 1, side A (both speaking). See also McKay, "Sex and Skin Cancer."

51. Conn, recording C1491/34, tape 1, sides A and B; tape 2, side A. Although Dugas received a Kaposi's sarcoma diagnosis that spring, his lymph nodes were also swollen, and Conn recalled him thinking that he had lymph node cancer.

Many cancer patients report profound changes in their self-identities following their diagnoses; the disease, for some, becomes "inscribed" into their life histories.[52] Dugas appears to have undergone a similar transformation from this point. He became focused on acquiring a new medical vocabulary, discovering and researching treatment options, and adjusting to the self-perceived role of "cancer patient." In the year prior to his seeking care from doctors Alvin Friedman-Kien and Linda Laubenstein in New York, Dugas had ample time to read widely, establish his own views of his disease, and resist the widespread notions of the time of cancer being a mysterious and deadly invader, one perhaps invited by patients' flawed character or their moral failures.[53]

In Vancouver, Ray Redford recalled that Dugas phoned him in the second half of 1981 to say that he was one of the gay men in New York receiving chemotherapy for "gay cancer." Redford was very worried about his ex-lover, despite reassurances from his friends "that it was not serious as it was 'only skin cancer.'"[54] His concern was echoed by one of Dugas's contemporaries in New York, who had received a KS diagnosis that June. In an interview, this man described how KS patients "share[d] a great need for psychological support . . . [and] to share our questions, our feelings and our pain." As gay men who were perhaps facing death, he emphasized what they required for recovery: "Hope, the will to live, these are important aspects of the healing process."[55] Redford would later recall how Dugas continued to draw important support from his fellow KS patients in New York.

To prepare for his own battle with cancer, Dugas shaved his head by the spring of 1981, in anticipation of the hair loss that chemotherapy would bring.[56] A studio portrait taken around that time shows a serious, soulful Dugas, with shadowed eyes staring hauntingly at the camera lens and at the viewer (see fig. 6.2). A mustached lip forms a gentle smile that is in tension with the serious expression of his eyes. Always one to lead in fashion and to poke fun at stereotypes, Dugas has his bald head boldly encircled by a thin band of leopard-print fabric—a nod to

---

52. Cynthia M. Mathieson and Henderikus J. Stam, "Renegotiating Identity: Cancer Narratives," *Sociology of Health and Illness* 17, no. 3 (1995): 302.

53. Susan Sontag, *Illness as Metaphor* (New York: Farrar, Straus and Giroux, 1978).

54. Ray Redford, "Notes for Richard McKay," document attachment in e-mail to author, October 7, 2010; see Ray Redford, "Reminiscences," Epilogue.

55. Lawrence Mass, "Cancer as Metaphor," *New York Native*, August 24, 1981, 13.

56. Ray Redford, e-mail message to author, January 7, 2008.

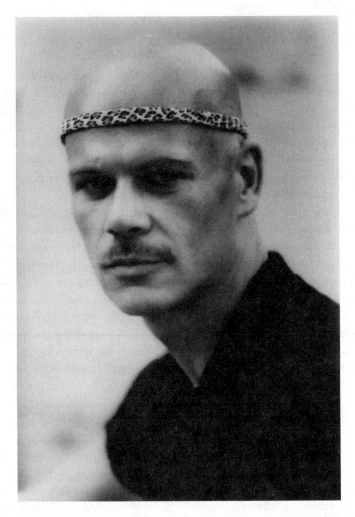

FIGURE 6.2 Gaétan Dugas, 1981; black-and-white photograph, 15.3 × 22.8 cm, scanned image e-mailed to author in January 2008, from Personal Papers of Ray Redford, Vancouver. (Every attempt has been made to locate the appropriate rights holder of this photograph of Gaétan Dugas. If you are the rights holder, or have information about this anonymous work, please contact the author so that proper attribution may be granted in subsequent editions of this book. Reproduced with permission from Ray Redford and from Richard A. McKay, who holds rights to the digital image.) Although the photograph appears to have been professionally produced, no copyright markings appear on the verso. There, according to Redford, who had received the photo in the mail, Dugas had written: "All my affection to you Ray, Gaetan [/] June 1981." It is possible that Dugas's choice of the leopard-print fabric, while representing a nod to fashion and his enjoyment of nonstandard gender displays, was also a playful reference to the spots of his Kaposi's sarcoma. It is difficult to say: the band may also have been a strategic mask for a lesion. The band's

FIGURE 6.2 (*continued*)
pattern highlights the photograph's narrow depth of field, as it travels on a gentle descent from full definition at the flight attendant's forehead to a more blurred haze by his left ear. The band's emphasis on the sphericity of Dugas's head draws support from the photographer's lighting choices, with front and rear illumination from above helping to give rounded shape and smooth texture, and to separate it from the blurred, patchy, and nondescript background. In this photograph, as in his circular representation in the cluster study diagram, Dugas occupies no discernable place. This portrait of Gaétan Dugas, confronting a cancer diagnosis, is far removed from the image of the jet-setting fun lover constructed by Shilts, a verbal image confirmed by the photograph of his tanned and muscular body, which reached millions of readers and television viewers across North America in 1987 (see figs. 4.2, 4.3, and 4.5–4.7).

the trend in animal print that was en vogue in early 1981—a daring accessory brightening the traditionally serious image of a cancer patient.[57] The seriousness of Dugas's expression hints at the challenges he would face as KS became a growing concern in North America's gay communities, amid the mounting realization that "gay cancer" was symptomatic of a far more deadly underlying condition.

Uneven Terrains of Knowledge

Stuart Nichols, a New York–based gay psychiatrist, wrote in the fall of 1982 about the urgent needs facing those who had been diagnosed with AIDS. "This illness is especially terrifying because there is little medical understanding of AIDS and no presently effective treatment for it. The emotional adjustment to such an illness goes beyond what has been described for other life-threatening diseases, even in otherwise healthy young adults, in that it frequently necessitates an immediate disruption in one's lifestyle with a loss of supportive relationships and a reliable social network." He described a support group that he ran for AIDS patients and articulated the "enormous needs for reassurance and information" that new patients felt. "They should be given straight answers, without hedging, from the medical doctors," he stated, "and if questions are not answerable, they should be told so clearly." Nichols warned that "misleading information, even slight differences of opinion among doctors, has dramatic impact among patients, intensifying panic, inflaming suspicions, and diverting valuable energy into unnecessary struggles."[58]

57. "Notes on Fashion," *New York Times*, June 16, 1981, B14.
58. Stuart Nichols, "For Patients, For Ourselves," *New York Native*, October 11, 1982, 15.

Against a backdrop of ever-shifting scientific hypotheses about the disease, health activists in lesbian and gay communities across North America raised the alarm about the serious health crisis between 1981 and 1983. Concerns about KS and the other unusual conditions affecting gay men mounted in New York City through the rest of 1981, with a concentration of cases and deaths that was initially unmatched in other cities with large gay populations. After quiet murmurings of a health problem and gradual efforts by physicians and health officials to alert gay men, San Francisco awoke to the health scare in the summer of 1982, just as the acronym "AIDS" began its ascendancy to become the preferred umbrella term for the syndrome. Though many followed these developments through the gay press and news from friends, members of Canadian gay communities in Vancouver and Toronto experienced their own more gradual awakenings in 1983. Typically, gay physicians sounded the alarm, alerted through their various professional and personal networks of developments in New York and later in San Francisco and other cities. They held community health fairs and information forums, often in concert with other community members interested in sexual health. From these initial efforts emerged local AIDS organizations which sought to offer assistance to the afflicted, raise funds to increase awareness and levels of research, and provide public education.[59] Looking back on his work to raise awareness in San Francisco, the dermatologist Marcus Conant likened his role to that of Cassandra, foretelling that "all hell's going to break loose," a message that frequently went unheeded in the early months.[60]

Many of the early efforts focused on helping physicians identify patients with KS, a relatively unknown condition, as well as other AIDS-related diseases, and to warn sexually active gay men to be careful about the partners they slept with, in case the condition was sexually transmissible. Hamstrung by a lack of research, most of the efforts focused on raising awareness and prevention, with very little practical information provided to those who were diagnosed with AIDS. In the absence of treatment, or even certainty about whether AIDS was rooted in an environmental, infectious, or genetic cause, the easiest answer to provide—

59. Silversides, *AIDS Activist*, 29–41; Epstein, *Impure Science*, 53–66.

60. Marcus Conant and Joseph Robinson, interview with author, San Francisco, July 27, 2007, recording C1491/10, BLSA (Conant quotation at tape 1, side A).

stop having sex—was often the most difficult for many people with AIDS to put into practice.[61]

Some of these individuals would lament the lack of consensus and expertise. Philip Lanzaratta was a New York man with KS who was diagnosed in October 1981, received treatment from Friedman-Kien and Laubenstein at New York University (NYU) Medical Center, and was a member of Nichols's support group. Given their shared physicians and early diagnoses, it is likely that he was among Dugas's extended network of fellow KS patients. In early 1982, Lanzaratta described the discontinuities in treatment in New York City, expressing the serious concerns he and other patients felt that, "with all the establishments and people involved," results and information were not being shared: "My feeling is that patients must ask all the questions that occur to them: What? Why? How long? Are there *alternatives*? Certainly all KS patients should realize that, along with the AID (acquired immunodeficiency) and GRID (gay-related immunodeficiency) patients, we are all white rats in one laboratory or another being tested, probed, and monitored."[62] Lanzaratta's comments, which categorized KS, AID, and GRID patients separately, indicate that the patients themselves were not convinced that their conditions were linked, a historical diversity obscured by their subsequent grouping under the AIDS umbrella from late 1982 onward. Indeed, in mid-1982 their doctors were still trying to demonstrate that the conditions were connected by a common underlying dysfunction.[63] As one friend later recalled, Dugas would distinguish his condition from those who became sick very quickly and died from pneumonia. He would say, not without reason, "I'm not like them. I don't have that."[64]

Handwritten notes that Randy Shilts recorded in 1986 indicate that Dugas had experienced fever and noticed "swollen [lymph] nodes since

61. For example, a letter to the community from Gay Men's Health Crisis and published in the *New York Native* (October 25, 1982, p. 20) summarized the information that was to be published in a future educational leaflet. It advised sick men to "PLAY FAIR YOURSELF! If you know or think or suspect that you have any disease you could give to someone else, don't risk the health of others by having sex. Wait until your doctor tells you it's safe."

62. Philip A. Lanzaratta, "Why Me?" *Christopher Street*, April 1982, 15; emphasis in original.

63. Alvin E. Friedman-Kien et al., "Disseminated Kaposi's Sarcoma in Homosexual Men," *Annals of Internal Medicine* 96, no. 6, part 1 (1982): 693–700.

64. Tivey, September 7, 2008, recording C1491/44, tape 1, side B.

Jan[uary 19]80." In May of that year, he had had a biopsy test performed on a spot by an ear, nose, and throat specialist based in Toronto. The two pages of notes in question list Montreal addresses for Dugas's residence and employer, details of his referral by a local San Francisco walk-in medical group, and his birth date and social insurance number. They indicate that in July 1981 Dugas had begun seeing dermatologist Alvin Friedman-Kien at NYU, where he had been put on a regime of VP-16 (etoposide), a common chemotherapy drug. He had tried discontinuing chemotherapy in January 1982 and promptly developed ten new lesions. By the time Dugas saw Marcus Conant—"Marc saw April 1 '82," the notes indicate—he had not experienced any *pneumocystis* pneumonia, though he had endured *Shigella* for a six-month period.[65] The early treatment regimen for KS was time-consuming and exhausting. Lanzaratta wrote of the large amounts of time devoted "to receiving chemotherapy (three days a month), weekly blood tests, shots, and an endless battery of other tests."[66] A friend of Dugas would later tell Shilts in an interview that the flight attendant in 1982 "looked terrible on chemotherapy," like "death warmed over," and that he had "lost hair [and] weight." This description accords with the self-image Dugas presented in his January 1982 letter. Nonetheless, his friend continued, Dugas's "attitude carried him through"; he was "always hopeful" and "kept saying he would beat it."[67]

Bill Darrow, the US CDC investigator, caught up with Dugas later, on April 23, 1982, when he flew to New York City to carry out further follow-up for the Los Angeles cluster study (as discussed in chapter 2).[68] As he did with all the early cluster cases, Darrow filled out the man's in-

---

65. "Gaton Dagus [*sic*]," handwritten notes, ca. 1986, 1–2, folder 23, box 34, Shilts Papers. One plausible source for these notes is Marcus Conant, the San Francisco–based dermatologist who was one of the earliest US campaigners for AIDS awareness and who saw Dugas as a patient in April 1982. However, the dermatologist emphatically denied that Shilts could have seen Dugas's patient records; Conant and Robinson, recording C1491/10 (Conant observation at tape 1, side A).

66. Lanzaratta, "Why Me?" 16.

67. "Simon," interview notes, p. 3, Shilts Papers.

68. "Trip Report—New York City, April 23, 1982," William Darrow to KSOI Task Force Chairman, memo, folder: KSOI: Cases and Contacts in New York City, Darrow Papers. Shilts reversed the order of Dugas's meetings with Darrow and Conant in *Band*, pp. 136 and 137–38.

formation onto a 3–by-5-inch card with his CDC patient number (57).[69] The card provides further details about Dugas's life, particularly about his movements in the United States. As Patient 57, Dugas reported that he had moved temporarily to New York City in 1981 for treatment, staying with a friend who lived several blocks north of Washington Square Park until February 1982. At that point, Patient 57 had moved to San Francisco, where he shared a house with a friend at the southern edge of the Pacific Heights neighborhood. The card also recorded that Patient 57 had 250 sex partners in 1979, had encounters with "blacks" and "in Europe," and confirmed sexual contact with five of the CDC's reported cases. Darrow wrote that the flight attendant was "very co-operative and will continue to help us"; indeed, the card was overflowing with information. Darrow noted that Patient 57 "consented to having his name used and picture shown to other cases."

Of particular interest to Darrow were his visits to New York City and Los Angeles, the emerging focal points for the epidemic. Dugas, as Patient 57, estimated that he had made one hundred or more overnight visits to each city since 1974, the year he began flying for Air Canada. Having drawn on colleagues and gay listings books to build a comprehensive list of gay establishments in New York, Los Angeles, and San Francisco, Darrow patiently led the man through the entries, noting any that he had attended.[70] Male, physically attractive, and white, Dugas was able to glide past the racially and physically discriminatory entrance requirements operating at many of these institutions and which drew protests during this period.[71] In New York City, he spent much of his spare time in lower Manhattan, enjoying visits to the East Village's Club Baths and the New St. Mark's Baths, the Western-themed Boots and Saddle bar on Christopher Street, and the leather-welcoming Anvil on West Fourteenth Street. He also spent many nights at the 12 West disco in Greenwich Village and in the subterranean shadows of the Mineshaft private members' sex club. In Los Angeles, Dugas's favorite nightspots were the Blue Parrot and the leather-friendly Eagle on Santa Monica Boulevard,

69. "Patient 57," cluster card [lined paper card summarizing data for patient in the cluster study], Darrow Papers.

70. William Darrow to Pauline Thomas, 25 February 1982, folder: KSOI: Cases and Contacts in New York City, Darrow Papers.

71. Clendinen and Nagourney, *Out for Good*, 494–96.

the Studio One disco on Lapeer Drive, and the city's most popular bath-house, West Hollywood's 8709 Club. Starting in February 1982, he had been spending more time in San Francisco, concentrating his attention on the Castro and Folsom Street areas. His preferred Castro hangouts were cruisy venues including the Midnight Sun, Moby Dick, and Bad-lands. He enjoyed dancing at the Haight's I-Beam disco but more fre-quently attended South of Market's Trocadero Transfer, and often ended up nearby at the Hothouse at Fifth and Harrison or in the Club Baths at Eighth and Howard.[72]

During their hour and a half meeting, Darrow avoided speaking pre-scriptively about Dugas's sexual activity. Although the investigator had written his doctoral dissertation on how using condoms reduced the spread of sexually transmissible infections among heterosexuals, he re-frained from advising Dugas on the possibility of using protection. For his work, Darrow knew that he depended on the cooperation of the gay community. He feared that by making suggestions about using con-doms—a measure associated at the time almost exclusively with birth control—he risked being ridiculed by the people with whom he needed a strong rapport. Darrow recollected of his conversation with Du-gas, "I did not tell him to change his lifestyle, his behavior. I gave him no orders. I said, 'Your life is your private life. We don't know enough now to say that it is sexually transmitted. I have to tell you we could be wrong, I could be wrong, but this is what we suspect.'" He recalled that the flight attendant was "dumbfounded" by the suggestion that his can-cer might have been caused by sex and that Dugas appeared to receive Darrow's suggestion as a moral pronouncement on his lifestyle.[73] De-spite the lack of evidence to support the theory of sexual transmission at the time, Shilts's history would later suggest that Darrow was "surprised

72. Gay establishment listings for New York, Los Angeles, and San Francisco, Case 57, folder: KSOI: Cases and Contacts in New York City, Darrow Papers. Edward Hooper also drew on these records in *The River*, 67.

73. Darrow, recording C1491/21, tape 1, side B. Dan Turner recalled to Shilts that his oncologist, Paul Volberding, had suggested in May 1982 that he begin using condoms; "Dan Turner 1-13-86," interview notes, January 13, 1986, p. 12, folder 3, box 34, Shilts Papers. In November 1982, the Southern Californian Physicians for Human Rights orga-nization was one of the earliest to recommend that gay men use condoms to decrease the transmission of viruses potentially linked to the syndrome. A more widespread discussion of condom use within the gay community took place in the spring of 1983; see Silversides, *AIDS Activist*, 31; Patton, *Inventing AIDS*, 42.

that Gaetan hadn't thought of it before," and it would be from this date that the story of his willful transmission of the virus would often be measured.[74] In contrast to Shilts's version, Darrow gave an account of this meeting to the authors of *The Truth about AIDS*—a book which Shilts used as a reference for his history. In it, the CDC official noted that the man "felt terrible" at the prospect of "having made others sick. . . . He had come down with Kaposi's but no one ever told him it might be infectious."[75] The book also quoted Dan William, a gay physician in New York, who suggested that Dugas was "living proof of the single-agent theory." William reached this view by midsummer 1982 when the evidence suggested to him that a single sexually transmissible agent was at work.[76] As we shall see, the flight attendant, like Mary Mallon decades before him, would find it difficult to give credence to a new medical theory that used his own body as its strongest evidence.

When Shilts described Dugas's confrontation with a panel of speakers at a public meeting organized by AIDS Vancouver in March 1983, he dismissed the flight attendant's reaction as "almost a textbook case of denial and anger."[77] Marcus Conant, in an interview, also suggested that this resistance to doctors' advice was denial.[78] Yet the reductive notion of denial—which implies one's resistance to accepting an obvious truth—makes little allowance for the existence of alternative views, expressed by many, of the available evidence of the time. For example, from late 1982 onward, two New York men with AIDS, who were also members of Nichols's support group, articulated a significant alternative theory to the notion that AIDS was caused by a single virus. Michael Callen and Richard Berkowitz, who copublished a popular safe-sex booklet in early 1983, were heavily influenced by the work of their physician, Dr. Joseph Sonnabend, who endorsed a multifactorial approach to disease causation. The theory suggested that the immune suppression in gay men was not caused by a new virus but by a systemic overload of sexually transmitted diseases (STDs), particularly the repeated reinfection

---

74. Shilts, *Band*, 136.

75. Fettner and Check, *Truth about AIDS*, 86; annotated copy in folder 23, box 34, Shilts Papers.

76. Dan William, "If AID Is an Infectious Disease . . . A Sexual Syllogism," *New York Native*, August 16, 1982, 33.

77. Shilts, *Band*, 247.

78. Conant and Robinson, recording C1491/10 (Conant suggestion at tape 1, side B).

of cytomegalovirus (CMV).[79] Among the theory's appealing qualities was the prospect it offered for patients to regain their weakened immune function if they reduced their exposure to infections.[80] "AIDS is a new syndrome and there are NO authorities," declared Callen and Berkowitz in a paid November 1982 advertisement in the *New York Native* for their Gay Men with AIDS group. "We believe that it is crucial for us to begin to share with others like ourselves our personal experiences in getting treatment." They urged sick men to educate themselves "by going outside the gay press. Get as broad a view and as many different opinions as possible." The advertisement also stated, in block capital letters, that "SOME IMMUNOSUPPRESSED GAY MEN WHO HAVE STOPPED INDISCRIMINATE SEX ARE BEGINNING TO SHOW SIGNS THAT THEIR IMMUNE SYSTEM IS HEALING."[81]

In an article summarizing an NYU conference on KS that took place in mid-March 1983, a journalist for the *Medical Post* reported the results of Bijan Safai, chief of dermatology at the Memorial Sloan Kettering Cancer Center, who was treating KS patients with "total skin electron beam radiation." Seventeen of his twenty patients so treated had enjoyed complete remission for forty-eight months (the other three died within four months). "Despite the ugly purple-colored tumors and extensive treatments," the journalist quoted Safai as saying, "plus a large loss in patient self-esteem once the diagnosis has been made," half of his KS patients "go back to their previous promiscuous lifestyle and acquire a new lesion."[82] Based on this summary, one can draw at least two conclusions: first, a number of men with KS in New York continued to have sex; and second, it appears that some medical practitioners viewed returning to a "promiscuous lifestyle" as being a sufficient cause for a recurrence of cancer. Following this logic, one might imagine KS patients of the time, like Dugas, finding in such studies evidence to support the immune overload theory.[83] This interpretation of the evidence, in turn,

79. Berkowitz and Callen, *How to Have Sex in an Epidemic*, 5–9.

80. Joe Wright, "'Only Your Calamity': The Beginnings of Activism by and for People with AIDS," *American Journal of Public Health* 103, no. 10 (2013): 1790.

81. Gay Men with AIDS, "A Warning to Gay Men with AIDS," *New York Native*, November 22, 1982, 16. See also Epstein, *Impure Science*, 58–66.

82. Mark Fuerst, "'Shell-Shocked' Gays Told 'Wear Condoms': Homosexual Practices Linked to Kaposi's Risk," *Medical Post*, April 19, 1983, 8.

83. For example, when interviewing gay men with AIDS in 1984, Lon G. Nungesser, who himself had KS, asked Arthur Felson how he thought he had "caught AIDS." This

could sustain the view that one's skin cancer was not contagious. By reducing one's sexual contacts and attending to other sources of immune stress, one could decrease one's own chances of a recurrence of cancer, without having to abstain from sex.

Such a perspective was moving in opposition to the growing scientific consensus that a single agent, likely a virus, caused AIDS. It was not, however, beyond the pale. In October 1983, Edward Brandt, the US Assistant Secretary of Health, inquired about this possibility to Jeffrey Koplan, the chair of the Public Health Service Executive Committee on AIDS, after having read a September supplement to the *Medical Tribune* called "Facing AIDS Today." After reviewing the article, which profiled Callen and Berkowitz and their claims of having improved their immune function after reducing their exposure to viruses and other infections, the committee's response was clear. It concluded "that the impression of clinical improvement in AIDS after lifestyle alteration is anecdotal at best and certainly affected by a desire for cure in persons with a seemingly fatal illness."[84]

Christos Tsoukas, a Montreal-based physician, also attended the NYU KS conference in March 1983 where Safai had presented his results. Two months later, Tsoukas encountered Dugas on rounds at the Montreal General Hospital. He was intrigued by Dugas's KS, the first case he had ever seen, and was struck by his patient's strongly held belief that his cancer could not be sexually transmitted. Although he acknowledged that it had not yet been proven that AIDS was caused by a virus, the physician felt sufficiently concerned to contact Linda Laubenstein, whom he had met at the NYU conference: "I was intrigued by the Kaposi's and the treatment that he was getting because we were seeing

New Yorker, who was part of an emerging person with AIDS (PWA) empowerment movement, provided a multifactorial explanation, attributing his personal health crisis to a combination of dietary, stress-related, and sexual risks, even acknowledging the possibility of a genetic component. "I believe I came down with the illness because I was a highly stressed, drug-abusing, sexually active man who was nutritionally insufficient and who was psychologically insufficient. I may have had a minimum amount of genetic predisposition." See Lon G. Nungesser, *Epidemic of Courage: Facing AIDS in America* (New York: St. Martin's Press, 1986), 6.

84. "Facing AIDS," in "Sexual Medicine Today," a supplement to *Medical Tribune*, September 14, 1983, 9–16; attachment to note from Edward Brandt to Jeffrey Koplan, October 7, 1983, and reply from Koplan to Brandt, October 19, 1983; AIDS Tracer M, folder: (1983 Sept.–Oct. FL 2 of 2), box 1, AIDS Correspondence (TRACER) archives, National Library of Medicine, Bethesda, MD.

other people with Kaposi's and I wanted to find out what was going on in New York. So I remember calling up to speak to Dr. Laubenstein, and she talked to me and then for certain things that I wanted to know she referred me to the nurses that would care for him, and the funny part was that . . . the nurses in New York nicknamed him 'The Vector.'"[85]

The nurses' reference to Dugas as an agent of transmission echoes a concern that motivated Callen and Berkowitz to develop and promote a new sexual ethics, one that emphasized a responsibility for one's own health and that of one's partners. "We must recognize," they wrote in a widely cited *New York Native* article in November 1982, "the self-hating short-sightedness involved in knowingly or half-knowingly infecting our sexual partners with disease, only to have that disease return to us in exponential form."[86] Berkowitz recalled in a memoir that they had been prompted, in part, by the attitude expressed by Philip Lanzaratta at their support group.[87] For parts of his book, Berkowitz drew on tape-recorded conversations with Michael Callen, transcripts of which can be found in Callen's archived personal papers. In one, Callen is recorded as saying, "I brought up the subject of sex and Phil Lanzaratta said yes, I still go to the baths, I worked all those years on my body and I'm still attractive, the lighting is such that there's this spot on my leg . . ." The phrase is left unfinished, but the implication is that the lesion remained unnoticed in the bathhouse's low light levels. Though describing Lanzaratta as "a complete sweetheart," Callen recalled being struck by the "coldbloodedness" of the man's reply to Callen's question about the possibility of transmission: "It's every man for himself, they've probably all got it anyway, one of them gave it to me and if they're there they're taking the same chance I took."[88] Although they were initially disturbed by Lanzaratta's remarks, Callen and Berkowitz ultimately recognized some of his sentiments in their own thinking and among many of the men who attended bathhouses. Troubled, they decided to reframe the conversation.

85. Tsoukas, recording C1491/30, tape 1, side A. See also Shilts's notes from his interview with Laubenstein: "Dr Linda," p. 2, folder 10, box 34, Shilts Papers.

86. Callen and Berkowitz, "We Know Who We Are," 29; Berkowitz and Callen, *How to Have Sex in an Epidemic*, 15.

87. Berkowitz, *Stayin' Alive*, 137–38.

88. "SONY XB-60 Microcassette—side a," p. 7, folder 250, box 9, Callen Papers.

In summary, there was a tension at play during this period, between some health workers, who were gradually becoming convinced that AIDS was caused by an as-yet-undiscovered virus, and significant numbers of gay men who wanted more proof of transmission prior to making dramatic adjustments to their lives. Many of the latter believed that making concessions before being presented with such evidence would create personal hardship and irrevocably undermine their hard-won political gains from the previous decade.

Rumors and Hostility

In July 1983, *Time* magazine noted ominously, "The AIDS reaction has its dark side. The gay culture is awash with rumors of unnamed victims who are purposely trying to infect as many others as possible."[89] This story built on a May 1983 article by Arthur Bell in New York's *Village Voice*. Bell stated, "Many AIDS victims, particularly those in advance[d] stages, literally live at the baths, not only in Manhattan, but in San Francisco and Los Angeles. In orgy rooms, dark hallways, and dimly lit cubicles, scars and lesions go undetected. The rationale (if there is one) among spreaders is 'I'm going to die anyway. I may as well go down happy.' Or worse: 'Somebody gave it to me, after all.'"[90]

Bell, in turn, had built his story, at least in part, from a remark from Richard Berkowitz, who was frustrated that the *Village Voice* refused to publish his and Callen's writing about AIDS. Berkowitz recalled, with regret, a conversation with Bell wherein he had exaggerated the motivations of men from his AIDS support group who continued to attend the baths without disclosing their health status. Hoping that he might generate more concern, he recounted, "I told Arthur Bell, and I had nothing to base it on, that there were gay men who were going to the baths because it was so dark they could have sex with people without anyone seeing their lesions. And Arthur reported it as fact [*chuckling*] in one of his columns. And I'm like, 'Oh Jesus, you know? I shouldn't have made up that little lie.' [*Speaking loudly*] *But I was so angry and frustrated that*

---

89. John Leo, "The Real Epidemic: Fear and Despair," *Time*, July 4, 1983, 58.

90. Arthur Bell, "AIDS Update: Love with the Proper Stranger," *Village Voice*, May 10, 1983, 16–17.

they wouldn't publish our writing, you know, that I wanted to do whatever I could, and I regret it. I really regret it."[91]

From mid-1982 onward, these stories circulated orally—through face-to-face interactions and telephone conversations—and more traceably in print.[92] They bore strong similarities to fears that traveled easily in much older epidemics. One flash point emerged in San Francisco between August and December 1982, as the cluster study directed attention to the possibility of a sexually transmissible agent and as the city's newly founded Kaposi's Sarcoma Foundation intensified its public-education drive. Later, as fears mounted alongside rising case numbers, echoes of these stories sounded throughout 1983, with the aforementioned examples in *Village Voice* and *Time* in the spring and summer and others in New York and San Francisco later in the autumn. As the author of one letter to the *New York Native* wrote in October 1983: "There is a rumor abroad that some known victims of AIDS, a deadly disease apparently transmitted through sexual contact, continue to engage in promiscuous sex with uninfected strangers, apparently on the theories (a) that someone else gave it to them and they're going to repay the favor (never mind that no uninfected person gave AIDS to anyone) and/or (b) they're under a death sentence so don't give a damn what happens to anybody else but need to live live live until they die."[93] Shilts also wrote a newspaper article in November 1983 about Selma Dritz's efforts to ban people with AIDS from baths. He quoted the public health official as saying, "We kept hearing through *informal community channels* that some (AIDS patients) were going to the baths." She continued, employing similar explanations for this behavior: "We can understand that they're trying to get everything they can when they have a life-threatening disease, but they shouldn't be taking other people down with them."[94]

In Canada, Gaétan Dugas would find himself surrounded by rumors

91. Richard Berkowitz, interview with author, New York City, April 25, 2008, recording C1491/24, tape 1, side B, BLSA.

92. Andrew Holleran parodied some of these telephone rumors in his semifictionalized "Journal of the Plague Year," *Christopher Street*, November 1982, 15–21. Marcus Conant recalled phoning Alvin Friedman-Kien, for example, to discuss Dugas's local attendance of San Francisco bathhouses; Conant, "Founding the KS Clinic," 167.

93. L. Craig S[c]hoonmaker, "Local 'Phobe," letter to the editor, *New York Native*, October 24, 1983.

94. Randy Shilts, "Some AIDS Patients Still Going to the Baths," *San Francisco Chronicle*, November 15, 1983, 4; emphasis added.

in Vancouver in mid-1983. In addition to focusing on this Canadian city in *Band*, Shilts referred to "a gay newspaper in Edmonton" which had, by March 1983, "written a story about an airline steward with AIDS who was popping into Alberta and screwing people in the bathhouses."[95] Moving more or less chronologically, it is worth examining some of these examples in greater detail to evaluate their reliability, from the San Francisco flash point flaring in the second half of 1982 to the available evidence for Vancouver. Before doing so, however, it is necessary to address the example Shilts cited in the Edmonton gay newspaper.

Edmonton

Fine Print, the main newspaper serving Edmonton's lesbian and gay community during this time, had a short-lived existence, with seven issues published between February and October 1983. A review of the articles and correspondence during this period reveals some of the contradictory responses of community members as they began to pay more attention to an epidemic which had appeared, until then, to be confined to other cities. Jokes about KS and herpes being the marks of social outcasts and skeptical questions wondering whether AIDS might be a "grotesque extermination plot" would give way to efforts to provide information about the condition and raise money to fight the epidemic.[96] The city would not see a reported case until July 1984, and some residents believed Edmonton was too remote and cold to be affected.[97] Fears about the risks befalling "innocent individuals" in Edmonton would be at the heart of the story Shilts cited, though the item in question was not a news article.

In July 1983, a reader's letter was published in which he shared a "matter of great concern" told to him the previous month, concerning an incident that had taken place in May. Like Defoe's fictional narrator from *A Journal of the Plague Year*, he prefaced a dark story of disease transmission with the disclaimer that it might not be true. Indeed, the letter's

95. Shilts focuses on the Vancouver rumors in *Band*, 251, and refers to the Edmonton newspaper "story" in *Band*, 247.

96. For example, Grayson Sherman, "Oh Come All Ye Faithful," *Fine Print*, February 1983, 17; Brian Chittock, "AIDS: A Case of Homophobia," *Fine Print*, April 1983, 10–11; "GATE Sponsors Informational Program on AIDS," *Fine Print*, May 1983, 21; advertisement for July 18th Calgary AIDS Benefit, *Fine Print*, July 1983, 11.

97. Testimony of Michael Phair to the Krever commission on April 21, 1994, *Verbatim Transcripts of Commission*, 34:6810.

author expressed hope that the matter was not "just a rumour"—despite the suspicious sign that the story related to a friend of friends of friends, and despite acknowledging that "serious consequences" might occur if he was repeating an untrue tale. Yet the author felt compelled to risk this possibility to share his "anger and outrage" at the incident that his friends had related to him: "Friends of theirs had an out of town visitor from Vancouver stay over this past Victoria Day weekend. He promptly told them that he was a victim of and did have AIDS. Having a friend tell you that he or she has AIDS would be difficult for anyone; however this friend also told them that as someone had given him the disease it was not going to prevent him from enjoying life. An admirable attitude for anyone who is a victim of this presently incurable disease." Having built dramatic tension, the writer rapidly switched gears: "At this point my heart went out to him, until I was told that he went out to the bars and picked someone up; and also did more than have this fellow just spend the night." The author was outraged that this man may have "knowingly passed on his unfortunate illness to an innocent victim [who might] pass it on to others unknowingly, and so on." Emphasizing the dangers posed by such a malicious infected outsider, he continued, "Right here, right now might well be the beginnings of an epidemic some months or short years in the future. From most reports this horrible disease is showing little signs of abating and one reason may be because assholes like this guy needed to get his rocks off." The writer invited readers to share his view that "this person has a disgusting, sickening attitude, one that may indeed destroy many [people's] lives. Just because someone 'gave' AIDS to him." He ended his letter bleakly, asking, "Can we survive attitudes like these from within our own community?"[98]

Although the letter's contents provide a weak substantiation of Shilts's claim—a man with AIDS from Vancouver, perhaps Dugas, may have had a (possibly unprotected) sexual contact in Edmonton—the example is more useful in other ways. At a time when concern about AIDS was rising, and when little information was known locally in the absence of AIDS cases, one can interpret the author's decision to share the rumor as fulfilling several important functions. First, by narrating his story, he could make sense of how a distant threat might affect his com-

98. Keith Dennis, "Alberta Beef," letter to the editor, *Fine Print*, July 1983, 2, 22. A review of all issues published during this journal's run from February to October 1983 revealed this letter to be the sole item resembling Shilts's cited source.

munity: through the actions of a conscienceless stranger and not, perhaps, through the existing travel patterns and contacts of local residents that might link them sexually to other, more affected areas.[99] Second, in a time of confusion, sending a letter allowed the man to channel his uncertainty into action.[100] Third, some experimental psychologists hypothesize that by telling and listening to emotionally arousing stories, individuals trigger the release of endorphins that increase their ability to withstand pain and also increase their sense of communal bonding.[101] The letter writer, like others before and after him who would share stories of whose veracity they could not be certain, could *feel* better by doing so. Not only might he gain some physical and psychological relief, but by boldly asserting his moral expectations for shared behavior, he might also feel more of a sense of closeness with his fellow community members.

San Francisco

A sample of articles and letters appearing between January and December 1982 in the *Bay Area Reporter* (*BAR*), one of San Francisco's most widely read and sensational gay newspapers of the time, illuminates a similar range of community responses to the emerging syndrome: initial dark humor giving way to uncertainty, suspicion, and fear. During this year the city would see its total reported caseload rise to nearly 120, with initially infrequent notices about KS giving rise to sustained coverage.[102] In April 1982, Arthur Evans, a gay activist who frequently wrote to the editor under the pseudonym "The Red Queen," submitted a tongue-in-cheek letter, poking fun at the newspaper's recent multipart feature article about the Cauldron, an S/M (sadomasochism) club in the city's South

99. See Diane Goldstein's discussion on the prevalence of "stranger danger" in lay beliefs about AIDS, in D. Goldstein, *Once Upon a Virus*, 159–62.

100. For a compelling example of a historian making sense of the appearance of similar rumors in diverse locations, see Wim Klooster, "Slave Revolts, Royal Justice, and a Ubiquitous Rumor in the Age of Revolutions," *William and Mary Quarterly*, 3rd ser., 71, no. 3 (2014): 401–24.

101. R. I. M. Dunbar et al., "Emotional Arousal When Watching Drama Increases Pain Threshold and Social Bonding," *Royal Society Open Science* 3 (September 21, 2016): doi: 10.1098/rsos.160288.

102. Michelle Cochrane, *When AIDS Began: San Francisco and the Making of an Epidemic* (London: Routledge, 2004), 149.

of Market area. He explained that he had been inspired to set up a separate venue, named the Hanky, specializing in "snot." Evans ended the letter with a cryptic reference to CDC investigators: "They want to ask me some questions about a Mr. Kaposi."[103] Known for writing letters that criticized members of the city's leather and S/M communities for their approaches to sexual expression, it seems that the Red Queen was also impugning them with an association with the emerging epidemic of KS and pneumonia.[104] Some members of this subcommunity responded defiantly in kind: advertisements featuring a shirtless, mustached, and muscular man in full leather gear appeared several times throughout the first half of 1982, boldly promoting "BLACK PLAGUE WEDNESDAYS" at the Boot Camp Club near 8th and Bryant.[105]

Over the next few weeks the tone shifted, from one of humorous wordplay to more anxious expressions. In May, one prominent member of the Sisters of Perpetual Indulgence, a group of gay men working to promote gay men's sexual health, offered "a sick joke" to the editor, wondering "how Doctor Kaposi feels when he sees his name in blights."[106] On June 24, a brief reference to the cluster study appeared with the headline "Infections suspected in KS, Pneumonia." A week later, an anonymous correspondent offered "some unanswered questions that need to be answered" before he could believe that "gays brought this awful disease upon ourselves by our sinful lifestyles and drugs we consume as a culture." The writer described how "the so-called Legionnaires Disease" had spread through a ventilation system, related stories of the US government's and CIA's secret chemical and biological weapons testing, and cited Fidel Castro's recent fears of American attacks using "deadly viruses and bacteria weapons." After he noticed that several local bath-

103. The Red Queen, "S'not What You Think," letter to the editor, *BAR*, April 29, 1982, 8. Evans's reference to "snot," or nasal mucus, directly parodied the Cauldron's emphasis on "piss," or urine, which was highlighted in Gary Pedler, "The Caldron Part II: Interview with the Owners," *BAR*, April 22, 1982, 14-16.

104. Hank Trout, "S & M Distinctions," letter to the editor, *BAR*, July 1, 1982, 8. For the early perceived associations between the city's leather community and AIDS, see Gayle Rubin, "Elegy for the Valley of Kings: AIDS and the Leather Community in San Francisco, 1981–1996," in *In Changing Times: Gay Men and Lesbians Encounter HIV/AIDS*, ed. Martin P. Levine, Peter M. Nardi, and John H. Gagnon (Chicago: University of Chicago Press, 1997), 101–44.

105. See, for example, *BAR*, February 25, 1982, 25; June 10, 1982, 29; and July 8, 1982, 30.

106. Sister Boom Boom, "Sis Boom Bah," letter to the editor, *BAR*, May 20, 1982, 6.

houses kept their windows closed, he explained that "certain things began to connect. If the C.I.A. had developed a virus that could break down the immunity system of the body, what unwanted or undesired group of people would they test it on? . . . Call me crazy, but first answer my questions!"[107]

By the end of the summer, weekly reports on the "gay cancer" had made KS a common term for the newspaper's readers. Considerable uncertainty remained, however, as to what caused the cancer and whether it was linked to an underlying condition of suppressed immunity.[108] When Marcus Conant spoke to an overflowing crowd at a KS information forum held at the MCC Church in early August, his remarks were summarized for *BAR*'s readers: "The doctors don't know what causes certain Gay men to have lower than normal immune levels; they don't know how Gay men catch the diseases, and they don't know how to cure them." While the newspaper granted that "Conant said the 'best guess' on Kaposi's is that it's caused by 'some transmissible agent,'" it noted that lack of funds prevented further investigation. Accompanying this news item was an article about Acquired Immune Deficiency (AID), prepared by the Gay Men's Health Crisis of New York. In answer to the question of whether the immune deficiency could be treated, it noted that there was "no certain treatment for AID [but] there are treatments for the cancers and infections to which AID predisposes."[109]

Later that month, Paul Dague, a therapist counseling patients at the University of California–San Francisco (UCSF) KS clinic, received a KS diagnosis himself. A journalist described how "the rumor spread through the Gay community faster than the disease itself: A doctor who was treating Gay victims of KS now has it!" In an interview, Dague dismissed any possibilities of contagion through casual contact, emphasizing that he only spoke with patients and did not touch them. To his mind, the evidence for the cause of his KS was "inconclusive." While he echoed the remarks of his physician, Marcus Conant, that KS was "prob-

107. Name Withheld on Request, "KS Puzzles," letter to the editor, *BAR*, July 1, 1982, 8.

108. See, for example, Richard B. Pearce, "Gay Compromise Syndrome: The Battle Widens," *BAR*, July 8, 1982, 15; Gay Men's Health Crisis, "Another Epidemic: Acquired Immune Deficiency," *BAR*, August 5, 1982, 1, 5; "Virus Linked to Cancer Outbreak in Gay Community," *BAR*, August 26, 1982, 4.

109. Gay Men's Health Crisis, "Another Epidemic," 5.

ably sexually transmitted," his interviewer immediately countered with "the truth is, Paul freely admits, 'We don't know.'"[110]

Meanwhile, in the absence of reliable information, readers expressed concerns about the sexual activities of KS patients, some of whom they could identify by their visible lesions. A letter published in mid-September 1982 related a disclosure at an August 24 forum on AIDS hosted by the city's public health department. The writer explained that Jim Geary from the Shanti Project, a support organization serving gays and lesbians with life-threatening conditions, announced "that it has been brought to his attention that KS clients are being seen at the various baths and backrooms." The letter writer urged for the newspaper to "acknowledge this information so that we attending such places can at least make an aware choice as to our possible exposure."[111] The same author published a letter the following week, criticizing as "vague" the editor's September 9 discussion of the syndrome and asked again, "If the public health department lectures can expose the fact that men with KS are being seen at the 8th & Howard baths then why don't you honor any letters with this information? The public, *e.g.* gay brothers, should be aware and make choices as to their exposures to baths and glory holes." The author also suggested that "an open letter to KS men addressing their sexuality would be helpful."[112]

Jim Geary penned a lengthy response for the following week's paper. He started by stressing the tenuous nature of the sightings, stating, "The reports that a man with Kaposi's sarcoma was seen at the baths was rumored by several sources. I know of no KS client currently served by the Shanti Project who attends the baths." He went on to point out the difficulties these men faced upon diagnosis: many doctors were advising them not to engage in any sexual interactions—even kissing—except with an ongoing partner. This strategy might protect them from further infections, yet it also "radically and painfully alters their sexual expression." He continued, "There is also speculation that acquired immunodeficiency syndrome (not Kaposi's sarcoma) may be caused from a transmissible agent. The clusters of men who have this syndrome lends support to this speculation." Here, the rapid repetition of the word *spec-*

110. Konstantin Berlandt, "KS Therapist Contracts KS: Denies Any Connection," *BAR*, August 19, 1982, 1.

111. J. Claremont, "They Shoot Horses, Don't They?" letter to the editor, *BAR*, September 16, 1982, 8.

112. J. Clar[e]mont, "Vague," letter to the editor, *BAR*, September 23, 1982, 7.

ulation suggests Geary's lukewarm assessment of this claim and lays the groundwork for his letter's shift toward a conclusion that was more in keeping with the immune overload theory. The issue, for Geary, was not what risks the men with KS might present to him but rather "what am I doing in my own life that puts my health at risk." Whereas he had previously rationalized episodes of VD with the prospect of swift treatment, he now saw the risks of this view: "I have come to understand that repeated exposure to such infections is detrimental. For me it's not as simple as getting known carriers of possibly infectious diseases out of baths but in examining my own sexual patterns and in realizing the full implications of the risks I take." Geary stated that he respected and admired the men he knew with KS, whom he counted "among the most strong, caring and socially conscious persons I know." Rather than "an open letter to persons with KS addressing their sexuality," as Claremont had suggested, Geary believed that it was "far more necessary to address such a letter to ourselves and to await our own answers."[113]

Bobbi Campbell, a local nurse who had received a KS diagnosis in October 1981 and had since been writing articles about his experience for a rival gay newspaper, applauded Geary's letter with his own a week later. He emphasized that "doctors and scientists have clues, not hard facts about AIDS," and that "if anything is transmissible, it is likely to be immune deficiency, not KS." He conveyed the most recent information that if a virus was the root cause, it was likely to be the sexually transmitted CMV, which was already common in the community. "Immune deficient persons shouldn't be socially shunned as pariahs," Campbell argued. "We have more to fear from contacts with you than you do: your minor illnesses could be serious to our weakened conditions."[114] Hank Wilson, one of the nurse's friends, would later recall that Campbell himself continued to attend the baths during this period, "all the way up until he got sick." Wilson pointed out that he did not know whether his friend "was doing X, Y, or Z in the baths"; nonetheless, the "physical presence [of people with KS] alone could get some people upset."[115]

---

113. Jim Geary, "Who Should Look at Whom," letter to the editor, *BAR*, September 30, 1982, 7.

114. Bobbi Campbell, "KS Exposure," letter to the editor, *BAR*, October 7, 1982, 10. See also J. Wright, "'Only Your Calamity,'" 1788–98.

115. Hank Wilson, interview with author, San Francisco, July 22, 2007, recording C1491/08, tape 2, side A, BLSA. Wilson died in 2008.

The autumn weeks saw further confusion and concern. One man with KS, writing on behalf of others with the disease, requested that the newspaper's writers "report the best information you can obtain, checking all facts and labeling any speculation or hearsay as such. Rumor and falsehood are nearly as dangerous to the health of our community as the diseases themselves."[116] One front-page article reported that the death rate from AIDS was much higher than previously thought, and a reader's letter advised against kissing friends "until we can rule out this as a means of transmitting the virus involved with the AIDS epidemic."[117] An October gathering of researchers at UC Medical Center received extended coverage, a journalist noting at one point that "one Gay man with Kaposi's sarcoma [was] reported to have had sexual contact with eight men who later came down with AIDS diseases"—an anonymized reference to Dugas and the LA cluster study, which also carried an implied direction of source and spread. Still, the root causes for AIDS remained undetermined; though poppers were considered less likely to be the single cause of immunosuppression, an agent transmitted through anal intercourse might also be at work, as might the antibodies produced in reaction to "sperm deposited time after time in the rectum."[118] Parasites, too, were raised by researchers and column writers as a promising lead in this rapid succession of explanations.[119] In the same November edition that carried news of the UC Medical Center conference, *BAR* editor Paul Lorch invoked ideas from Toronto's *Body Politic*, cautioning against "allowing the medical profession to define, [restrict], pathologize us."[120]

A very unusual letter from "The Fungus Queen" appeared in mid-November 1982. In a gloss, Lorch acknowledged that it was difficult to judge "where fact leaves off and fantasy takes over." The writer described a recent visit to a public sex facility where, "in the dimly lit shad-

116. Jerry Badurski, "Covering KS," letter to the editor, *BAR*, September 16, 1982, 7.

117. Wayne April, "AIDS Mortality Higher Than First Thought," *BAR*, October 14, 1982, 1; Keith Stanton, "Hugs Instead of Kisses," letter to the editor, *BAR*, October 14, 1982, 6.

118. Richard B. Pearce, "'AIDS' Topic of Local Conference: Causes, Spread, and Possible Cures Discussed," *BAR*, November 4, 1982, 2.

119. Karl Stewart, "A Full Knight," *BAR*, December 23, 1982, 29; Richard B. Pearce, "Parasites and Immune Suppression: An AIDS Connection?" *BAR*, December 30, 1982, 4.

120. Paul Lorch, "The Cast [*sic*] against Fear," *BAR*, November 4, 1982, 6; *restrict* spelled "restruct" in original.

ows," "a very pretty blond, about 30 and not much more, maybe less, reached out and held my arm for a long time it seemed, must have been three minutes or more." Suddenly, the writer realized with horror that the blond's "hands were half eaten away by athlete's foot. I broke contact and ran away to the sink, and soaped away." The Fungus Queen explained that using fungal cream on one's hands for long periods of time could lead to the body absorbing its elements, "wip[ing] out your immune system. . . . No defense, and on comes all disease and maybe lots of death too for many gay souls, and nobody knows how it happens; it's the 'Gay Disease' they say." The Fungus Queen finished sardonically: "If you're lucky, you only give the doctors lots of money and live to repeat it all again, never knowing how the vicious circle in all ignorance works, between the 'Immune Deficiency' and the 'New Gay Disease' and the masochistic pain lovers who enjoy the hot burning pain of half-eaten hands, touching hundreds each month, working for the doctors and the undertaker."[121]

This fascinating submission articulates and parodies the fear and rumors that had descended on San Francisco's gay community, by apparently acknowledging the tale of a disease-carrying blond. By invoking athlete's foot, a relatively benign condition which one might easily contract by attending bathhouses, the author may have been commenting on the extreme paranoia of the times. That being said, medical researchers at the October UC Medical Center conference had listed fungal infections as one of several types of opportunistic infections, two of which would allow a physician to diagnose AIDS.[122] The infections were also difficult for those with compromised immune systems to fight off; indeed, according to one of Dugas's friends, fungal infections were one of the reasons that Dugas would later substantially reduce his casual sexual contacts when he moved to Vancouver.[123] By suggesting that the underlying cause of this disease may have been due to the overapplication of a prescribed drug, the Fungus Queen's letter cast a net of suspicion over the medical community as well.

This climate could prove unsurprisingly hostile to people with AIDS; men with KS, whose lesions threatened to render them visible, may have

121. The Fungus Queen, "Fungus," letter to the editor, *BAR*, November 18, 1982, 8.

122. Pearce, "Local Conference," 13.

123. Noah Stewart, interview with author, Vancouver, September 3, 2007, recording C1491/19, tape 1, side B, BLSA.

felt particularly vulnerable. Paul Lorch, the editor of the *Bay Area Reporter*, wrote a lurid article in December 1982 about a twenty-nine-year-old man who hanged himself in Golden Gate Park after being diagnosed with a KS lesion in his mouth. According to Lorch's unpleasant account, for the previous year and a half the dead man "had been spending four to five nights a week at the 8th and Howard baths [where] he took on all comers and was regarded as hot sex."[124] Meanwhile, the man's suicide note, printed alongside the article in a macabre editorial decision, speaks of unbearable pain, pressure, and loneliness. "I am weak," the man wrote, "and no one to touch, to hold, to cry on." Lorch would later controversially endorse suicide as a reasonable response to an AIDS diagnosis and dismiss gay people with AIDS as offering little to their community apart from their "calamity."[125] Randy Shilts would later write of a "stranger" approaching Dugas on the streets of the Castro in the fall of 1982 and threatening him with violence if he did not choose to leave town. The man declared, "I know who you are and what you're doing."[126] By this it was implied that Gaétan was the rumored individual deliberately infecting others with his "gay cancer" in the bathhouses. But how could a stranger be certain of this, unless he felt emboldened by stories in circulation?[127]

Within this powder keg of tension, it is difficult to determine how much, if any, Dugas's actions contributed to these rumors, or whether the rumors simply stuck to Dugas because of his visible KS. It is conceivable that the rumors in San Francisco were also linked in part to the scale-up of public education in that city. In July 1982, the Kaposi's Sarcoma Research and Education Foundation set up a telephone hotline and began printing informational brochures; by November, it had distributed nearly twenty-five thousand copies of the brochure, and the office continued to be "barraged by phone calls and information requests."[128] Conant congratulated the foundation's director for his team's "excellent job" in establishing the hotline and putting on community forums, noting that these had "met with excellent success and have been responsible

124. Paul Lorch, "KS Diagnosis, Takes Life," *BAR*, December 23, 1982, 1, 15.

125. J. Wright, "Only Your Calamity," 1792.

126. Shilts, *Band*, 208.

127. It is logical to assume that if this man was a stranger, he was acting based on—at best—secondhand information.

128. "Foundation Program Activities," Rick Crane to Board of Directors, 15 November 1982, folder 10, carton 2, SFAF Records.

for identifying patients with Kaposi's sarcoma." Conant may have been mistaken, however, when he added that the foundation's efforts had succeeded in "allaying the fears and hysteria that is occurring in New York and which could so easily have occurred in San Francisco."[129]

Conant recalled being told by Frank Jacobsen, who oversaw the KS Foundation's hotline, that the phones would "*literally* light up" with callers relaying stories of a man with a French accent having sex in the city's bathhouses. According to these callers, the man would tell his partners after sex that he had gay cancer.[130] The aggregation of the hotline's call statistics into monthly totals and a complete absence of references to problematic patients with KS in the organization's records from that period prevent the interrogation of this claim. It seems possible that Dugas, not believing his KS to be contagious, might have remained quite calm if asked by a sexual partner during postcoital bathhouse conversation about one of his skin lesions. Furthermore, the erotics of bathhouse interactions often discouraged conversation before sexual contact.[131] However, to someone in Dritz's or Conant's position at that time—physicians who had been working for many months with the hypothesis of a sexually transmissible agent—such calmness could easily have been misinterpreted as an act of malice.[132]

According to Shilts, who drew a great deal of information for his book from Dritz, whom he held in high esteem, "it was one of the most repulsive things Dritz had heard in her nearly forty years in public health."[133] In a 1992 oral history interview, Dritz recalled her single encounter with the flight attendant, which Shilts dates to November 1982: "I knew that Gaetan Dugas was still in town. I couldn't get to him, but I put word out, 'If you see Gaetan Dugas, let him know I want to see him.' He came up. I

---

129. Marcus Conant to Rick Crane, 11 November 1982, folder 32, carton 2, SFAF Records.

130. Conant and Robinson, recording C1491/10 (Conant recollection at tape 1, side A), emphasis on recording; Conant, "Founding the KS Clinic," 165–67.

131. For descriptions of sexual interactions at bathhouses in New York and San Francisco in 1984, some without a verbal exchange until after physical contact, see Lucio Castigliano, "My Night at the Baths," *NYN*, January 30, 1984, 1, 21, 23; Michael Helquist and Rick Osmon, "Sex and the Baths: A Not-So-Secret Report," *Journal of Homosexuality* 44, no. 3/4 (2003): 153–75.

132. Cochrane, *When AIDS Began*, 85–86.

133. Shilts, *Band*, 200. The author's handwritten dedication in Dritz's personal copy of *Band* clearly articulates his view: "To Selma Dritz—a hero in this story"; Dritz Papers.

told him, 'Look, we've got proof now.' I didn't tell him how scientifically accurate the information was. It wasn't inaccurate, but it wasn't actually scientifically proven. I said, 'We've got proof that you've been infecting these other people. You've got AIDS, you know. We know it's transmissible now, because you're transmitting it.'"

Dugas did not believe Dritz, and she recalled that he told her to mind her own business and that he could do what he wanted with his life. She continued, recounting their exchange, "'Yes, but you're infecting other people.' 'I got it. Let them get it.' I said, 'You've got to cut it out!' 'Screw you.' He walked out. I never saw him again." Dritz conceded that Dugas was only "presumptive proof" that AIDS was "transmissible from an infected person directly to the uninfected person."[134]

It seems likely that Dugas reacted to Dritz's attempts to overstate the current evidence for transmission. In addition, he was almost certainly influenced by the strongly defiant articles emerging from his former home city of Toronto that month, published in the *Body Politic* and reprinted in the *Bay Area Reporter*. Spencer Macdonell, an acquaintance of Dugas, explained in an oral history interview the perceived threat to the flight attendant's identity:

I'm sure Gaétan heard it as probably them telling him to stop being queer, okay? Because at that time [*speaking slowly*] *that's how most fags saw themselves. Sucking dick and getting fucked is what made you queer*, and if you stopped doing that you might as well be a straight boy. And I think that was how he interpreted it and, if he threw it back in their face that was what he was throwing back in their face, you know, "No, I'm not going back in the closet for you, not for nothing."[135]

Macdonell's view finds support from a June 1983 article by writer Richard Goldstein, more than half a year after Dritz's confrontation with Du-

134. Selma E. Dritz, "Charting the Epidemiological Course of AIDS, 1981–1984," 35–36, oral history interview conducted in 1992 by Sally Smith Hughes, in *The AIDS Epidemic in San Francisco: The Medical Response, 1981–1984, Volume I*, Regional Oral History Office, Bancroft Library, University of California, Berkeley, 1995, Online Archive of California, 2009, http://content.cdlib.org/ark:/13030/kt2m3n98v1/. The author met with Selma Dritz and her daughter in 2007, a year before her death, but the effects of a stroke prevented a full interview. Her 1992 oral history interview with Hughes remains the best source.

135. Macdonell, recording C1491/27, tape 2, side A; emphasis on recording.

gas. The *Village Voice* reporter described a situation facing gay men that was every bit as challenging: "No wonder so many gay men feel caught between hysteria and paralysis. Who can distinguish fact from metaphor when the clinical data are so scant and suppositional? If one were to devise a course of action based on incontrovertible evidence alone, there would be no conclusion to be drawn. Should I screen out numbers who look like they've been around? Should I travel to have sex? Should I look for lesions before I leap? How do I know my partner doesn't have the illness in its (apparently protracted) dormant stage?" Though Goldstein's remarks were likely intended to describe the difficulties experienced by those hoping to avoid falling ill, they would have been just as valid for articulating the challenges of those who were already sick. Goldstein struggled to answer a friend who asked him, "Why can't you people just fuck less?" He ventured that "for many gay men, fucking satisfies a constellation of needs that are dealt with in straight society outside the arena of sex. For gay men, sex, that most powerful implement of attachment and arousal, is also an agent of communion, replacing an often hostile family and even shaping politics. It represents an ecstatic break with years of glances and guises, the furtive past we left behind."[136] As Goldstein's words made clear, many gay men—whether already sick or among the worried well—balked at the prospect of reducing their sexual connections, let alone abstaining from sex.[137]

Vancouver

By early 1983, and no doubt in partial response to the hostility he experienced in San Francisco, Dugas had moved to a full-time Vancouver residence. He lived downtown in a tenth-floor apartment by the ocean on Pacific Street, in the midst of the city's growing West End gay district. At this time, when so little information had been disseminated locally about the disease, Dugas represented the first person with KS whom many gay

136. Richard Goldstein, "Heartsick: Fear and Loving in the Gay Community," *Village Voice*, June 28, 1983, 12.

137. In a survey of sexually active gay men in San Francisco conducted in November 1983, researchers found that of the respondents who had three or more sexual partners the previous month, more than two-thirds agreed with the statement, "It is hard to change my sexual behavior because being gay means doing what I want sexually." See Leon McKusick, William Horstman, and Thomas J. Coates, "AIDS and Sexual Behavior Reported by Gay Men in San Francisco," *American Journal of Public Health* 75 (1985): 495.

Vancouverites would meet. He endured a great deal of fear and resentment in his new community, particularly after publicly identifying himself as a KS patient at the first public forum of AIDS Vancouver, the recently formed community-based organization, on March 12, 1983.[138]

As the evidence will show, it is difficult to determine whether Dugas attracted stories due to his particular actions, public knowledge of his illness, or his refusal to disappear from public life. Nonetheless, it seems clear that his evolving fashion preferences reinforced his outsider status. Gone were the carefully styled Marilyn Monroe locks from years past. By donning leather gear and riding a motorcycle around Vancouver, Dugas presented a more hard-edged masculinity and invoked a strong linkage to S/M culture. As the anthropologist Gayle Rubin has demonstrated, leather functioned as a cultural marker that could be read in many ways, whether to "signal merely a passion for motorcycles . . . [,] indicate an interest in sexual and social interactions among men with masculine personal styles, or announce a preference for some variety of 'kinky sex.'"[139] Since, from 1982 onward, men who wore leather were more readily associated with risky sex and AIDS, Dugas's stylistic self-presentation would have amplified any perceived risk that he posed to his communities. The recollections of one man, who sang in the Vancouver Men's Chorus, support this explicit linkage: "A friend was visiting from Toronto and Gaetan pulled up on his motorcycle. My friend, knowing my type, said to me, 'Stay away from him, there are stories in Toronto that he has some strange sickness.' Only later did I learn that he had been pegged as Patient Zero."[140]

The local gay press did not record Dugas's arguably overstated outburst at the AIDS Vancouver public meeting in March as significant at the time. Instead, the pages of the *Vancouver Gay Community Centre News* presented two articles that described the forum from opposing viewpoints.[141] The first, Fred Gilbertson's "Forum Fans Fears," argued

138. A description of this meeting can be found in Shilts, *Band*, 246–47.

139. Rubin, "Elegy for the Valley of Kings," 101–44, quotation on pp. 103–04.

140. Bill Monroe, e-mail to author, January 4, 2008. Another acquaintance who met Dugas in New York City circa 1980 linked him to men he thought "were into S and M and stuff like that"; Stewart, recording C1491/19, tape 1, side A.

141. Based on a decision taken at the February 11, 1983, AIDS Vancouver meeting, the "regular media" was not contacted in advance of the forum; see "AIDS Vancouver—February 11, 1983," in *AIDS Vancouver: Exhibits of the British Columbia Hearings, March 1994—Commission of Inquiry on the Blood System in Canada* (Ottawa: The Com-

that it had failed to answer basic questions about AIDS, and "may have done us harm . . . by exhorting us to make life style adjustments on an unproved supposition." Gilbertson made no reference to Dugas, while specifically mentioning another man by name. Greg Cutts was a gay activist and producer for *Gayblevision*, the local lesbian and gay television program, who enjoyed close connections to San Francisco and to Los Angeles, where his spouse, Troy Perry, was the spiritual leader of the Metropolitan Community Church. Cutts, Gilbertson wrote, "relentlessly pressed the panel on the number of sex partners question." The panel, observed the author, appeared to have difficulty replying with a definite answer to Cutts's questions, acknowledging that the "'infection agent' [was] an assumption. 'Last year AIDS was caused by poppers,' [Cutts reportedly said,] 'this year it is caused by promiscuity.'"[142] Clearly, Dugas was not the only one to question the motives or wisdom of the medical "experts," a fact that Shilts acknowledged but downplayed in his book.

Gilbertson's skeptical report was accompanied by a rebuttal from David Myers, who noted that "the analysis presented in the preceding article differs from most of the opinion presented by the guest speakers at the AIDS symposium." Myers included quotes from Dr. Stephen Sacks, who had outlined the apparent similarities between hepatitis B and AIDS; from Paul Popham, describing AIDS in New York City; and from Dr. Michael Maynard, who listed the following risk-reduction strategies:

1. Decrease the number of different sexual partners cutting out anonymous one-time sex.
2. Reduce the number of contacts of anal or oral-anal sex.
3. Don't get involved with someone whose health you're not sure of.
4. Do not use intravenous drugs or get involved sexually with people who do.
5. Get a lot of rest, make sure you have adequate nutrition, decrease stress, get exercise and cut down on your use of drugs, recreational or prescription.

mission, 1994), vol. 49, tab B21; copy consulted at the Sir James Dunn Law Library, Dalhousie University.

142. Fred Gilbertson, "Forum Fans Fears," *Vancouver Gay Community Centre News (VGCCN)*, April 1983, 41–43; copies of this periodical are held at the British Columbia Gay and Lesbian Archives in Vancouver. After Cutts died suddenly and unexpectedly less than three months after the AIDS Vancouver forum, a report in the *Body Politic* raised questions of suicide. See Kevin C. Griffin, "A Community Mourns BC Activist's Death," *Body Politic*, July/August 1983, 10; Nancy Wilson and Jeri Ann Harvey, "Profile: In Memorium," *Journey*, June/July 1983, 6–7, 31, https://issuu.com/mcchurches/docs/1983-june-july-journey.

Maynard was also quoted by Myers in an attempt to convince the audience of the possibility that the AIDS-causing agent—if it existed—might
spread in Vancouver. The physician noted that there was thought to be
a latency period of at least eighteen months before people would display symptoms. As quoted by Myers, Maynard stated, "We already have,
we believe, at least six people in Vancouver with AIDS. During that 18
months a person is probably contagious."[143]

Paul Popham and Bob Tivey, both of whom Shilts interviewed with
regard to this event, seem to have viewed Gaétan Dugas's conduct at the
forum as characterized by strong anger and denial. Another witness's
recollection presents a substantially different possibility, one of defiant
public disclosure to his fellow community members. Alan Herbert, who
would go on to join AIDS Vancouver and eventually served as its chair,
recalled:

> He stood up, wearing a cape, pushed forward a moveable seat in front of him
> so he could put one foot up on it, then stared at the "Five AIDS Docs" as
> they were called, and bitterly posed the question: "So I've got this disease
> you're talking about . . . what are you going to do about it." The audience of
> the West End Community Centre went silent, everyone turned to look at this
> man, "a person with AIDS"—many still called it GRID [gay related immune
> deficiency]. Of course the answer, which followed an uncomfortable silence,
> was that "there is nothing we can do for you."[144]

Readers are invited to compare these men's descriptions with video recorded that evening, segments of which were recently made available online as part of AIDS Vancouver's thirtieth anniversary activities.[145] In
the only known surviving audiovisual footage to capture Dugas, the man
speaks during the question-and-answer session with a measured, serious,

143. Quotations from Myers, Sacks, and Maynard in David Myers, "Doctors Warn
Gays," *VGCCN*, April 1983, 43–44.

144. Alan Herbert, e-mail message to author, June 5, 2008. Refer also to Alan Herbert, interview with author, Vancouver, June 11, 2008, recording C1491/28, tape 1, sides A
and B, BLSA.

145. Don Durrell, Don Larventz, and Barry Spillman, *A Gablevision Special on
A.I.D.S.*, television program first broadcast April 2, 1983 (Vancouver: Video Out Distribution, 2013), DVD. See also an edited compilation video of Dugas's questions from the *Gayblevision* broadcast, along with some of the doctors' responses: AIDS Vancouver, "30 30
AIDS Vancouver: 1983–The Forum," 2013, http://3030.aidsvancouver.org/1983/.

and sometimes pleading tone.[146] His comments repeatedly expressed his concerns about fears directed toward people with AIDS or displaying related symptoms, and, with a strong parallel to the experiences of Mary Mallon, he pressed the doctors for information on how they could confirm that someone was a "carrier."

Dugas suggested that "you shouldn't fear someone who has AIDS or has symptoms of AIDS, because there is no specific reason why you should get in contact with AIDS, with an infectious agent." Regarding people with AIDS having lovers, he asked the panel, "What is the warning you are giving to people?" He observed of the risk-reduction guidelines, "It seems like there is a kind of a fear towards those people here, that, who could have the symptom or did have the symptom, or did have the disease, you should fear those people. But," he finished tentatively, "you should, you know, not necessarily fear those people?" He asked whether, since the new hepatitis B vaccine was developed from samples donated by gay men, individuals receiving the vaccine were at risk of exposure to AIDS.[147] And he pushed for more certainty about diagnosis, asking, "If you think you may have or you could be a concerned person with AIDS, if you present yourself to doctor, what kind of test could you ask him to be undertaken in a manner to confirm if you are possibly a carrier or not?"

Popham replied that, although nothing could be proved, an infectious agent was likely involved and that if he was an AIDS patient, he would disclose his health status to any sexual partners. Sacks responded that there was "not one shred of evidence" that the vaccine might cause the syndrome. Maynard, while describing the types of tests doctors could run to test for immune function, acknowledged that there was no way to "check whether or not you've been exposed to AIDS. That test simply

146. Though this raises the possibility that some of those present later conflated Cutts's anger with Dugas's presence in their memories, one must also bear in mind that the original video may have been substantially edited before it aired on Vancouver's *Gayblevision* television show.

147. Durrell, Larventz, and Spillman, "Gablevision Special." One might interpret the question Dugas raised regarding the hepatitis vaccine as suggestive of a growing paranoia. At the same time, however, it may simply be an indication of his close attention to current debates, since from late 1982 through the middle of 1983 a number of observers had ventured the possibility of infection via this route. See, for example, Michael S. Gottlieb et al., "UCLA Conference: The Acquired Immunodeficiency Syndrome," *Annals of Internal Medicine* 99 (1983): 208–20.

does not exist."[148] Brian Willoughby, a family physician and fellow panelist, later recalled gesturing at this point to Geoff Mains, the event's moderator, to somehow remove Dugas from the microphone. If the man continued to ask the panel his "valid questions"—"for which," Willoughby acknowledged, "there were not answers"—the physician feared it would "undo any good" that the session had achieved.[149]

Following Dugas's very public announcement of his health status, Ray Redford related that, "despite being harassed by others at the bars and told that he should stay home," his friend and former lover continued to go out publicly, albeit less frequently. Redford admired Dugas's determination "to stand up for himself, to be himself. This same, fighting spirit was evident when he went to the beach and made no attempt to disguise or cover up his [KS] lesions, defiantly staring back at those who stared at him."[150] Another friend, seen walking with Dugas along Vancouver's waterfront, was later approached by a stranger and told, "You shouldn't be seen with that man. You're going to ruin your reputation. He has AIDS."[151] Bob Tivey, who became friends with Dugas through support activities with AIDS Vancouver, recalled going out for a social drink at Neighbours, a local bar, and seeing people there treat Dugas like a "pariah."[152] "People were afraid, they just got out of his way. These were other gay men *moving* when they saw him coming."[153]

Dugas's fellow flight attendant Richard Bisson remembered hearing rumors about his friend: "I heard stories around Gaétan that came from people here in Vancouver . . . [about] his behavior at the baths—you've probably already heard about that, I suspect. I had a hard time believing that . . . he was actually having sex with people despite the fact that he had been diagnosed [with] HIV. The idea seemed to be that he didn't believe that he could be contagious or that indeed their assessments were correct, that it was transmissible." Acknowledging his own uncertainty, Bisson ventured that, if his friend did continue to have sex, he attributed his actions to "being human." And, he continued, "it's like a girl getting pregnant, you know what I mean? I think it's just as much the responsi-

148. Durrell, Larventz, and Spillman, "Gablevision Special."

149. Willoughby, recording C1491/18, tape 1, side A.

150. Redford, "Reminiscences," Epilogue.

151. Kevin Brown, interview notes, 1986, p. 7, folder 23, box 34, Shilts Papers.

152. Tivey, interview notes, pp. 4–5, folder 23, box 34, Shilts Papers.

153. Tivey, September 7, 2008, recording C1491/44, tape 1, side B; emphasis on recording.

bility of the partner to take measures, so I can't really out and out blame Gaétan for that."[154]

Ultimately, such expressions of anger and discrimination may have had less to do with whether Dugas was attending bathhouses locally and more with his relatively visible presence in the gay community. Noah Stewart, a typesetter and health activist who was a founding volunteer for AIDS Vancouver, later described some of the paranoia of the time. His comments evoke the aftermath of the public forum, where worried men were encouraged to be alert to their own health and that of their sexual partners. They may have viewed a man with KS, using makeup to mask his lesions, or sharing his experiences with other local patients, as engaging in deceptive behavior aimed at evading their risk-reduction efforts: "[Was Vancouver] swirling with rumors? *Absolutely*. That Gaétan was lurking in Stanley Park, infecting people; that Gaétan was disguising himself, . . . that Gaétan was teaching people how to disguise themselves—*ridiculous* things. Just idle gay gossip, essentially. And I don't . . . think I heard any of these things more than once, from any individual. . . . It was a bunch of scared people making up stories, and I think even they realized it."[155]

Physician–Patient Conflicts

It is without question that Dugas's behavior provoked some physicians. As we have seen, in 1982 his decision to continue attending the baths clashed with Alvin Friedman-Kien and Marcus Conant, and he shared a fiery confrontation with Selma Dritz. In Vancouver, he sought treatment from at least three physicians whose practices served the city's gay male population: Michael Maynard, a founding member of AIDS Vancouver; "Dr. X," an unnamed gay physician; and finally Brian Willoughby, who, like Maynard, was also closely involved with AIDS Vancouver. Of these three, the first two doctors certainly found themselves challenged

154. Bisson, recording C1491/38, tape 1, side B.

155. Stewart, recording C1491/19, tape 1, side B; emphasis on recording. Stanley Park is a large forested urban park adjacent to downtown Vancouver. In 1983, much like today, the park was a key cruising ground for gay men and had been a site of sexual encounters for at least two generations; Macdonell, recording C1491/27, tape 1, side A. The reference to disguises is most likely an interpretation of the fact that Dugas continued to use makeup to mask the KS lesion on his nose.

by their patient, while the third was able to adopt a more sympathetic perspective.

Noah Stewart recalled that Maynard, his own physician and a man whom he considered to act with consummate professionalism, surprised him one day with a remark about Dugas. He and Maynard were discussing AIDS in Vancouver when Stewart mentioned that he had recently run into Dugas on the street. The two men recognized each other from attending the same parties in Manhattan several years previously, a period when Stewart divided his time between Toronto and New York. They stopped to talk, and it was during this conversation that Dugas had mentioned that Maynard was his doctor. As Stewart recalled, "I remember this quite well because it was the only time that [Michael] ever said an unprofessional thing in my presence. He said, 'Honest to God, I don't know what to do for the guy, but a sterile revolver is at the top of the list.' And I said 'What? What are you talking about?' And he said, 'As near as I know, this guy is the one that's spreading that disease locally.'"[156]

Evidently, Maynard believed that Dugas posed a sexual risk to other Vancouver men in Vancouver's gay community. In retrospect, this would seem to disregard the close travel links that many gay Vancouverites enjoyed with San Francisco and Los Angeles, other cities with more established epidemics.[157] At the time, however, the short hypothesized incubation period fit with Maynard's fears that his patient was largely responsible for Vancouver's emerging epidemic. Maynard's suspicions were not supported by Stewart, who recalled that "I knew every single person that had AIDS in Vancouver at that point in time, and for the most part I knew where they got it. And they didn't get it from Gaétan."[158] While on one level Stewart's statement still presupposed a short incubation period for the disease, the point remained that many gay men in Vancouver shared practices that put them at risk of becoming infected with the etiological agent for AIDS.

Evidence about the interactions between Dugas and his second Vancouver physician, "Dr. X," come from an unusual source: court decisions from 1990 and 1991 where the unnamed doctor was found guilty

156. Stewart, recording C1491/19, tape 1, side A.

157. Martin T. Schechter et al., "The Vancouver Lymphadenopathy-AIDS Study: 1. Persistent Generalized Lymphadenopathy," *Canadian Medical Association Journal* 132 (1985): 1273–79.

158. Stewart, recording C1491/19, tape 1, side A.

of professional misconduct for having sex in 1985 with a male patient, one whom he had that day diagnosed as having antibodies to AIDS.[159] According to the 1990 case record, the physician did not deny having sex with his patient but invoked an unusual historical justification for his behavior: "In 1983 Dr. X was made aware of the seriousness of the spread of AIDS when he became the Vancouver physician for Gaetan Dugas. Dr. X had tried to convince Mr. Dugas not to engage in unsafe sex, but had failed." The case record noted parenthetically that "Gaetan Dugas was the French Canadian flight attendant who is believed to have spread the AIDS virus into many cities in North America in 1983." The decision reported that "this experience had weighed heavily on Dr. X," and it worried him when in 1985 another patient tested positive and "announced that he would not practice safe sex." Apparently fearing "he might be dealing with another Mr. Dugas," the doctor argued that, through his unconventional actions, he was trying to show his patient that he would not be rejected sexually if he disclosed his status and used protection. "Further," the case record explained, Dr. X "believed that if he did not engage in sex with the complainant that evening, that the complainant would leave with the intention of concealing the fact that he was infected and inflict the virus on numerous innocent victims."[160]

At first glance, this example might read as straightforward evidence that Dugas had refused to practice safe sex in 1983. Yet one wonders how the physician could have been certain that his efforts with this man had failed. Also, the imbalance between the naming of Dugas, a dead patient and for several years an infamous public figure, and the anonymity afforded to the accused physician, is striking. In this precarious legal situation, the medical professional had every reason to emphasize the outlandishness of Dugas's historical behavior. For him to justify an extreme breach of his own professional ethics, the stakes for the extenuating circumstances needed to be exceptionally high.

Dr. X was punished for his error in judgment by being suspended from practice for a year. Maynard, too, would later stand accused of professional misconduct for having sex with his patients. Though he denied the charges, in 2003 he resigned from the British Columbia College of Physicians and Surgeons and agreed never to resume practicing medi-

---

159. X. v. College of Physicians and Surgeons of British Columbia [1990] B.C.J. no. 1316, and [1991] B.C.J. no. 2410.

160. Ibid.

cine.[161] Marcus Conant, the San Francisco dermatologist, reflected on the intense pressures faced by gay physicians within North America's gay communities during the early years of the epidemic. He recalled that "the number of young men who had AIDS who would try to seduce their doctor was legion. I mean you would have these beautiful young men who literally were saying, 'I'll do anything if you'll keep me alive.' And . . . it was a challenge for young physicians, I'm sure, to realise that this was not affection, this was not sexual interest, this was desperation."[162] Other physicians would acknowledge the blurring of professional and personal boundaries during these years, as well as the moral distancing they occasionally established between themselves and their patients to protect against their own feelings of vulnerability as gay men.[163] Though a small minority subsequently found themselves accused of abusing their positions of power, it is worth emphasizing that the period was an exceptionally difficult one for gay patients and physicians alike.

Brian Willoughby, the third Vancouver physician to take Dugas as a patient, recalled a conversation with the flight attendant near the end of summer 1983, when he realized that the man might be experiencing conflict with his current physician. Shortly thereafter, Dugas became Willoughby's patient. Reflecting on Dugas's sexual activity, whether he took precautions, and whether he advised others about the possible risks, he acknowledged that he couldn't be certain. "But I do know this, that came from a *different* patient, a patient who had sex with him, with Gaétan, and who was also my patient by then, who had been negative, and became positive in a manner that is compatible with [acquiring] it from Gaétan, although certainly he could have acquired it from someone else. As we became aware of this I reflected on some of what [I'd] heard, and thought, 'Well, gee, maybe it's true.'" And yet Willoughby recalled that both Dugas and this individual independently said that it was the latter man, not Dugas, who chose to forgo using condoms: "I'm not sure, I mean one can always fault Gaétan in that circumstance, saying, "Well you shouldn't . . ." you know? But I'm not sure how strongly I would choose to fault him, under such a situation. Because it would still have been in the timeframe when there was no absolute proof that this was

161. Pamela Fayerman, "AIDS Doctor Faces Permanent Ban: Michael Maynard Is Accused of Sexual Misconduct," *Vancouver Sun*, March 6, 2003, A1.

162. Conant and Robinson, recording C1491/10 (Conant quotation at tape 1, side A).

163. Bayer and Oppenheimer, *AIDS Doctors*, 113–18.

a virus and that this was the mode of transmission."[164] As one of Willoughby's other patients, Kevin Brown, explained to Shilts in an interview in 1986, "When you're that pretty and p[eo]pl[e] push it hard on you[,] you put some resistance but they push and push!"[165]

Willoughby remembered Dugas to have been a "bright" and "thoughtful" patient, and "very co-operative."[166] He recalled that they attempted a course of low-dose radiation therapy that succeeded in treating the KS lesion on Dugas's nose, though it left another on his arm unaffected.[167] Willoughby could not associate the patient he knew with the accounts of deliberate transmission described in Shilts's book, and he took issue with the description offered by physicians including Friedman-Kien and Conant of the flight attendant being a sociopath. Willoughby preferred instead to view Dugas's challenge as one of a patient demanding strong evidence for medical hypotheses:

> I think there would be some people who work within public health who would take his aggressive questioning of what we knew versus what we thought, and the suggestion that we should act on what we know, not what we think, to verge on being sociopathic, that I could accept. But I'm not sure that fulfills the criteria for sociopathy, and I'm not a shrink but I would bet a lot of the people who made the statement weren't psychiatrists either. And that's just their view, that this man *should* have been more cautious, and a failure to do so was sociopathic.[168]

Shifts in medical authority and a rise in patient activism in the late twentieth century would lead to physicians being challenged more than ever. In this regard, perhaps *sociopathic* is an extreme articulation of *non-*

164. Willoughby, recording C1491/18, tape 1, side A, BLSA; emphasis on recording.

165. Kevin Brown, interview notes, 1986, p. 5, folder 23, box 34, Shilts Papers.

166. Willoughby, recording C1491/18, tape 1, sides A and B.

167. Willoughby, recording C1491/18, tape 1, side A.

168. Willoughby, recording C1491/18, tape 1, side B. Willoughby's comments were echoed by a Toronto psychologist, Rosemary Barnes, who had been involved as a counselor with the AIDS Committee of Toronto (ACT) in the early 1980s. She noted that the casual application of the term *sociopath* "completely disregards" the framework in which such a diagnosis was meant to function and in some cases "it's just a way of saying something nasty about someone because you're mad about what they've done." She believed it also disregarded "other ways of understanding what might have been happening for him." Rosemary Barnes, interview with author, Toronto, September 5, 2008, recording C1491/43, tape 1, side B, BLSA.

compliant, the term most frequently used to refer to such patients. Although the term *sociopathic* is now obsolete in professional parlance, its ability to stigmatize remains strong, particularly when used by other physicians.[169]

Adjustments

Meanwhile, Dugas attempted to deal with the annoying consequences of recurrent opportunistic infections. Stewart remembered the flight attendant's propensity for taking vitamins, an immune system treatment touted throughout the gay press in the early 1980s as a possible palliative aid for AIDS patients, and a regimen adopted by other early persons with AIDS (PWAs). In addition, Dugas was having throat difficulties, and so he obtained a hand mixer to make soothing milk shakes.[170] He remained close with other members of his cohort of early "gay cancer" patients from Friedman-Kien and Laubenstein's practice and grieved on learning that one of his friends had died.[171] Returning to work for a few months beginning in summer 1983 also meant interacting with colleagues and passengers in the immediate aftermath of a widely publicized scientific article that speculated that AIDS could be transmitted through casual contact.[172] At least one colleague chose not to fly with Dugas for fear that he might be contagious or spit in passengers' food.[173] Another remembered attending a recertification session where the two had to share a mannequin to practice artificial respiration. Recalling the uncertainty over whether an AIDS-causing agent might be easily transmitted via the mannequin, the woman made sure to take her turn first.[174]

169. Jenny L. Donovan and David R. Blake, "Patient Non-Compliance: Deviance or Reasoned Decision-Making?" *Social Science and Medicine* 34, no. 5 (1992): 507–13; Jeremy A. Greene, "Therapeutic Infidelities: 'Noncompliance' Enters the Medical Literature, 1955–1975," *Social History of Medicine* 17, no. 3 (2004): 327–43.

170. Stewart, recording C1491/19, tape 1, side A. Dugas mentions that he "overdose[d]" on these in his January 1982 letter to Redford. In the absence of effective treatment, the gay press emphasized the importance of vitamins; see, for example, Donald E. Dickenson, "Your Immune System and Nutrition," *Advocate*, January 20, 1983, 33–41.

171. Redford, "Reminiscences," Epilogue.

172. See also Tiemeyer, *Plane Queer*, 180–83.

173. Female flight attendant, e-mail to author, July 19, 2008.

174. Female flight attendant to author, incident related in recording C1491/26, tape 1, side B.

For someone as socially outgoing as Dugas had been, and who valued his physical appearance, the appearance of a disfiguring KS lesion on his face was significant. One work colleague recalled that "his appearance was really important to him, and that's one of the things that was so tragic about the disease was that as soon as he started having [visible lesions] he isolated himself, he went home, he didn't stay in touch with anyone." She felt that "there were a lot of people that worked with him that would have loved to reach out and support him when he was ill, and he didn't want anyone to see him."[175] Bisson remembered the time when he discovered the lengths that his friend would feel compelled to take to conceal the lesions: "I remember helping him with his makeup at one point . . . I just said, 'You know your rouge is just a little too much here,' so I brushed it off and saw . . . what he needed to deal with . . . once this had kind of taken over." Bisson could not blame his friend for wanting to cover up his lesions with makeup. "I mean," he reflected, "everybody wants to present their best face."[176]

It seems highly likely that, in light of the negative attention he drew, Dugas experienced a sense of persecution during this time. He was being pressured to stay out of sight and away from the beaches, bars, and bathhouses that would normally have formed key parts of his social support system, not to mention being asked to abstain from the sexual activity which had for years been a key source of fulfillment.[177] Furthermore, he apparently felt that he could not escape from the CDC's apparently all-seeing gaze. This sense of feeling tracked by the CDC was likely compounded when members of the organization contacted him to arrange a plasma donation in summer 1983.[178] Stewart recalled that "the CDC

175. Dunn, Watson, and Miller, recording C1491/26 (Watson quoted at tape 1, side A). Dugas's friend and colleague, Desiree Conn, had a similar recollection about another Air Canada flight attendant with visible KS lesions. She suggested that he and Dugas may have been "very, very self-conscious of it, and they didn't want anybody to see them like that because they were such good-looking men"; Conn, recording C1491/34, tape 1, side A.

176. Bisson, recording C1491/38, tape 1, side A.

177. Gaynor and Metcalfe, recording C1491/35 (observation made by Gaynor at tape 1, side A); Levaque, recording C1491/47, tape 1, side B.

178. In finalizing the Worobey et al. collaborative *Nature* paper in 2016, it became apparent that Shilts had provided a misleading date for this donation, which he included with events from May 1982; *Band*, 157. The journalist's notes from his interview with Harry Haverkos illuminate the source of this error, which points to a vulnerability of the journalist's data-gathering approach, one which was heavily reliant on interviews. The CDC investigator initially mentioned "Patient Zero" in the context of the challenges scientists faced

scared him. They were acting like he was Typhoid Mary . . . that's what I gathered from how he felt about it, and he didn't want anything further to do with them. He wanted to live in Vancouver, he wanted to be quiet, and the thing is that he was not cutting a sexual swath through the local population. That is *just not true*."[179]

There is evidence to suggest that the flight attendant substantially curtailed his sexual activity while in Vancouver. Stewart contended that Dugas slowed down over time, echoing the guidance that someone with a compromised immune system had more to fear from a casual liaison than his healthy partner:

> Gaétan was aware that if he had sex with strangers he would pick up opportunistic infections that would be dangerous to himself. And that's not a big stretch right? Like . . . if you keep coming down with thrush . . . sooner or later you put two and two together and you think, "Well, Christ, you know, I had five guys at the tubs last night, maybe that has something to do with it." And he was sick and tired of being treated for opportunistic infections. It's not fun. . . . We were the generation that if you got the clap, well, you know, that was just a series of shots, and you had to possibly restrict yourself for six weeks but, the stuff that he was dealing with was not the clap, you know, it was worse and more annoying—like fungal infections in your toenails and stuff like that. He just got sick of dealing with it, and he just essentially stopped doing that stuff.[180]

In an unofficial capacity, Stewart also assisted Dugas's efforts to redirect his sexual energy with the use of a new technological development: the videocassette recorder. Prices had dropped sufficiently in recent years to make this technology newly affordable for the general public. This shift also opened up a new market for pornographic home videotapes. Stewart recognized that it would likely be difficult for people with AIDS to face being denied any sexual outlet, and he encour-

---

in establishing viable cultures of virus—"trying to grow LAV"—in late 1983 and early 1984. Haverkos then moved backwards in time, briefly, to 1982 to provide context about the Los Angeles cluster study, before continuing with his account of the man's later plasma donation. Shilts did not catch this time switch as he wrote his notes; "Harry Haverkos," interview notes, p. 4, folder 29, box 33, Shilts Papers.

179. Stewart, recording C1491/19, tape 1, side A; emphasis on recording.

180. Stewart, recording C1491/19, tape 1, side B.

aged Dugas's pornography consumption by loaning him his own video-tapes. Stewart then provided this service to later PWAs through AIDS Vancouver, all as part of a multifaceted approach to reducing casual sex and the possible chance of transmission. In this regard, too, Dugas was like other early men with AIDS, looking for creative ways to find other sexual outlets.[181]

Even if Dugas decreased his sexual activity dramatically during 1983, his visible presence in the community spawned rumors that concerned AIDS Vancouver. The organization's worries about Dugas were captured in Shilts's book, which noted that, less than a month following their informational forum, its board members wondered, "Why would anyone do what Gaetan was doing?"[182] Amid plans for incorporation, promotional activities, fund-raising, and volunteer concerns, the April 4, 1983, meeting minutes end with a final point regarding "AIDS victims": "There was some discussion about what to do regarding AIDS victims such as Gaetan. Our 'hands are tied' legally. Instead, it is necessary to change the attitude. Counsellors should be available to those who need them. Michael [Maynard] will contact Gaetan."[183] While one might surmise that the necessary "change in attitude" would be directed at Dugas, Stewart later interpreted the meeting minutes differently, remembering that each sentence of the minutes represented a succinct précis of lengthy discussions. He recalled that it was the attitude of the rest of the community toward "AIDS victims" that needed to be changed, that they could not simply bully a person with AIDS into staying at home.

Minutes from the meeting of June 20, 1983, make another reference to Dugas, though this time a bit more discreetly through the use of his initial. By this point the organization had grown somewhat and was seeking

181. See, for example, Philip Lanzaratta, "Surviving AIDS," *Christopher Street*, October 1984, 35. Also, Helen Schietinger, a nurse at the San Francisco KS Clinic, described to a reporter an evolution in acknowledging PWAs' need for sexual expression, as opposed to widespread medical advice in 1982 to halt all activity; see Michael Helquist, "What to Expect at the KS Clinic," *Coming Up!* March 1983.

182. Shilts, *Band*, 262.

183. The minutes of this meeting were not included in the Krever commission's public evidence, possibly because they named a person with AIDS. The copy which Shilts gathered during his hurried 1986 Vancouver visit is available, however, in his professional papers; "Meeting: April 4, 1983," AIDS Vancouver meeting minutes, folder 23, box 34, Shilts Papers.

to fill what was quickly emerging to be a gap in the provision of support services and education. It had a number of subcommittees, and there was a team devoted to supporting "AIDS victims" and their friends. In a discussion regarding the volunteer support group, Bob Tivey, the organization's counselor, "expressed concern that G., an AIDS victim, has returned to Vancouver and has been seen in circulation. The question is: How do we get him out of circulation given that there is no legal quarantine option?" One committee member suggested a "campaign of persuasion," though this approach was deemed "to be futile if not actually counterproductive, since it would reinforce G.'s paranoia and sense of persecution." Announcing the man's name in public would put AIDS Vancouver at risk for libel. "The most credible alternative," the group decided, "was felt to be an attempt at diversion by appealing to G.'s personal sense of responsibility to the community."[184]

This final option was eventually chosen and proved to be effective. Dugas was approached and recruited into a peer education scheme—a "Buddy program" based on models used at other North American AIDS organizations—in which he took part. When the controversy over the "Patient Zero" story erupted in 1987, Michael Welsh, the support coordinator for AIDS Vancouver in 1983, defended Dugas's name, recalling that Gaétan had "frequently offered support to other sufferers." Furthermore, "he tried to educate people about AIDS. He was always very sociable—he brought a lot of levity to the experience and helped to make it less negative."[185] More recently, Welsh recalled a walk he took with Dugas and some other AIDS support group members along the city's seawall around Stanley Park on a beautiful day in the summer of 1983. The support group meetings at this point were informal and small—the mix of people with AIDS, support workers, and a facilitator totaled fewer than a dozen individuals—and often took place in people's downtown apartments in the city's West End. On this day, with a comment similar to Dugas's friend Richard Bisson, Welsh pointed out a smudge that he saw on Dugas's nose, before realizing that it was a lesion covered with makeup. "Oh!" the flight attendant responded, with grace and quick humor, "It's not what you think it is!" To Welsh, this exchange

184. "Meeting: June 20, 1983," minutes, in *AIDS Vancouver: Exhibits of the British Columbia Hearings*, vol. 49, tab B21.

185. Welsh quoted in Anne Steacy and Lisa Van Dusen, "'Patient Zero' and the AIDS Virus," *Maclean's*, October 19, 1987, 53.

summed up Dugas's easy nature in that environment: very much part of the group and willing to share his experiences.[186]

End of Life, Death, and Remembrance

Stewart had introduced Dugas to an ex-boyfriend of his, the male model with whom, Shilts wrote, "Gaetan had managed to nurture a torrid love affair."[187] Since Stewart and his ex lived in adjacent apartments and were still friendly, Stewart would often see Dugas when the French Canadian came to visit his new lover. The model also sold marijuana, which his new partner enjoyed smoking, and Dugas would often come over to spend time and chat with Stewart as he relaxed.

Stewart made use of Dugas's unusually long experience of living with his condition by asking him questions about how he had dealt with various AIDS-related issues. Stewart thought that he was the only member of the AIDS Vancouver board who could speak comfortably with Dugas, and that Dugas was a valuable resource in terms of his experience as a patient. Through this peer sharing, Dugas was perhaps most able to help other people with AIDS. As Stewart and Redford each recalled, in view of his declining health, Dugas told them that he had made arrangements for an early death. He had designated the recipient of his Air Canada pension and arranged for the cleanup of his apartment as well as the posthumous distribution of his belongings. His advice was useful to Stewart, who was beginning to counsel an increasing stream of people with AIDS, many of whom were receiving their diagnoses at a very late stage of the disease. This problem was echoed elsewhere in the unfolding early history of AIDS in North America, where diagnostic limitations and an incomplete understanding of the natural history of the disease resulted in many people with AIDS being diagnosed and then dying within weeks.[188] Stewart later explained one of AIDS Van-

186. Michael Welsh, telephone interview with author, March 22, 2013.

187. Shilts, *Band*, 439. Readers may wish to compare this description of Dugas's "torrid love affair" with the article Shilts himself wrote in May 1983 about the decrease in partner numbers and resurgence of monogamous relationships among gay men in San Francisco in response to AIDS; Randy Shilts, "How AIDS Is Changing Gay Lifestyles," *San Francisco Chronicle*, May 2, 1983, 1.

188. Douglas Elliott also emphasized the rapid decline of many individuals diagnosed in this period; Elliott, recording C1491/39, tape 1, side B.

couver's less-publicized efforts to assist those who progressed rapidly toward death, which he credited to Dugas:

> AIDS was taking people very suddenly in those days, right? And so, one of things that we ended up doing a lot of was, I ended up with a sort of a bucket of house-keys that people would deposit with me and say, "OK, you know, if I die, go over to my place and clean out the porn and the dildos." Right? Cause you know the next person into that apartment is liable to be your mom, who has to empty it out, right, and they didn't want that to happen. And since I was providing the porn in the first place, they used to make sure that I went over there and got rid of it.[189]

Stewart said that Dugas's advice made him "work harder" to encourage newly diagnosed people with AIDS to address the "loose ends" in their "personal lives that were going to be left dangling when they died. Because he had tied all his off."[190]

Dugas also benefited from his interactions with Stewart and in assisting others with AIDS education. In Stewart's opinion, Dugas's loneliness was an important motivator for his eventual involvement, however loose, in AIDS Vancouver's outreach activities. As an AIDS patient with visible KS lesions, Dugas was enduring acute social deprivation, particularly after many years of intense sociability and being accustomed to occupying the center of attention in group situations. By offering guidance and advice, whether to Stewart or others, Dugas was able to take part in an exchange that allowed him to make use of his humor and interact with others. His former lover Redford recalls going to a dance at a local Vancouver gay bar, "likely in the summer of 1983, and seeing [Dugas] there with his boyfriend, dancing with great joy and abandon, barechested, his shirt rolled up and held high above his head, whirling in the air between his outstretched arms, his whole body lost to the music. He was a compelling figure, beautiful and brave—still very, very young, defiant in the face of disease and death just as he had always been defiant in the face of all that had threatened to limit his joy in life."[191] If the date of this recollection is correct, then Dugas appears—at certain points, at least—to have reached an entente with his disease and his community.

---

189. Stewart, recording C1491/19, tape 1, side A.
190. Stewart, recording C1491/19, tape 1, side B.
191. Redford, "Reminiscences," Epilogue.

Over the previous years, Dugas had moved home to be with his family during periodic bouts of acute sickness. One of his sisters would take time off to nurse him while he was at home, and she did so in secret because of fears that she would lose her job if this activity became known.[192] In January 1984, Dugas's condition worsened once more, and the following month he planned to return to Quebec again.[193] Redford recalled their last evening together: "I invited him to the house for dinner on the night before he left and we all had a good visit, but it was a different, very quiet and reflective Gaétan that night. I can remember him sitting on the couch, listening to the tick tock of my old wall clock, talking about how peaceful and beautiful the sound was, and thanking us [Redford and his partner] over and over for the evening. When I drove him home, we were very quiet, both near tears, both of us realizing, I think, that we wouldn't see each other again."[194]

Dugas rejoined his supportive family the next day. Within a few weeks, his health deteriorated and he returned to Quebec City's Centre hospitalier de l'Université Laval. There, he received visitors when he could and spoke regularly with friends by phone. One day when Redford called, a relative answered the phone and explained that the family had assembled for the administration of last rites. Redford's friend died shortly afterward, on March 30, 1984. A memorial service was held three days later and was attended by family members, friends, and colleagues from Air Canada.[195] Both the obituary, which described Dugas as "agent de bord" (flight attendant), and a personalized memorial card encapsulated the joy Dugas took from his career and lifestyle (see fig. 6.3).

Shortly after Dugas's death, Noah Stewart contributed a reminiscence about his friend to *Angles*, a local Vancouver community newspaper. He did not identify Dugas by name, "to preserve his anonymity and in order to respect the wishes of his family." "Nevertheless," Stewart

192. Wadden, e-mail.

193. The recollections of "Simon" (interview notes, p. 6, Shilts Papers) and Brian Willoughby (recording C1491/18) accord with this date.

194. Redford, "Reminiscences," Epilogue.

195. "Simon" described a "big" funeral to Shilts, interview notes, p. 9. Elaine Watson recalled hearing that an Air Canada base manager attended the funeral along with other company employees. Watson and another female flight attendant who had been Dugas's roommate coordinated the collection of written reminiscences from their colleagues in a book that they sent to his family; Dunn, Watson, and Miller, recording C1491/26 (Watson recollection at tape 1, side B).

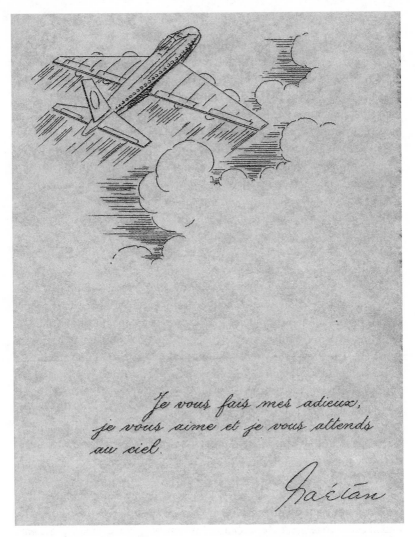

Je vous fais mes adieux,
je vous aime et je vous attends
au ciel.

Gaétan

FIGURE 6.3 Front cover of Gaétan Dugas's memorial card, dated March 30, 1984; thermographic print with raised silver ink on cream paper, 11.4 × 15.5 cm; copy in author's personal collection, gifted by Ray Redford and reproduced with permission from Dugas's surviving family members. The signed inscription reads, "Je vous fais mes adieux, je vous aime et je vous attends au ciel." ("I bid you my farewells, I love you and I await you in the sky.") In text and image, Dugas's parting message to his friends and family exudes the love of flight he had experienced for much of his life. It is possible that Dugas himself produced the sketch used for this print. The religious connotations of this image would have resonated in the wider Catholic community of his hometown, and were drawn out further through the text, with *adieux* also signifying "to god" and *au ciel* meaning "in heaven." The careful preparation evident in creating this personalized card also attests to Noah Stewart's recollection of one lesson Dugas had taught him and others at AIDS Vancouver: the importance of having one's affairs in order before departing on one's final journey.

continued, "his story will be familiar to many in the city." His submission bears reprinting at length:

My friend had had AIDS for a long time, longer, even, than we have had the name AIDS for the disease which finally took his life. He contracted a disease that alerted physicians to the fact that something was seriously wrong with his immune system when we were still calling the mysterious disease GRID, gay-related immune deficiency. Then, after travelling for a time, he settled in Vancouver and continued to work at his profession.

A year or so ago, when AIDS Vancouver put on its first forum, he was in the audience. I hadn't yet met him at that point but I had certainly heard his name. AIDS Vancouver was in its formative stages. None of us knew with any accuracy just what it was that we were faced with. The disease itself was a mystery. The society surrounding the disease seemed on the brink of an explosion, in which direction no one knew. Fear and hysteria were being transmitted from person to person, fanned by the uncaring "news"-creating media. Although I had agreed to devote some time to helping people affected by AIDS, I had not yet met anyone who had the disease. Then I met my friend.

I had heard his name, of course. In the councils of AIDS Vancouver, we had discussed what sort of assistance we might offer this man who, it later turned out, was quite capable of proceeding without assistance. And a number of well-meaning people, having learned his name and the fact he had AIDS, were busily informing the community of his condition.

As the unofficial specialist in social issues surrounding AIDS, I have often been asked if I have found any verifiable stories of prejudice against people with AIDS. Generally, I reply that in Canada at least, no one to my knowledge has been denied employment or housing on the basis of their medical condition. More subtly, though, the only prejudice I have actually experienced has been from the gay community itself. At the time I met my friend, the rumours were flying. He had been seen in a back-room bar, he had been seen picking up a stranger in a bar, he had been doing all sorts of things to deliberately communicate his disease to the uninformed. He should be quarantined, said some. Other suggestions were less polite. And all of them were based on fear, ignorance and hysteria.

After we got to know each other better, we discussed the rumours about his activities. First off, he pointed out a very interesting idea that the underinformed tend to overlook. If he had indeed been picking up strangers in bars, he would have been endangered by the chance of acquiring any disease which that person had, even unwittingly. We all carry the activating agents of many diseases dangerous to people with AIDS, with no difficulty to ourselves. Since my friend had come to this realization, he had stopped having sexual contacts.

"Why the rumours?" I asked. He had dealt with this before. He saw it as a kind of projection of the fears of the gay community. We imagined the worst thing that could happen and then acted as if it were so. Over the past year, as we grew to know one another better, the rumours became less frequent and less hysterical. I'd like to think that the gay community mastered its collective fear of the unknown dangers of AIDS.

Why am I bringing up this topic? Because my friend fought his disease. He fought the manifestations of AIDS with every bit of willpower at his command (which was considerable will). He changed his habits and his lifestyle to preserve his precious life. And at the same time, he fought the ignorance and fear of the people around him, meeting it with good sense and information.

He would have been embarrassed if I had referred to him as a symbol of the strength that people can find within themselves to meet extraordinary challenges. Before his illness, he was a gay man much like you or I, with the same desires and human failings. When AIDS entered his life, he mobilized his energies to fight. And I sincerely believe—and find it profoundly comforting—that he fought every inch of the way. He found life very precious. His indomitable will never gave up. Even at the very end of his life, when his body had been overwhelmed beyond his power to control it, he did not stop to relax, to die without resistance to a force which was too strong for him. My friend never quit. He only died.[196]

* * *

In addition to the meanings suggested in previous chapters, the term "Patient Zero" can be read to mean the complete nullification of a patient's perspective. This interpretation seems highly appropriate, given how Dugas's lived experience has been overwritten by the fictionalized character popularized in *And the Band Played On*. Evidence gathered from contemporary sources across North America yields a far more nuanced perspective of the most demonized person with AIDS of all time.

196. Noah Stewart, "A Friend's Death," *Angles*, May 1984, 17; it was also reprinted in the next month's issue. Stewart did not mention his written submission during the 2007 interview. He had forgotten about it until the author forwarded him a copy in July 2010. In the final paragraph, *embarrassed* corrected from "embarassed" in original.

Instead of a relentless, immovable killer, an image perpetuated by much of the media coverage that followed the publication of Shilts's book, we have witnessed the difficult struggles of a young patient during a turbulent time of fear, rumor, and changing information. Early suggestions that AIDS patients should abstain from sex would have jarred with Dugas's pride—not shame—in a gay identity expressed through sexual connection. The evidence suggests that Dugas did continue to have sex through the spring and summer of 1983. Nonetheless, the contemporary medical and scientific uncertainties, the tumultuous rumors, the changing ethical landscape of the North American communities he navigated, and the difficulties he faced in his day-to-day life all make it difficult to maintain that to do so was the act of a sociopath. Supporting, as Dugas most likely did, a multifactorial explanation for his illness, he would have believed that it was as much up to others as to himself to reduce numbers of sexual partners and prevent reinfection with other diseases. The fact that he reduced his sexual contacts, became involved in AIDS Vancouver's support efforts, and remained close to friends and family near the end of his life confirms that there are a multitude of ways to view Gaétan Dugas's experiences of the early North American AIDS epidemic. In the end, it is only by laying the notion of "Patient Zero" to rest that we can come close to appreciating what his own views may have been.

Zero Hour

Making Histories of the North American AIDS Epidemic

zero hour, n. 1. The time at which a military operation is scheduled to begin.
2. The time at which a person feels at his or her lowest.
3. The hour from which a new cycle of time is measured.[1]

In gentle defiance of the impending rain, a crowd steadily filled Toronto's Cawthra Square Park on the evening of June 24, 2014, gathering for the city's thirtieth annual candlelight AIDS vigil. Out-of-town visitors attending the World Pride festivities on Church Street helped swell the crowd's numbers, many carrying an umbrella in one hand and an unlit candle in the other. As darkness fell, lights illuminated the triangular concrete pillars of the city's AIDS memorial, each one adorned with simple plaques engraved with the names of Toronto residents who had died in the epidemic—more than 2,700 in total, listed by year of death. The semicircular sweep of the memorial served as an amphitheater for the ceremony, embracing a small artists' stage faced by hundreds of audience members. As the ceremony began at 9:00 p.m., a short but intense downfall of rain drew a blossoming of umbrellas, rainbow blooms which, with the end of the cloudburst, gradually withered and folded away. The event hosts—Barbara Hall, a former city mayor, and Henry Luyombya, a Ugandan-born Canadian citizen and AIDS activist—introduced a series

---

1. *Oxford English Dictionary Online*, s.v. "zero hour," accessed February 5, 2017, http://www.oed.com/view/Entry/413123.

of performers from around the world and reflected on the global nature of the pandemic and its enormous human and social cost.[2] As the artists completed their acts in succession, murmurs of disapproval spread through the audience, as some of those present were so moved by the performances that they forgot or ignored organizers' requests to withhold applause. More sanctioned audience participation came when candle lighters, individually and in small groups, appeared on stage and lit their candles, each reciting short lines into the microphone to illuminate their actions:

I light this candle as a symbol of hope.
I light this candle as a symbol of compassion.
I light this candle as a symbol of understanding.
I light this candle as a symbol of peace.
I light this candle as a symbol of faith . . .

Imagining a simple, traceable cause for disease epidemics is a human response that dates back many centuries in Europe and North America. Often coupled with the assumption of a short incubation period, humans have long believed that sickness can be traced to events and moments of contact with other individuals, especially those transpiring within their recent memory. When faced with the fearsome prospect of contagion, past peoples regularly ascribed malicious motives to those whose circumstances, traits, or behaviors had already marked them as different. The responses thrown up by the unexpected and devastating return of epidemic disease in the late twentieth century often revealed an uncanny resemblance to precedents established in the distant past. This book is intended as a contribution toward understanding the appeal of these responses—an intervention to clarify how and why, in the particular case of "Patient Zero," events followed a certain trajectory during

2. Hall had enjoyed strong support from the many members of the city's lesbian and gay communities for many years and as early as 1987 marched in the annual pride parade. Weeks after the 2014 candlelight vigil, the city of Toronto renamed Cawthra Square Park in her honor. See Andrea Houston, "Ford to Pass on Pride, but Barbara Hall Shows Longstanding Solidarity," *Daily Xtra*, June 21, 2011, http://www.dailyxtra .com/toronto/news-and-ideas/news/ford-pass-pride-barbara-hall-shows-longstanding -solidarity-5088; "Park Renaming to Honour Former City of Toronto Mayor, Barbara Hall," City of Toronto, July 14, 2014, http://wx.toronto.ca/inter/it/newsrel.nsf/bydate/ 52ED80777CB64FAB85257D150057C547.

the early years of the North American AIDS epidemic, and indeed why they might again—if left unchecked—follow a similar path in future epidemics. From this understanding—indeed, from this zero hour—I very much hope that a new cycle of compassion can follow.

This book began with a misleading medical dictionary entry for the term *patient zero*, which stated that the US Centers for Disease Control (CDC) identified this individual as the man who introduced HIV to North America and who directly infected nearly fifty other people. Similarly, although suggesting that the tale was a "myth," for many years the history page of a widely consulted AIDS reference site simplistically explained that "Patient O" was "mistakenly identified in the press as 'Patient Zero.'"[3] These explanations were both incorrect and inadequate. The media's role in disseminating the term and the story that carried it is undeniable and important to recognize. However, solely focusing on the media implies that scientific knowledge is initially "pure" before an imperfect diffusion through the media's filters results in a contaminated product. Such a model fails to recognize, for example, the "microprocessing" of the CDC investigators, whose informal discussions shifted a term from its initial descriptive and abbreviatory function (the letter *O*) to one intensely infused with cultural significance and multiple interpretations (the numeral or word *zero*). As one sociologist of science has aptly noted, "Scientists often dismiss the way their work is appropriated by the media as oversimplified and distorted. But the relationship between science and culture is far more complex. For science itself is a cultural product—a form of knowledge shaped by social assumptions. Indeed, many of the values expressed in popular rhetoric draw support from the promises generated by scientists and the language they use to describe their work."[4] Regarding the way in which CDC investigators presented the example of "Patient 0," readers may be divided in their interpretation of one HIV researcher's comments: "He represented a great example, and that's how he got written up as. And calling him 'Patient 0' made it sound like the whole epidemic started with him, which was mis-

3. Annabel Kanabus and Sarah Allen, and updated by Bonita de Boer, "The Origin of AIDS and HIV and the First Cases of AIDS," AVERT, updated May 12, 2005, http:// web.archive.org/web/20050527223015/http://www.avert.org/origins.htm. A review of website captures gathered between 2000 and 2016 on the Internet Archive indicates that this account was first posted in May 2005 and remained in place until September 2015.

4. Nelkin, "Promotional Metaphors," 30.

leading. Did it bother anybody? I don't think so. The purists would be upset, but most of us would say, 'Get the message out. If you have to . . . take a person as an example to herald the fact that this is sexually transmitted [and] you'd better be careful—it's fine.'"[5] These remarks notwithstanding, we must acknowledge the impact of professional practices, personal worldviews, and chosen terminology in the work of scientists—and maintain similar awareness when interpreting the work of policy makers, journalists, and historians, among others. And we must also remain aware of the long-standing cultural narratives that weave their way through this work and through the matrices of our shared socially constructed reality.

* * *

. . . I light this candle as a symbol of love.
I light this candle as a symbol of diversity.
I light this candle as a symbol of justice.
I light this candle as a symbol of solidarity.
I light this candle as a symbol of strength . . .

Many people interviewed for this book explained the attention focused on "Patient Zero" as a simple expression of a universal human desire to blame someone else for misfortune. Given the centuries-old examples of individuals and groups appropriating and recirculating stories and images about disease spreading to make sense of epidemics, it should not be surprising that these impulses emerged in the early 1980s in response to AIDS. An unexpected turn, perhaps, was the speed with which this novel manifestation of an old and widely held cultural trope—that individuals with disease may try to spread it deliberately to the uninfected—was adopted in several American legal texts of the late 1980s with little empirical support. One reason for the swift uptake of Randy Shilts's characterization of Gaétan Dugas as "Patient Zero" appears to be its simplicity, which offered a far more clear-cut example of deliberate infection than some cases before the courts in 1987. In this manner, the way in which many readers readily accepted the "Patient Zero" story is suggestive of the broad appeal of neat, uncomplicated

5. Jay Levy, interview with author, San Francisco, July 16, 2007, recording C1491/05, tape 1, side A, BLSA.

answers. Given this simplicity, there was also no reason to expect that the term "Patient Zero" would remain solely associated with AIDS or, for that matter, with infectious disease. With an efficient means of production and distribution behind it, and encapsulated as an infectious and easily digested phrase, "Patient Zero," the idea, has since traveled widely to new metaphorical and fictional settings. An infected computer used to launch a malicious attack on a network, the first financial institution to fail in a collapse, or a jihad-fixated bioterrorist who infects himself with a killer strain of zombie plague—all of these examples have inherited the title.[6] Mostly, users employ the phrase to denote the origins of an interconnected problem and, to a lesser extent, to signal some degree of blameworthiness.[7]

Other countries have produced variations of the "Patient Zero" story in their own national histories of AIDS origins, devoting close attention to the sexual contacts of the first detected cases.[8] These stories deserve further investigation and comparison to the North American version, as well as some skepticism, given the evolving understanding of HIV infection and the inherent limitations of disease surveillance systems in detecting an infectious disease that takes years to manifest symptoms. In some cases, the American story was explicitly exported, as with the president of the American Medical Association's uncredited recycling

6. Abhishek Kumar, Vern Paxson, and Nicholas Weaver, "Exploiting Underlying Structure for Detailed Reconstruction of an Internet-Scale Event" (paper presented at the fifth ACM SIGCOMM Conference on Internet Measurement, Berkeley, CA, October 19–21, 2005), https://www.usenix.org/legacy/event/imc05/tech/full_papers/kumar/kumar.pdf; Luke Mullins, "Rep. John Mica on Fannie/Freddie Special Prosecutor," *The Home Front* (blog), *US News and World Report*, October 29, 2008, http://money.usnews.com/money/blogs/the-home-front/2008/10/29/rep-john-mica-on-fanniefreddie-special-prosecutor.html; Jonathan Maberry, *Patient Zero* (New York: St. Martin's Griffin, 2009).

7. The success of Malcolm Gladwell's *The Tipping Point: How Little Things Can Make a Big Difference* (New York: Little, Brown, 2000), which likened social change to infectious disease epidemics, has no doubt helped further popularize the term. Gladwell, who included Dugas among a group of highly sexually active men who "aren't like you or me," drew on Shilts's misguided characterization of Dugas as "Patient Zero" to explain that "these are the kinds of people who make epidemics of disease tip" (Gladwell, *Tipping Point*, 19–22).

8. Paula Treichler, *Theory in an Epidemic*, 355–56. For example, South Africa's first diagnosed AIDS case in 1982 was identified as a "white, homosexual air steward"; Iliffe, *African AIDS Epidemic*, 43. Grmek describes the homosexual contacts of "the Soviet Union's 'Patient Zero,'" the "first known patient" in that country; Grmek, *History of AIDS*, 191–92.

of Shilts's story in Kobe, Japan, or in Germany, where *Der Spiegel* (the *Mirror*) reproduced excerpts of Shilts's book, along with a picture of Dugas identifying him as an "AIDS-spreader."[9] Stories and pictures of "Patient Zero" could also illuminate more complicated transnational tensions. A Montreal newspaper used the tale to link that city's hosting of the 1989 World AIDS Conference to broader geopolitical frameworks. The *Gazette* reported that Dugas's photo, labeled "Patient Zero," was hanging in a university teaching hospital in Lusaka, Zambia. This, the journalist explained, was suggestive of the view that Canada "gave AIDS to the world."[10] The example further illustrates how the idea traveled and was adopted and incorporated into increasingly global tides of blame. Further research may illuminate whether the story cross-pollinated with accusations of deliberate spreading of HIV that circulated across areas of Africa in the late twentieth and early twenty-first centuries. The authors of an article describing the results of a continent-wide fictional story-writing competition noted the concerning frequency of depictions of people living with HIV (PLWH) as "vengeful individuals out to infect as many people as possible." One competition judge in Madagascar is quoted as saying that it seemed that in some stories "the only thing that many PLWH do is run around getting revenge by spreading HIV."[11]

The "Patient Zero" angle became firmly ensconced as a reporting formula in novel outbreaks of infectious disease. When paranoia was growing about newly emerging diseases such as Ebola in the 1990s, journalists sought out information about the first known case subject, calling that individual "patient zero."[12] Indeed, it was during this period that *Mosby's Medical Dictionary,* the medical reference text, first added a definition for the term. The global outbreak of severe acute respiratory syndrome (SARS) in 2003 reinforced this trend, with extensive media attention focused on its earliest known case. Much was written about

9. James W. Jones, "Discourses on and of AIDS in West Germany, 1986–90," *Journal of the History of Sexuality* 2, no. 3 (1992): 450.

10. David Johnston, "Africans Asking: Did Canada Give AIDS to World?" *Montreal Gazette,* June 3, 1989, A9.

11. Kate Winskell and Daniel Enger, "A New Way of Perceiving the Pandemic: The Findings from a Participatory Research Process on Young Africans' Stories about HIV/ AIDS," *Culture, Health and Sexuality* 11, no. 4 (2009): 464.

12. Sam Kiley, "Third Nun Dies as Zaire Tracks Down Killer Virus," *Times* [London], May 13, 1995, 17.

the man who infected an elevator-load of people at Hotel Metropole in Hong Kong, with some reports describing him as "patient zero" without explaining the genesis of the term.[13] Although in this instance the multinational investigative teams employed an alphabetical system for their reports, referring to this "index patient" as "patient A," others did not follow suit.[14] A published account of two SARS outbreaks in Canada, one in Toronto and the other in Vancouver, assigned the label "patient 0" to the primary case in each city.[15] It seems that no media description of a response to an outbreak is now complete without including an account of health authorities' attempts to locate "the first patient to contract the virus—the 'index patient' or 'patient zero, in epidemiological terms.'"[16]

Critics have emphasized how a focus on the person-to-person spread of infectious disease, a narrowed vision encouraged by the "Patient Zero" story, might obscure other, equally important factors contributing to the spread of infection. If infectious disease affects the poor disproportionately, and at faster rates, is there not a significant cost to spending increasing sums of money targeting individuals, rather than allocating resources to concrete, community-enhancing measures? Highlighting the one can draw attention away from the wider ecosystem.[17] As the epidemiologist Andrew Moss suggested with regard to the early AIDS epidemic in San Francisco, "It's not a matter of one—*one*—one time. It's a matter of what's going on when it gets there." He explained that "whoever brought the virus to San Francisco—not him [Dugas], but somebody—brought it to a population of fifty thousand gay men with an *extremely* high rate of 'sexual partner turnover,' as we say in the busi-

13. Peter Washer, "Representations of SARS in the British Newspapers," *Social Science and Medicine* 59 (2004): 2561–71.

14. T. Tsang et al., "Update: Outbreak of Severe Acute Respiratory Syndrome—Worldwide, 2003," *MMWR* 52 (2003): 241–48, https://www.cdc.gov/mmwr/preview/mmwrhtml/mm5212a1.htm.

15. Danuta M. Skowronski et al., "Coordinated Response to SARS, Vancouver, Canada," *Emerging Infectious Diseases* 12, no. 1 (2006): 156.

16. Shannon Brownlee et al., "Horror in the Hot Zone," *US News and World Report*, May 22, 1995, 57. I explored this material in more detail in my M.Sc. dissertation: Richard Andrew McKay, "The Emergence of the 'Patient Zero' Concept in the North American AIDS Epidemic" (MSc diss., University of Oxford, 2005).

17. Wald, *Contagious*, 267; David S. Barnes, "Targeting Patient Zero," in *Tuberculosis Then and Now: Perspectives on the History of an Infectious Disease*, ed. Michael Worboys and Flurin Condrau, 49–71 (London: McGill-Queen's University Press, 2010).

ness. When you *drop* a sexually transmitted virus in there—you're going to have a lot of disease, and many people were eligible for that role. Because people are coming from here to New York *all the time*, you know, and wherever else in the world."[18] The tendency to focus on the individual, as opposed to the group, may continue in the future, however, since investigators now have the ability to trace infections through molecular epidemiologic technologies with capabilities far outreaching those available to researchers investigating Kaposi's sarcoma and opportunistic infections in the early 1980s.[19]

Although there is, among some journalists, an awareness of the risky oversimplifications involved in using the term "Patient Zero" and in framing a story around such an individual, this cannot be said for the profession at large.[20] When a public health reporter suggested in 2008 that "nobody would dare use that term any more," he was perhaps optimistically discounting its popularity with readers and its frequently illusory ability to explain a phenomenon.[21] During the coverage of the H1N1 epidemic in Mexico in 2009, the narrative was predictably resurrected when reporters announced that they had discovered "Patient Zero" of the epidemic, in the form of five-year-old Édgar Hernández. Although fortunately in this case the child survived, the anguish and confusion of the Dugas family's experience can be read in the words of Hernández's mother, María, who faced swarms of international reporters in the weeks following the announcement of the outbreak. "Some people are saying my boy is to blame for everyone else in the country getting sick," she told reporters, confronted with the full force of a media narrative searching for its main villain. "I don't believe that. I don't know what to think."[22] A similar response came in 2014 from the Guinean father of a dead two-year-old boy. The child was identified by name in the media as "Patient Zero"—"the first traceable person to have contracted the disease"—of the Ebola outbreak that ravaged several western African countries in 2013 and 2014.[23] While grieving the deaths of his son, daughter, and

18. Moss, recording C1491/09, tape 1, side B; emphasis on recording.

19. Barnes, "Targeting Patient Zero," 49–71.

20. See Treichler, *Theory in an Epidemic*, 213.

21. André Picard, interview with author, Toronto, September 4, 2008, recording C1491/42, tape 1, side B, BLSA.

22. María Hernández quoted in Marc Lacey, "From Édgar, 5, Coughs Heard Round the World," *New York Times*, April 29, 2009, A1.

23. Adam Withnall, "Ebola Outbreak's 'Patient Zero' Identified as a Two-Year-Old

partner, the man endured months of probing photographs and questions from international journalists seeking to commoditize the epidemic's "ground zero" and first known case. "It wasn't Emile that started it," he explained through an interpreter, pushing back against the blame which infused the explanations for the outbreak's emergence. "Emile was too young to eat bats, and he was too small to be playing in the bush all on his own."[24] As long as this uncritical reporting formula remains unchallenged, it is a foregone conclusion that relatives of early cases in future outbreaks will be hounded in their grief.

* * *

... I light this candle as a symbol of for all those who have died of HIV/
  AIDS so that we may honor them.
I light this candle as a symbol for all those affected by HIV/AIDS so that we
  may remember them.
I light this candle as a symbol for all those living with HIV/AIDS,
  particularly long-term survivors, so that we may celebrate them.

Composing this epilogue, and structuring it explicitly around a recent instance of ceremonial remembrance, offers me an opportunity to reflect on my personal experience of writing a history of the North American AIDS epidemic. The process from conception to completion of this book, like many works of history that begin in graduate study, has lasted more than ten years, during a period spanning the third and fourth decades since the epidemic's initial recognition in 1981. I have been on this journey from the ages of twenty-seven to thirty-eight (and counting), and much longer if one sets the zero hour from my false-positive HIV diagnosis in 2000. The journey has seen me move between North America and Europe. At several points in my research, as I visited San Francisco,

Boy from Guinea Named Emile Ouamouno," *Independent* [London], October 28, 2014, http://www.independent.co.uk/news/world/africa/ebola-outbreaks-patient-zero-identified -as-a-two-year-old-boy-from-guinea-named-emile-ouamouno-9823513.html.

24. Misha Hussain, "Hunger and Frustration Grow at Ebola Ground Zero in Guinea," Reuters, March 3, 2015, http://uk.reuters.com/article/us-health-ebola-guinea -village-idUKKBN0LZ1R220150303; Suzanne Mary Beukes, "Ebola in Guinea: Finding Patient Zero," *Daily Maverick* [Johannesburg, South Africa], October 27, 2014, http:// www.dailymaverick.co.za/article/2014–10–27-ebola-in-guinea-finding-patient-zero/# .V_zWNTsefB4.

New York, and Los Angeles, and returned home to Vancouver, I was struck by the parallels between my peregrinations and those of Randy Shilts and Bill Darrow before me, and Gaétan Dugas before them. Thinking particularly of Shilts and Dugas, I could not help but notice the similarity in our ages, and by the very different yet intertwined ways in which AIDS had consumed our energies and attention during each of our young adulthoods. To be sure, researching and writing a history, of what was in the 1980s and '90s too often a cruelly fatal disease, is in no way comparable to living with the corporeality of an untreated HIV infection. Nonetheless, spending more than a decade in the intimate study of the lives and deaths of mostly young men my own age has taken an undeniable emotional toll, and my life has been profoundly marked by this experience. At times I would halfheartedly quip that, while some might respond to the shock of a false-positive HIV test by seeking therapy, I undertook a history doctorate to make sense of it instead. At a certain point, though, I stopped making this joke when I realized that it masked a deeper truth. Bundled up in my intellectual work was a kind of emotional displacement; buried beneath my attempts to write a compassionate history of AIDS lay a deep, residual sense of vulnerability about the possibility of becoming infected myself. Thus, one reflection to emerge from this experience is the notion of historical research as a process of self-exploration, of engrossing—yet inherently limited—self-therapy.

One common interpretation of the term "Patient Zero" has been that of an individual occupying a central and seemingly prominent position in a network. In this sense, then, Gaétan Dugas has undeniably been "Patient Zero" for an eclectic chain of historians using the idea as they purposefully made sexual histories of various kinds to make sense of the North American AIDS epidemic.[25] Darrow, David Auerbach, and their colleagues at the CDC unintentionally forged the term as they reconstructed sexual networks of early cases and postulated modes of transmission. Shilts and Michael Denneny fashioned a chronology of the American epidemic to highlight the epidemic's heroes and villains and bring about political change; they deployed the idea of "Patient Zero" to animate and publicize it. John Greyson turned the notion on its head in an homage to the impatient spirit and vitality of direct AIDS activ-

25. In writing this section, I was influenced by Jeffrey Weeks's democratic description of creating sexual histories in *Making Sexual History* (Cambridge: Polity Press, 2000), 1–14.

ism. Meanwhile, Douglas Elliott saw an opportunity to restore geography where it had been absent: he used the idea to unsettle the notion that public health information flowed as it should have done during the 1980s between the United States and Canada, and between provincial and federal Canadian health authorities. Furthermore, in doing so, he sought to put "on the record" a history of lesbian and gay communities that had too often been overlooked or deliberately silenced. Now in my turn I have employed the idea of "Patient Zero" as an organizational thread to draw together a diverse series of personal and institutional histories. In this way, another reflection that comes to mind in reviewing the idea's wide-ranging uses and travels is that of a certain intellectual promiscuity, an interdisciplinarity that, to me, fully suits a history of the disease that launched "an epidemic of signification."

A final organizing reflection on this experience is one that conceives of researching and writing contemporary history as a process of enriching intergenerational mentorship. As I learned through my own real-world experience and subsequent historical investigations, gay communities have long wrestled with aging and intergenerational interactions. Particularly in the highly sexualized bars like those I frequented as a younger man, and which have for decades featured as prominent community meeting spaces, it was difficult for many gay men of disparate generations to strike up acquaintanceships, particularly those of a non-sexual kind. Among many reasons for gratitude, therefore, I would like to highlight the opportunities my research generated for me to interact with an older generation of gay men. These exchanges of information, often in the form of oral history interviews but also through interactions with volunteer archivists and history enthusiasts, have expanded my horizons of personal possibility and in some cases led to valued friendships. Though I often felt that I was the beneficiary of these exchanges, occasionally I was able to reciprocate in kind. After having closely studied the interview notes Shilts compiled when he was researching his book in 1986, I was fortunate to be able to reinterview some of the same individuals more than twenty years later and, in one or two cases, to reunite them with a lost memory. When I met with Bob Tivey in 2008, for example, he had forgotten the anecdote he shared with Shilts and which is described in chapter 3 of this book, where Dugas thanked Tivey for giving him "a normal day." Since Tivey had strived in his support work to treat Vancouver's early diagnosed persons with AIDS with dignity and respect, he said that he had for years "hung on to" Dugas's remark—"like a gift"—until it eventually slipped beyond his recollection.[26] At moments like these, I felt rather like a time-traveling intermediary—reviving, redistributing, and cocreating memories from decades past.

Working on a history of AIDS, I was always cognizant that I was speaking to a generation of survivors. In interviews, emotions were never far below the surface, and even the most assured speakers would trip up with little warning. I came to understand that many interviewees steeled themselves for the emotional journey of our discussions, only too aware of the feelings that they kept contained, and knowledgeable of the pain which was likely to surface as they reminisced. Yet most insisted on carrying on. Spencer Macdonell, having lost most of his friends to the AIDS epidemic, explained this sense of duty, even as his emotions came close to choking his words. "*Phwwwwww* [*exhaling deeply*] so Goddess has left me here for a reason. I'm here to—yeah, I'm here to remember. And probably a few other things too but, but that's the one that—that's the one that's important. That's the one that [*voice breaking*] *phwwwwwwwwww* [*exhaling slowly and deeply*] helps keep me going on bad days."[27] Similarly, Richard Berkowitz told me he felt compelled "to bear witness" to his dead friends and to "mak[e] history by remembering it." He explained that "by talking about it, it's like you honour the people that you knew who died [and] you kind of bring them back to life for a moment in the stories." Researchers, too, felt a strong desire to pass on their experiences; "I want you to know . . ." was the prefix to several of Bill Darrow's recollections.[28] I am grateful to all of the survivors who trusted me with their memories, and who mentored me in the broader history of North America's lesbian and gay communities and the epidemic that so devastated them.

At a certain point during the Toronto candlelight vigil, audience members were asked to say aloud the names of those they knew who had died of AIDS. It was at this moment, as those around me began recit-

26. Tivey, September 7, 2008, recording C1491/44, tape 1, side B; tape 2, side A.

27. Macdonell, recording C1491/27, tape 1, side B. Macdonell drew a military analogy in our interview: "A line combat unit is deemed ineffective [*voice breaking*] after it's had fifty percent casualties. I lost sixty percent of my friends" (ibid.).

28. Berkowitz, recording C1491/24, tape 1, side B; Darrow, recording C1491/21, tape 1, side B.

ing names, that I experienced a humbling and rather painful realization of the disconnect between historical research and living memory. After all my travels, all my research, and all my writing, I could name only one individual I knew personally who had died of AIDS: one of my sister's schoolteachers. Following an initial silence, I eventually offered *Gaétan Dugas*—whose name was, of course, inscribed nearby on one of the memorial's plaques—and a moment later, *Randy Shilts*. On one level, as a historian, I knew these latter two individuals intimately—much better than my sister's teacher. Yet on another, there was a significant divide separating my own expert historical knowledge of AIDS from the lived experiences of gay men of the era before highly active antiretroviral therapy, men like Dugas, like Shilts and Denneny, like Greyson and Elliott, and like the dead Toronto poet and activist Michael Lynch, the founder of the Toronto AIDS memorial, who had cried out in mourning "these waves of dying friends."[29] In this moment, I viscerally felt the historian's lament: no matter how close one may draw to understanding the past—even the recent past—in some very important ways it will always escape one's reach.

With this experience in mind, I have chosen to end my book with a survivor's account, written by a man deeply affected by the epidemic and who is exceptionally well placed to offer a final reflection. Ray Redford e-mailed me in August 2007, after a friend of his in San Francisco learned of my doctoral research into the history of the idea of "Patient Zero." This friend read a letter I had written to an LGBT newspaper in the Bay Area promoting my research project and seeking interviewees.[30] Redford explained that he and Dugas had been lovers in the early 1970s and that he later remained friends with the flight attendant until Dugas's death in 1984. At an early stage in our correspondence, Redford indicated his preference for contributing a written reminiscence instead of a recorded interview, not wanting his choice of spoken words on the day to forever color impressions of his friend and former lover. At his request, I sent him a list of questions in late December 2007, as suggestions to structure his recollections.[31] He e-mailed me a draft of his notes in early

29. From Lynch's poem "Cry," quoted from Silversides, *AIDS Activist*, 106.

30. Richard A. McKay, "'Patient Zero' Research," letter to the editor, *San Francisco Bay Times*, July 5, 2007.

31. The following are the questions I sent to Redford in December 2007:

1. When and where were you born?
2. Where did you grow up and go to school?

January 2008, along with some scanned photographs. In October 2010, Redford sent me a revised version of his reminiscences; it is this final contribution that appears here in its entirety. Sensitive, caring, and often very moving, Redford's prose helps restore Dugas's memory to a realm from which it has long been publicly denied: the intimate space of a loving relationship.

Ray Redford's Reminiscences

I was born in Vancouver in 1947.

I grew up on northern Vancouver Island, mainly in Campbell River. I left Campbell River in 1965 to attend UBC [the University of British Columbia]. While I have returned to Campbell River for summer jobs and family visits, Vancouver has been my home since 1965.

---

3. What brought you to Vancouver?
4. Can you tell me about your experience coming out?
5. Can you describe the popular gay spots in Vancouver in the 1970s and early 1980s?
6. In the 1970s, was it common for gay men in Canada to travel to American cities with large gay populations (i.e., New York, San Francisco, Los Angeles)?
7. How and when did you meet Gaétan?
8. Can you describe your first meeting?
9. Was Gaétan living in Vancouver at that time?
10. Did he discuss wanting to be a flight attendant with you?
11. Did he tell you any stories about his travels and/or working for Air Canada? Life growing up in Quebec? His relationship with his family?
12. Can you describe your relationship with Gaétan and how it changed over time?
13. When was the first time you heard that he was sick?
14. Did he ever discuss his illness with you?
15. Were you aware of rumours of any sort about him (or other people with AIDS) circulating in Vancouver?
16. Do you remember when you first heard about AIDS? What did you think caused the disease? Do you remember there being confusion about its cause?
17. In the early 1980s, what sources of information did you trust to provide accurate information about this disease?
18. Did you attend the first AIDS Vancouver information forum in March 1983 at the West End Community Centre? If yes, what do you remember of it?
19. Were you ever contacted by Randy Shilts? Were you aware that he travelled to Vancouver in 1986 to interview local men about Gaétan?
20. Do you remember the first time you heard the term "patient zero"? Was it in connection with Gaétan? What did (and does) the term mean to you?

I was lucky to be born into a wonderful family. My parents were a good match, a happy couple totally committed to home and family. Because this family was such a comfortable, safe place to be, I didn't really go through the usual teenage rejection of family for friends. I often felt more comfortable at home than in the teenage social scene. At school, possibly because I was a very strong student in a streamed academic class, I was not taunted by other students for being different. I knew I didn't have the same interests as most boys and didn't feel any excitement dancing or dating girls, but I didn't feel outcast or particularly lonely, in part because of my family, but also because I had one very close friend with whom I spent all my spare time when I was at school or in town. Of course, he turned out to be gay as well, but, at the time, it was never discussed.

Coming out was a long process, mainly the result of my shyness and social insecurity in the larger world, not my horror or revulsion about being gay. I was fortunate to be coming of age just when the world was opening up and liberalizing, when it was cool to be different and adventurous.

Coming across a copy of the *Young Physique* in a magazine store the summer after grade 12 really began my sexual awakening. The following September, I decided to hike down to the beach below our residences at UBC. The trail led directly to what was then the gay section of Wreck Beach. I returned later with a friend who announced that he thought these men were homosexual. Excited and intrigued, and always a good student and an avid reader, I went to the UBC library and found shelves of books (both fiction and nonfiction) on homosexuality. I read most of them. In a sense, being gay was a revelation (a late one) to me, an explicit explanation of my "difference," not something that I had hidden for years and finally allowed to escape. The difficulty in coming out was not from internal shame, but on how to do it—alone. I wanted to meet others, but didn't know how. I knew that I could not talk about it with my friends, but that just made me desire a different world with new friends; I did not want to live in the closet.

I began buying more physique magazines and, when I learned that there were gay trails in Stanley Park, I would sometimes drive there on Sunday afternoon. My first sexual encounters were there, but I tended to find the men I met too old, too different. I wasn't running from my homosexuality as much as I was running from this realistic version of it. This pattern of secret exploration continued for 2–3 years. In my third year at

UBC, I was in an English Honours seminar taught by a very dynamic, out gay man who became a very positive role model for me, though I was too shy to talk to him directly about being gay. In 1969, I met a student a couple of years older who took me out for the first time—to the B&B Club on Richards Street.

When I began graduate work, I was determined that the secrecy would end. I told my friend from high school, who had become a room-mate, that I would not live with him the next year unless I could be open about my life. Within a few months he was out as well and we were going downtown together. It was a small world, but it felt safe and exciting and I never really worried about anything except finding true love.

In the late 1960s, the main gay club (I can't remember the name) was on Hastings Street, which had no appeal for me, though I did find myself driving through the neighbourhood. In 1969, when I first went out, the main club was the B&B at 1369 Richards (later to become the Playpen South). I soon gravitated to a new club, Faces, on the corner of Robson and Seymour, which had a more "hippy" image and played newer music. The Castle and Ambassador pubs were also popular spots, but I was not a great drinker or smoker and I didn't feel comfortable there. You could not stand up with a beer, but had to sit at a table and it was just too dif-ficult a scene for someone as shy as I. There were also steam baths, but I was also too shy and self-conscious for that scene, and felt it was too focused on sex. For me, it was an innocent time, full of possibility and hope mixed with anxiety and impatience.

All the clubs in those days were "bottle" clubs, meaning that you could only drink the liquor that you brought. You paid a cover charge to get in, checked your liquor at the bar, and then went to mix or dance. A key change to the gay scene was the opening of the Gandy Dancer in 1975 in a huge, beautiful space with a liquor licence and pulsating, disco music. Other clubs that I can remember from that time were the Playpen Central, the Playpen North, Neighbours, and Thurlow's. In the 1980s just before AIDS hit Vancouver, the big club on the weekends was John Barley's in Gastown.

These early years were a heady time—most people went out on at least one night of the weekend and very quickly the clubs felt less like clubs and more like huge, friendly parties where you could easily meet people from all socioeconomic backgrounds. It seemed a world free of elitism, a scene that just kept opening up and getting better and, being young, and almost always with a lover, I was having a great time.

For men in Vancouver, the big party magnet was definitely San Francisco, though it was also common in those days to head to Seattle and Portland for the weekend. Most people soon had friends in Seattle and/or Portland and weekend visits became regular occurrences. I had met a man from San Francisco and would visit there at least twice a year.

I first saw Gaétan at Faces in May 1972. I was with my best friend and a man I was in a relationship with and so only looks were exchanged. Gaétan stood out in the crowd partly because of his good looks, but also because of his cutting-edge, extreme style—bleached blond hair and clothing that was tight and bright and worn with casual insouciance. In a Vancouver gay scene that was just beginning to open up, Gaétan was something new—a man flamboyantly and defiantly and happily gay, seemingly unconcerned about what others thought.

We actually met him a few days later (May 24th to be exact) when we were all at Wreck Beach. He and his friend Jacques had come to Vancouver to learn English in a UBC summer program and were staying in the residences on the top of the hill. We visited and exchanged phone numbers. It was an awkward time because of the intense and immediate attraction between Gaétan and me and the fact that my current partner also liked Gaétan very much. My relationship had been teetering a little already; Gaétan was the catalyst that pushed it over the edge.

By the middle of the summer, Gaétan and I were in love and together, though, of course, he had to return to Quebec. That was the beginning of a tumultuous, intensely passionate affair that was only finally over in early 1975. We were, in most respects, opposites, but there was no questioning our passion for each other. Looking back over my life, I realize that I am most attracted to those who are different from me, that my quiet, secure childhood and cautious, analytical brain made those who were wilder and freer most attractive to me. As in the Joni Mitchell song, I am, I suspect, "afraid of the devil, but attracted to those ones who ain't." Conversely, I think that Gaétan was attracted to my consistency and dependability.

Of course, in every respect, the relationship was doomed from the start—by youth, by our differences, by the burgeoning sexual freedom of the times, and by distance. I don't recall the sequence of events exactly, but know that he was here some again in the fall of 1972; that I visited him and his family in Quebec in December 1972; that he was here again for a few weeks in January 1973; that a job was arranged for him here in early 1973 that fell through. In May 1973, I flew to Winnipeg to meet him as he drove west and he lived here for a few months working as a hairdresser. I drove back to see him in Quebec in October 1973. It was a confusing time—when he was here, he missed his family and friends and Quebec, and, I think, felt stifled within the monogamous expectations of the relationship; when he was away, he missed me and worried I would meet someone new. It was a time of easy promiscuity and yet, despite the distance, we both (me especially) held each other to impossible 1950s standards of fidelity. Lies, cheating, pain, and recrimination became part of the relationship. I was working full-time as a welfare case worker, trying desperately to finish my master's thesis, considering the possibility of moving to Montreal, and, ultimately, feeling overwhelmed and occasionally depressed by it all.

Gaétan had determined early on that he wanted to be a flight attendant and that was a major impetus for the original trip to learn English in Vancouver. Although I am not fluent in spoken French, I had studied it in university, and can remember helping him with his letters of application to Air Canada—enough that he credited me with getting him through the first door to the program. When he was accepted for training, we were happy, assuming that all would be solved, that he would be based in Vancouver with lots of opportunities to return to Quebec. All of this happened in 1974. After his training, however, he was based in Toronto and, as we gradually saw less and less of each other, both began to move on, though still with many phone calls and visits in an attempt to keep things going. Only later did Gaétan confess to me that he had actually requested Toronto because the flights were better and, I suspect, because he wanted some freedom and fun. When things really began to fall apart, he did arrange a transfer to Vancouver, but it was too late: too much distance and distrust had developed, and our attempt to live together then was disastrous. He moved out into his own apartment in early 1975 and, I think, shortly later transferred back to Toronto or Montreal. Later that spring, I began a short relationship with another man, then left for Europe in the fall, returning in December. On my first visit to the Gandy Dancer on January 3, 1976, I met the man who would become my lover and partner until he died in May 1993. Gaétan did fly in one night in the spring of 1976, and wanted us to try again, but I was in love with a new man and was surprised to find that I could, for the first time, say "no" to Gaétan.

After that, I had no contact with Gaétan until 1980 or 1981 when he called while here on a layover. He wanted me to visit him in his hotel room, but my lover didn't want that and so we only visited on the phone. There may have been other calls during this period, but I don't recall hearing from him again until he phoned, sounding distraught and lonely, to tell me that he had "gay cancer" and was having chemotherapy treatment. Up until this point, I had only read a tiny article in the paper about the mysterious cancer that had shown up in gay men in New York. I was astonished to learn that Gaétan was part of this group. I was very worried, though some of my friends assured me that it was not serious as it was "only skin cancer." I can remember sending Gaétan encouraging letters. I have a card that he sent me in January 1982 when he is feeling depressed about the loss of hair (say he feels like an "alien") and is responding to an invitation that I had sent him to come and visit us. I had obviously sent him a picture of my lover and he comments on how handsome he is.

I think that he moved to San Francisco shortly after that . . . and sometime soon after moved back to Vancouver where he rented an apartment on Pacific Street. He became a good friend to both me and my lover to the extent that they sometimes went off to movies and shows together when I wasn't interested. They shared the same sense of humour and Gaétan quickly became a part of our life. I was so impressed then by how much Gaétan had grown up, by how supportive he was of my relationship, how strong he was about his health situation, and by how much joy he could still bring to life. Gaétan had a rare ability to live in the moment and to look for and focus on what was humorous and entertaining in that moment.

I remember, after one medical setback, holding him in his apartment and him telling me that he wasn't afraid of being dead; he was just scared of dying. He never expressed any great sense that life had been unjust; he just seemed determined to make the best of whatever time he had left. Early on in our relationship, I had suggested to Gaétan that he might feel differently about something (I can't remember what) when he was forty; he told me then that he simply couldn't imagine being forty. I don't think he ever really expected a long life.

In Vancouver, Gaétan did continue to go out, but not frequently. He seemed happier to do simple things—go for a ride on his motorcycle, go the movies, come visit for lunch, go to the beach with us. I think he was a little tired of the gay scene, still willing to play it, but longing for a secure relationship, a lover. He did develop a relationship with a new man, though I could tell he wasn't really in love. I remember his sadness when he learned of other men in his New York medical group dying and also his upset and anger when someone phoned him from Los Angeles and accused him of killing his partner.

I was somewhat aware of the controversy about Gaétan going out and continuing to be sexually active, but we and our friends were very dismissive of people who thought he should hide. My partner's sister had phoned and warned us to keep him out of our house, but we were repulsed by her, not him. Good people, we felt, do not shun the ill. We accepted him without hesitation or fear into our lives. It's also important to remember that the consensus at this point was that AIDS was the result of the collapse of an overburdened immune system. Cancer—and Kaposi's sarcoma was still the major definitive marker of the illness—was not, we all knew, contagious. If people were changing their lifestyles as a result of AIDS, it was to limit the number of partners and amount of party drugs, not to change what they did with those partners. I do remember telling a friend of people being afraid to be with Gaétan and him telling me, "I'd sleep with him." Certainly, some people were afraid, but most of us thought that fear was baseless and wrong.

In the fall of 1983, he started to feel very ill and, I think in December, decided to return home to Quebec for a visit. I invited him to the house for dinner on the night before he left and we all had a good visit, but it was a different, very quiet and reflective Gaétan that night. I can remember him sitting on the couch, listening to the tick tock of my old wall clock, talking about how peaceful and beautiful the sound was, and thanking us over and over for the evening. When I drove him home, we were very quiet, both near tears, both of us realizing, I think, that we wouldn't see each other again.

I did talk regularly to Gaétan in his final weeks in Quebec, the last time when he was very ill in hospital after some kind of operation as a result of his MAI [mycobacterium avium intercellulare] infection in his lungs. My last call to his room was answered by a relative who told me that they were all gathered there for the administration of the last rites. . . .

After he died, I worked with his friend, David Durnin, to clear the apartment and distribute some of his belongings as he had requested. As he had requested, I also wrote a letter of thanks to Air Canada for giving him a job that he loved and for treating him with respect and patience.

Gaétan didn't give me a lot of information about his youth, but I do think that he was harassed a fair amount for being gay. He spoke about aggressively and physically fighting those who taunted him. I think what many people took for arrogance was simply another instance of Gaétan determined to stand up for himself, to be himself. I remember early in our relationship that I had expressed some reservation about his dress; he met me later that day in full gay regalia . . . telling me, without words, that he would be who he was. This same, fighting spirit was evident when he went to the beach in 1983 and he made no attempt to disguise or cover up his Kaposi's sarcoma lesions, defiantly staring back at those who stared at him. While I wasn't there, he also told me how he had stood up alone to speak of his experience and needs at a gay meeting downtown. I assume this must have been the meeting in 1983.

As I have said, despite being harassed by others at the bars and told that he should stay home, Gaétan did continue to go out and be himself while in Vancouver, though I'm sure that those responses, plus changes within him, were why he went out less and less and with far less joy. I don't know how he dealt with his AIDS status when he met strangers, but it wasn't something he could easily have hidden as his legs and torso had many KS lesions. Certainly, the man he was in a relationship with was well aware of his health situation. As a gay man, Gaétan was completely imbued with the spirit of Stonewall, stronger and braver than many who were so critical of him. That spirit led him to embrace the sexual revolution in all its fullness; it also gave him immense strength when that whole world turned around on him and he was left so alone, not yet thirty, his beauty suddenly marked by lesions that seemed to signal death. Somehow, he kept himself together, fought on to be who he was and live as he wanted to live.

Gaétan also told me that he was adopted. He had met his birth mother, though they were not close. In my visit with the family in 1972, he seemed a very integral and popular member of his adopted family—a particular favourite of his mother, who seemed totally supportive of his gay sensibility—lavishing praise on his flamboyant clothes and interested in his shelves of cosmetics and creams. She and the whole family were very welcoming to me and we slept together in a guest room upstairs.

I first read about AIDS in the paper. My mother was far ahead of her time in her knowledge of nutrition and health. She had stressed to us very early the importance of disease prevention, the risks of catching disease from strangers, the dangerous side effects of too much medication, and the importance of staying healthy by minimizing exposure

to disease. I had been very critical of the carelessness with which Gaétan and my friends in San Francisco—in fact most gay men—took antibiotics and dealt with STDs. Even doctors seemed to view STDs as amus-
ing hiccups in life. Several of my friends had contracted hepatitis from
sex and many were frequently taking antibiotics for a variety of other
infections. I knew the lifestyle was unhealthy, and had been very wary;
my first assumption was that AIDS was caused by the breakdown of the
immune system, the cumulative effect of the generally unhealthy lifestyles of liberated gay men. All the expert advice early on was to limit
the number of partners to reduce the strain on the immune system. My
view only changed when I read an article by Larry Kramer in the *Advocate*, which, for the first time, suggested that AIDS was a communicable
disease, that the issue was likely not how many partners, but what you
did with those partners.

In the 1980s, AIDS information was very confusing and contradictory. The medical establishment seemed at odds with alternative views
expressed in gay papers or articles in the alternative press. People were
nervous of dangerous, debilitating drugs, such as AZT, suddenly being prescribed to gay men. It was a time of great anxiety and not a little paranoia; almost everyone felt in the dark and argued for their versions of the light. I think it was especially hard for gay doctors who had
been trained to believe that they could solve almost all medical problems, only to be confronted with something that they knew almost nothing about and that was killing their friends and patients.

I was never contacted by Randy Shilts and never read his book,
though have read about it. I was not aware that he was in Vancouver in
1986.

I think that I first read about "Patient Zero" in reviews of *And the
Band Played On*, but I'm not sure. I remember seeing a movie at a gay
film festival, *Zero Patience*, which provided a reasonably accurate view
of Gaétan's family. I never seriously considered that Gaétan was "Patient Zero," though I'm sure, given the times, that he did help to spread
the virus. But Gaétan was no different than the vast majority of gay men
then. If he had more partners than most, it was only because his personality, looks, and job made that easier for him than for others. Gaétan was no ogre and no saint . . . just a young man exploring the world
as it opened up for him in his twenties. Like almost all gay men who had
grown up lonely in a homophobic world, he found being desired and attractive intoxicating and there seemed no reason not to make the most

of all the love and joy suddenly available to him. While he certainly couldn't remain sexually faithful to me, and lied to hide that from me, I never doubted the purity of his heart or the reality of his love; he was a generous lover, friend, and family member, a young man of immense charm with an intoxicating sense of humour, who took intense joy in making people laugh, whose smile was truly magnetic. I remember going to a T-Dance at John Barley's, likely in the summer of 1983, and seeing him there with his boyfriend, dancing with great joy and abandon, bare-chested, his shirt rolled up and held high above his head, whirling in the air between his outstretched arms, his whole body lost to the music. He was a compelling figure, beautiful and brave—still very, very young, defiant in the face of disease and death just as he had always been defiant in the face of all that had threatened to limit his joy in life.

Oral History Interviews

The author recorded fifty-two interviews—fifty in English and two in French—on audiocassette in 2007 and 2008. These recordings were later converted to digital files, and the English interviews were then transcribed by the author's mother, Jane McKay. Of the fifty-two interviews, agreement was obtained for fifty to be archived at the British Library, under the collection title Imagining Patient Zero: Interviews about the History of the North American HIV/AIDS Epidemic. The collection includes audiocassette tapes, digitized copies, and verbatim transcripts. All but one of the interviewees assigned their copyright in the recordings to the British Library; the author and Robin Metcalfe have retained their copyrights for the duration of their lifetimes, after which their rights are transferred to the British Library. All the recordings are cataloged on the British Library Sound and Moving Image catalog (http://sami.bl.uk) and can be accessed at the British Library, subject to any access restrictions requested by individual interviewees and the author.

Number	Date	Location	Interviewee
C1491/01	July 6, 2007	Los Angeles	Don Spradlin
C1491/02	July 6, 2007	Los Angeles	Zvi Howard Rosenman
C1491/03	July 10, 2007	San Francisco	George Rutherford
C1491/04	July 12, 2007	San Francisco	Daniel Detorie
C1491/05	July 16, 2007	San Francisco	Jay Levy
C1491/06	July 19, 2007	San Francisco	Rink Foto
C1491/07	July 19, 2007	San Francisco	Mervyn Silverman
C1491/08	July 22, 2007	San Francisco	Hank Wilson
C1491/09	July 24, 2007	San Francisco	Andrew Moss
Not deposited*	July 26, 2007	San Francisco	Selma Dritz
C1491/10	July 27, 2007	San Francisco	Marcus Conant & Joseph Robinson

Number	Date	Location	Interviewee
C1491/11	July 27, 2007	San Francisco	Paul Volberding
C1491/12	July 28, 2007	San Francisco	*Josh Lancaster*
C1491/13	July 28, 2007	San Francisco	Ken Maley
C1491/14	July 29, 2007	San Francisco	*Peter Roberts*
C1491/15	July 29, 2007	San Francisco	Ross Murray
C1491/16	August 28, 2007	Vancouver	Richard Mathias
C1491/17	August 28, 2007	Vancouver	Gordon Price
C1491/18	August 31, 2007	Vancouver	Brian Willoughby
C1491/19	September 3, 2007	Vancouver	Noah Stewart
C1491/20	January 8, 2008	Vancouver	Terry Twentyman
C1491/21	March 28, 2008	Miami	William Darrow
C1491/22	April 8, 2008	New York	Michael Denneny
C1491/23	April 14, 2008	New York	Larry Kramer
Not deposited†	April 24, 2008	New York	Alvin Friedman-Kien
C1491/24	April 25, 2008	New York	Richard Berkowitz
C1491/25	April 28, 2008	New York	Lawrence Mass
C1491/26	June 10, 2008	Vancouver	Barbara Dunn, Elaine Watson & Janice Miller
C1491/27	June 11, 2008	Vancouver	*Spencer Macdonell*
C1491/28	June 11, 2008	Vancouver	Alan Herbert
C1491/29	July 9, 2008	Montreal	Richard Morisset
C1491/30	July 9, 2008	Montreal	Christos Tsoukas
C1491/31	July 10, 2008	Montreal	Ross Higgins
C1491/32	July 10, 2008	Montreal	Norbert Gilmore
C1491/33	July 14, 2008	Montreal	Jean Robert
C1491/34	July 25, 2008	Halifax	Desiree Conn
C1491/35	July 31, 2008	Halifax	Rand Gaynor & Robin Metcalfe
C1491/36	August 1, 2008	Halifax	Eric Smith
C1491/37	August 19, 2008	Vancouver	Jacques Menard
C1491/38	August 21, 2008	Vancouver	Richard Bisson
C1491/39	August 27, 30 & September 6, 2008	Toronto	Douglas Elliott
C1491/40	August 30, 2008	Toronto	Erica Moghal
C1491/41	September 2, 2008	Toronto	John Greyson
C1491/42	September 4, 2008	Toronto	André Picard
C1491/43	September 5, 2008	Toronto	Rosemary Barnes
C1491/44	September 7 & 9, 2008	Toronto	Robert (Bob) Tivey
C1491/45	September 9, 2008	Toronto	Franco Polillo
C1491/46	September 10, 2008	Toronto	Horace Krever
C1491/47	September 11, 2008	Toronto	Pierre-Claude (Pedro) Levaque
C1491/48	September 14, 2008	Toronto	Ed Jackson
C1491/49	September 15, 2008	Toronto	Theresa Dobko
C1491/50	September 15, 2008	Toronto	Ron Rosenes

Note: Italic type denotes a pseudonym.
* The author and Debbie Dritz, Selma Dritz's daughter, jointly decided not to deposit the interview. Readers are encouraged to consult instead Selma Dritz's reminiscences in Sally Smith Hughes's *The AIDS Epidemic in San Francisco* at the Bancroft Library, University of California–Berkeley.
† A signed waiver was never returned, pending its review by New York University's attorney, thus the interview was not used for research purposes nor deposited.

Bibliography

Archival Materials

Canada

Halifax

Sir James Dunn Law Library, Dalhousie University

Exhibits of the Commission of Inquiry on the Blood System in Canada

AIDS Vancouver: Exhibits of the British Columbia hearings, March 1994, xlix.

Montreal

Bibliothèque et Archives nationales du Québec

Formulaire de mariages

Ottawa

Library and Archives Canada

Air Canada fonds

Canadian Association for Journalists, acc. 1990–0395

Census of Canada, 1911

Telephone directories

Quebec City

L'Aéroport international Jean-Lesage de Québec

Institutional records

Toronto

Canadian Lesbian and Gay Archives

Accession 2014–054

Records of the AIDS Committee of Toronto

AIDS Memorial Committee files

The Film Reference Library, Toronto International Film Festival Group

John Greyson Collection

Vancouver
British Columbia Gay and Lesbian Archives
Periodical clippings
Personal Papers of Ray Redford

United Kingdom
London
Personal and Professional Papers of Joseph Sonnabend

United States
Bethesda, MD
History of Medicine Division, Archives and Modern Manuscripts Collection, National Library of Medicine
AIDS Correspondence (TRACER) archives, 1982–1990. Office of the Assistant Secretary for Planning and Evaluation, US Department of Health and Human Services, MS C 607.
National Commission on Acquired Immune Deficiency Syndrome Records, 1983–1994, MS C 544.
Los Angeles
ONE National Gay and Lesbian Archives at the USC [University of Southern California] Libraries
Jim Kepner Collection
Miami
Personal and Professional Papers of William W. Darrow
New York City
Columbia Center for Oral History Archives, Rare Book and Manuscript Library, Columbia University in the City of New York
Physicians and AIDS Oral History Project
Reminiscences of Neil Schram, 1996
Reminiscences of Dan William, 1996
Lesbian, Gay, Bisexual and Transgender Community Center National History Archive
Michael Callen Papers
Manuscripts and Archives, New York Public Library, Astor, Lenox, and Tilden Foundations
Gay Men's Health Crisis Records
Karla Jay Papers
Lawrence Mass Papers
Providence, RI
John Hay Library, Brown University
St. Martin's Press Archive

San Francisco
  Gay, Lesbian, Bisexual, Transgender Historical Society
    AIDS Ephemera Collection
    Linda Alband Collection of Randy Shilts Materials
    Frank Robinson Papers
    Dan Turner Papers
  LGBTQIA Center, San Francisco Public Library
    Randy Shilts Papers (GLC 43)
  San Francisco History Center, San Francisco Public Library
    San Francisco Department of Public Health AIDS Office Records (SFH 4)
  Archives and Special Collections, UCSF Library and Center for Knowledge
    Management, University of California–San Francisco
    Marcus A. Conant Papers
    Selma E. Dritz Papers
    San Francisco AIDS Foundation Records
Simi Valley, CA
  Ronald Reagan Presidential Library
    Gary Bauer Files (OA19222)

Published Sources, Reports, and Dissertations

"AIDS: At the Heart of an Epidemic." *Pittsburgh Post-Gazette*, March 28, 1988, 14.

"AIDS Killed Cdn. In '79." *Medical Post*, October 4, 1988, 59.

"AIDS Patient Zero." *Seth McFarlane's Cavalcade of Cartoon Comedy*. Directed by Greg Colton. Beverly Hills, CA: 20th Century Fox, 2009. DVD.

"AIDS Vancouver—February 11, 1983." In *AIDS Vancouver: Exhibits of the British Columbia Hearings, March 1994—Commission of Inquiry on the Blood System in Canada*, vol. 49 Ottawa: The Commission, 1994.

AIDS Vancouver. "30 30 AIDS Vancouver: 1983– The Forum." 2013. http://3030.aidsvancouver.org/1983/.

Albrink, Wilhelm S., Samuel M. Brooks, Robert E. Biron, and Moses Kopel. "Human Inhalation Anthrax: A Report of Three Fatal Cases." *American Journal of Pathology* 36, no. 4 (1960): 457–71.

Allard, Lionel. *L'Ancienne-Lorette*. Ottawa: Éditions Leméac, 1979.

Altman, Dennis. *AIDS in the Mind of America: The Social, Political, and Psychological Impact of a New Epidemic*. Garden City, NY: Anchor Press, 1986.

Ammann, Arthur J., Diane W. Wara, Selma Dritz, Morton J. Cowan, Peggy Weintrub, Howard Goldman, and Herbert A. Perkins. "Acquired Immunodeficiency in an Infant: Possible Transmission by Means of Blood Products" *Lancet* 321, no. 8331 (1983): 956–58.

Anderson, Roy M., and Robert M. May. "Epidemiological Parameters of HIV Transmission." *Nature* 333, no. 6173 (1988): 514–19.

And the Band Played On. Directed by Roger Spottiswoode. HBO Pictures, 1993. Burbank, CA: Warner Home Video, 2004. DVD.

"And the Band Played On: Politics, People and the AIDS Epidemic." *Publishers Weekly*, September 11, 1987, 72.

April, Wayne. "AIDS Mortality Higher Than First Thought." *Bay Area Reporter* [San Francisco], October 14, 1982, 1.

———. "Doctors Brief 'Gay Leaders' On AIDS." *Bay Area Reporter* [San Francisco], April 7, 1983, 3, 18.

Arnim, [Bettina von]. "Les aventures d'un manuscrit." *Revue germanique* 9, no. 26 (1837): 149–85.

Arrizabalaga, Jon. "Medical Responses to the 'French Disease' in Europe at the Turn of the Sixteenth Century." In Siena, *Sins of the Flesh*, 33–55.

Arrizabalaga, Jon, John Henderson, and Roger French. *The Great Pox: The French Disease in Renaissance Europe.* London: Yale University Press, 1997.

Ashforth, Adam. "Reckoning Schemes of Legitimation: On Commissions of Inquiry as Power/Knowledge Forms." *Journal of Historical Sociology* 3, no. 1 (1990): 1–22.

Associated Press. "It's Waterloo Again for 'Napoleon,'" *Orlando Sentinel*, November 19, 1987, E8.

Astruc, John. *A Treatise of Venereal Diseases, in Nine Books; Containing an Account of the Origin, Propagation, and Contagion of This Distemper.* 2 vols. London, 1754. Facsimile, Eighteenth Century Collections Online digital library, http://find.galegroup.com/ecco/infomark.do?&contentSet= ECCOArticles &type=multipage&tabID=T001&prodId=ECCO&docId= CW108536016&source=gale&userGroupName=oxford&version=1.0&doc Level=FASCIMILE.

Auerbach, David M., William W. Darrow, Harold W. Jaffe, and James W. Curran. "Cluster of Cases of the Acquired Immune Deficiency Syndrome: Patients Linked by Sexual Contact." *American Journal of Medicine* 76, no. 3 (1984): 487–92.

Babineau, Guy. "The Prettiest One: Gaetan Dugas and the 'AIDS Mary' Myth." *XTRA! West* [Vancouver], November 29, 2001, 13–15.

"The 'Bacillus Carriers' of Enteric Fever." *Lancet* 171, no. 4410 (1908): 732–33.

Badurski, Jerry. "Covering KS." *Bay Area Reporter* [San Francisco], September 16, 1982, 7.

Baldwin, Peter. *Disease and Democracy: The Industrialized World Faces AIDS.* Berkeley: University of California Press, 2005.

Banaszynski, Jacqui. "Reporter Calls Accounting of AIDS a 'Mission.'" *St. Paul* [MN] *Pioneer Press Dispatch*, November 10, 1987, 1A, 4A.

Barnes, David S. *The Making of a Social Disease: Tuberculosis in Nineteenth-Century France*. Berkeley: University of California Press, 1995.

———. "Targeting Patient Zero." In *Tuberculosis Then and Now: Perspectives on the History of an Infectious Disease*, edited by Michael Worboys and Flurin Condrau, 49–71. London: McGill-Queen's University Press, 2010.

Batza, Catherine P. "Before AIDS: Gay and Lesbian Community Health Activism in the 1970s." DPhil diss., University of Illinois at Chicago, 2012.

Bayer, Ronald. *Homosexuality and American Psychiatry: The Politics of Diagnosis*. New York: Basic Books, 1981.

———. "AIDS, Privacy, and Responsibility." *Daedalus* 118, no. 3 (1989): 79–99.

———. *Private Acts, Social Consequences: AIDS and the Politics of Public Health*. New Brunswick, NJ: Rutgers University Press, 1991.

Bayer, Ronald, and Gerald M. Oppenheimer. *AIDS Doctors: Voices from the Epidemic: An Oral History*. Oxford: Oxford University Press, 2000.

Bell, Arthur. "AIDS Update: Love with the Proper Stranger." *Village Voice*, May 10, 1983, 16–17.

Bellefeuille, Roger. "Propagation du sida aux États-Unis: La famille de Gaétan Dugas fort affectée." *Le Soleil*, October 9, 1987, A3.

Bercaw, Charlotte. "Author Bemoans AIDS Travesties in Best-Seller." *Beacon-News* [Aurora, IL], November 15, 1987, A1, A5.

———. "Shilts Gets Grip on His Being, Then Worldwide Epidemic." *Beacon-News* [Aurora, IL], November 15, 1987, A5, A8.

Berco, Cristian. "Syphilis and the Silencing of Sodomy in Juan Calvo's *Tratado Del Morbo Gálico*." In Borris and Rousseau, *Sciences of Homosexuality in Early Modern Europe*, 92–113.

Berger, Leslie. "Nurse Battles City's TB Cases with Cunning Detective Work." *Washington Post*, August 11, 1982, sec. District Weekly, DC1.

Bergman, Lowell. "Patient Zero." On *60 Minutes*, CBS, airdate November 15, 1987. Online video, 14:01. https://www.youtube.com/watch?v=Sc7bYnH2Zpo.

Berkowitz, Richard. *Stayin' Alive: The Invention of Safe Sex; A Personal History*. Oxford: Westview Press, 2003.

Berlandt, Konstantin. "KS Therapist Contracts KS: Denies Any Connection." *Bay Area Reporter* [San Francisco], August 19, 1982, 1, 9.

Berridge, Virginia. "The History of AIDS." *AIDS* 7, Suppl. 1 (1993): S243–48.

Berridge, Virginia, and Philip Strong. "AIDS and the Relevance of History." *Social History of Medicine* 4, no. 1 (1991): 129–38.

Bersani, Leo. "Is the Rectum a Grave?" In *AIDS: Cultural Analysis, Cultural Activism*, edited by Douglas Crimp, 197–222. Cambridge, MA: MIT Press, 1988.

Besharov, Douglas J. "AIDS and the Criminal Law: Needed Reform." *State Factor* 13, no. 8 (1987): 1–8.

Beukes, Suzanne Mary. "Ebola in Guinea: Finding Patient Zero." *Daily Maverick*

[Johannesburg, South Africa], October 27, 2014. http://www.dailymaverick.co
.za/article/2014-10-27-ebola-in-guinea-finding-patient-zero/#.V_zWNTsefB4.

Bluestein, Ron. "Cries and Whispers of an Epidemic." *Advocate*, November 24, 1987, 52–53, 63–65, 67.

Boffey, Philip M. "Reagan Urges Wide AIDS Testing But Does Not Call for Compulsion." *New York Times*, June 1, 1987, A1, A15.

Books That Shaped America. Washington, DC: Library of Congress, June 25, 2012. Exhibition catalog. https://www.loc.gov/exhibits/books-that-shaped -america/overview.html.

Boorstin, Robert O. "Criminal and Civil Litigation on Spread of AIDS Appears." *New York Times*, June 19, 1987, A1, A16.

Borris, Kenneth, and George Rousseau, eds. *The Sciences of Homosexuality in Early Modern Europe*. New York: Routledge, 2008.

Boswell, John. *Christianity, Social Tolerance, and Homosexuality: Gay People in Western Europe from the Beginning of the Christian Era to the Fourteenth Century*. London: University of Chicago Press, 1980.

Bowman, Karlyn, Andrew Rugg, and Jennifer Marsico. *Polls on Attitudes on Homosexuality and Gay Marriage*. Washington, DC: American Enterprise Institute for Public Policy Research, 2013. http://www.aei.org/files/2013/03/ 21/-polls-on-attitudes-on-homosexuality-gay-marriage_151640318614.pdf.

Boyd, Nan Alamilla. *Wide-Open Town: A History of Queer San Francisco to 1965*. Berkeley: University of California Press, 2003.

——. "Who Is the Subject? Queer Theory Meets Oral History." *Journal of the History of Sexuality* 17, no. 2 (2008): 177–89.

Bradshaw, W. V. Jr. "Homosexual Syphilis Epidemic." *Texas State Journal of Medicine* 57 (1961): 907–9.

Brandt, Allan M. *No Magic Bullet: A Social History of Venereal Disease in the United States since 1880*. Expanded ed. Oxford: Oxford University Press, 1987.

——. *The Cigarette Century: The Rise, Fall, and Deadly Persistence of the Product that Defined America*. New York: Basic Books, 2007.

Brier, Jennifer. *Infectious Ideas: US Political Responses to the AIDS Crisis*. Chapel Hill, NC: University of North Carolina Press, 2009.

Brownlee, Shannon, Eric Ransdell, Traci Watson, Fred Coleman, and Viva Hardigg. "Horror in the Hot Zone." *US News and World Report*, May 22, 1995, 57–61.

Brown, Michael P. *RePlacing Citizenship: AIDS Activism and Radical Democracy*. London: Guilford Press, 1997.

Brown, William J. "Cluster Testing—A New Development in Syphilis Case Finding." *American Journal of Public Health* 51, no. 7 (1961): 1043–48

——. "Migration as a Factor in Venereal Disease Programmes in the United States." *British Journal of Venereal Diseases* 36, no. 1 (1960): 49–58.

Brown, William J., Thomas F. Sellers, and Evan W. Thomas. "Challenge to the Private Physician in the Epidemiology of Syphilis." *Journal of the American Medical Association* 171, no. 4 (1959): 389–93.

Brunvand, Jan Harold. *Curses! Broiled Again!* London: W. W. Norton, 1989.

Burak, Tim. "Books." *Seattle Gay News*, November 27, 1987, 26–29.

Burci, Gian Luca, and Claude-Henri Vignes. *World Health Organization.* The Hague: Kluwer Law International, 2004.

Bureau International des Expositions. "1967 Montreal." Accessed March 9, 2017. http://www.bie-paris.org/site/en/component/k2/item/102-1967-montreal.

Burri, Regula Valérie, and Joseph Dumit. "Social Studies of Scientific Imaging and Visualization." In *The Handbook of Science and Technology Studies*, 3rd ed., edited by Edward J. Hackett, Olga Amsterdamska, Michael Lynch, and Judy Wajcman, 297–317. Cambridge, MA: MIT Press, 2008.

Bury, M. R. "Social Constructionism and the Development of Medical Sociology." *Sociology of Health and Illness* 8, no. 2 (1986): 137–69.

Bussières, Ian. "Agent de bord exonéré d'avoir propagé le sida en Amérique : la famille de Gaétan Dugas soulagée mais amère." *Le Soleil* [Quebec City], October 31, 1987, 17.

Caen, Herb. "Use 'Em or Lose 'Em." *San Francisco Chronicle*, November 10, 1987, B1.

Callen, Michael, and Richard Berkowitz. With editorial assistance by Richard Dworkin. *How to Have Sex in an Epidemic: One Approach.* New York: News from the Front Publications, 1983.

———. With Richard Dworkin. "We Know Who We Are: Two Gay Men Declare War on Promiscuity." *New York Native*, November 8, 1982.

Campbell, Bobbi. "KS Exposure." Letter to the editor. *Bay Area Reporter* [San Francisco], October 7, 1982, 10.

Campbell, Duncan. "An End to the Silence." *New Statesman*, March 4, 1988, 22–23.

———. "Shilts Theory Is Nonsense!" *Capital Gay* [London], March 4, 1988, 1, 4.

Canaday, Margot. "Thinking Sex in the Transnational Turn: An Introduction." *American Historical Review* 114, no. 5 (2009): 1250–57.

"Canadian Blamed for Bringing Aids to US." *Times* [London], October 8, 1987, 11.

Canadian Press, "AIDS-Fearing Parents Plot Boycott." *Vancouver Sun*, October 9, 1987, A6.

"Canadian Said to Have Had Key Role in Spread of AIDS." *New York Times*, October 7, 1987, B7.

Carmichael, Ann G. *Plague and the Poor in Renaissance Florence.* Cambridge: Cambridge University Press, 1986.

Cassel, Jay. *The Secret Plague: Venereal Disease in Canada, 1838–1939.* London: University of Toronto Press, 1987.

———. "Private Acts and Public Actions: The Canadian Response to the Problem of Sexually Transmitted Disease in the Twentieth Century." *Transactions of the Royal Society of Canada* 4 (1989): 305–28.

Castigliano, Lucio. "My Night at the Baths." *New York Native*, January 30, 1984, 1, 21, 23.

Centers for Disease Control and Prevention (CDC). "Prevention of Acquired Immune Deficiency Syndrome (AIDS): Report of Inter-Agency Recommendations." *MMWR* 32, no. 8 (1983): 101–3.

Chancellor, John, and Walter R. Mears. *The News Business.* New York: Harper and Row, 1983.

Chang, Yuan, Ethel Cesarman, Melissa S. Pessin, Frank Lee, Janice Culpepper, Daniel M. Knowles, and Patrick S. Moore. "Identification of Herpesvirus-Like DNA Sequences in AIDS-Associated Kaposi's Sarcoma." *Science* 266, no. 5192 (1994): 1865–69.

Chauncey, George. *Gay New York: Gender, Urban Culture, and the Making of the Gay Male World, 1890–1940.* New York: Basic Books, 1994.

———. "'What Gay Studies Taught the Court': The Historians' Amicus Brief in *Lawrence v. Texas.*" *GLQ: A Journal of Lesbian and Gay Studies* 10, no. 3 (2004): 509–38.

———. *Why Marriage? The History Shaping Today's Debate over Gay Equality.* New York: Basic Books, 2004.

Chittock, Brian. "AIDS: A Case of Homophobia." *Fine Print* [Edmonton], April 1983, 10–11.

Christy, James V. Letter to the editor. *St. Petersburg* [FL] *Times*, November 8, 1987, Factiva (stpt000020011118djb802326).

Claremont, J. "They Shoot Horses, Don't They?" Letter to the editor. *Bay Area Reporter* [San Francisco], September 16, 1982, 8.

———. "Vague." Letter to the editor. *Bay Area Reporter* [San Francisco], September 23, 1982, 7.

Clendinen, Dudley, and Adam Nigourney. *Out for Good: The Struggle to Build a Gay Rights Movement in America.* New York: Simon and Schuster, 1999.

Clowe, John Lee. "The Changing World of AIDS: We Are All At Risk." *Vital Speeches of the Day* 59, no. 5 (1992): 135–38.

Cochrane, Michelle. *When AIDS Began: San Francisco and the Making of an Epidemic.* London: Routledge, 2004.

Cohen, Jon. *Shots in the Dark: The Wayward Search for an AIDS Vaccine.* New York: W. W. Norton, 2001.

Cohn, Victor. "Poll Shows Widespread Awareness, Misguided Fears About Disease." *Washington Post*, September 4, 1985, H7.

Coleman, James S. *The Adolescent Society: The Social Life of the Teenager and Its Impact on Education.* New York: Free Press, 1961.

Coleman, William. "Epidemiological Method in the 1860s: Yellow Fever at Saint-Nazaire." *Bulletin of the History of Medicine* 58, no. 2 (1984): 145–63.

——. *Yellow Fever in the North: The Methods of Early Epidemiology*. Madison: University of Wisconsin Press, 1987.

Colgrove, James. *Epidemic City: The Politics of Public Health in New York*. New York: Russell Sage Foundation, 2011.

"The Columbus of AIDS." *National Review*, November 6, 1987, 19.

Conant, Marcus A. "Founding the KS Clinic, and Continued AIDS Activism." Oral history interviews conducted in 1992 and 1995 by Sally Smith Hughes. In *The AIDS Epidemic in San Francisco: The Medical Response, 1981–1984, Volume II*. Regional Oral History Office, Bancroft Library, University of California–Berkeley, 1996. Online Archive of California, 2009. http://ark.cdlib.org/ark:/13030/kt7b69n8jn.

Condrau, Flurin. "The Patient's View Meets the Clinical Gaze." *Social History of Medicine* 20, no. 3 (2007): 525–40.

Conner, Susan P. "The Pox in Eighteenth-Century France." In *The Secret Malady: Venereal Disease in Eighteenth-Century Britain and France*, edited by Linda E. Merians, 15–33. Lexington: University Press of Kentucky, 1996.

Cooter, Roger, with Claudia Stein. *Writing History in the Age of Biomedicine*. New Haven, CT: Yale University Press, 2013.

Corbitt, Gerald, Andrew S. Bailey, and George Williams. "HIV Infection in Manchester, 1959." *Lancet* 336, no. 8706 (1990): 51.

Courte, Bernard. "The Spread of AIDS." *Maclean's*, November 30, 1987, 6.

——. "Un bouc émissaire." *Sortie*, February 1988, 7.

Crewdson, John. "Case Shakes Theories of AIDS Origin." *Chicago Tribune*, October 25, 1987, 1, 20.

Crimp, Douglas, ed. *AIDS: Cultural Analysis, Cultural Activism*. Cambridge: MIT Press, 1988.

——. "AIDS: Cultural Analysis/Cultural Activism." In Crimp, *AIDS: Cultural Analysis, Cultural Activism*, 3–16. .

——. "How to Have Promiscuity in an Epidemic." In *AIDS: Cultural Analysis, Cultural Activism*, 237–71.

——. *Melancholia and Moralism: Essays on AIDS and Queer Politics*. London: MIT Press, 2002.

——. "Randy Shilts's Miserable Failure." In *Melancholia and Moralism*, 117–28.

Crook, Tim. "Don't Attack Gilligan for Doing His Job." Letter to the editor. *Guardian* [London], September 9, 2003, https://www.theguardian.com/media/2003/sep/10/bbc.guardianletters.

Cross, Sue. "Jerry Falwell Calls AIDS a 'Gay Plague.'" *Washington Post*, July 6, 1983, B3.

Curran, James W., Harold W. Jaffe, Ann M. Hardy, W. Meade Morgan, Richard M. Selik, and Timothy J. Dondero. "Epidemiology of HIV Infection and AIDS in the United States." *Science* 239, no. 4840 (1988): 610–16.

Daly, Michael. "AIDS Anxiety." *New York* [Magazine], June 20, 1983, 24–29.

Damski, Jon-Henri. "The Victim Zero Story." *Windy City Times* [Chicago], October 22, 1987.

Darrow, William W. "AIDS: Socioepidemiologic Responses to an Epidemic." In *AIDS and the Social Sciences: Common Threads*, edited by Richard Ulack and W. F. Skinner, 82–99. Lexington: University of Kentucky Press, 1991.

———. "A Few Minutes with Venus, A Lifetime with Mercury." In *The Sex Scientists*, edited by Gary G. Brannigan, Elizabeth R. Allgeier, and A. Richard Allgeier, 156–70. New York: Addison, Wesley, Longman, 1998.

Darrow, William W., Donald Barrett, Karla Jay, and Allen Young. "The Gay Report on Sexually Transmitted Diseases." *American Journal of Public Health* 71, no. 9 (1981): 1004–11.

Darrow, William W., E. Michael Gorman, and Brad P. Glick. "The Social Origins of AIDS: Social Change, Sexual Behavior, and Disease Trends." In *The Social Dimensions of AIDS: Method and Theory*, edited by Douglas A. Feldman and Thomas M. Johnson, 95–107. New York: Praeger, 1986.

Davidson, N. S. "Sodomy in Early Modern Venice." In *Sodomy in Early Modern Europe*, edited by Thomas Betteridge, 65–81. Manchester, UK: Manchester University Press, 2002.

Davidson, Roger. "'The Price of the Permissive Society': The Epidemiology and Control of VD and STDs in Late-Twentieth-Century Scotland." In *Sex, Sin and Suffering: Venereal Disease and European Society since 1870*, edited by Roger Davidson and Lesley A. Hall, 220–36. London: Routledge, 2001.

Davies, D. S., and I. Walker Hall. "A Discussion on the Etiology and Epidemiology of Typhoid (Enteric) Fever: Typhoid Carriers, with an Account of Two Institution Outbreaks Traced to the Same 'Carrier.'" *Proceedings of the Royal Society of Medicine* 1 (1907–8): 175–91.

Defoe, Daniel. *A Journal of the Plague Year*. Edited by Louis Landa. Oxford: Oxford University Press, 1990.

De Gruttola, Victor, Kenneth Mayer, and William Bennett. "AIDS: Has the Problem Been Adequately Assessed?" *Reviews of Infectious Diseases* 8, no. 2 (1986): 295–305.

Delaporte, François. *Disease and Civilization: The Cholera in Paris, 1832*. Translated by Arthur Goldhammer. London: MIT Press, 1986.

D'Emilio, John. *Sexual Politics, Sexual Communities: The Making of a Homosexual Minority in the United States, 1940–1970*. Chicago: University of Chicago Press, 1983.

D'Emilio, John, and Estelle B. Freedman. *Intimate Matters: A History of Sexuality in America*. 2nd ed. New York: Harper and Row, 1997.

Dennis, Keith. "Alberta Beef." Letter to the editor. *Fine Print* [Edmonton], July 1983, 2, 22.

Deschamps, Marie-Marcelle, Daniel W. Fitzgerald, Jean William Pape, and Warren D. Johnson Jr. "HIV Infection in Haiti: Natural History and Disease Progression." *AIDS* 14, no. 16 (2000): 2515–21.

Des Jarlais, Don C., Samuel R. Friedman, David M. Novick, Jo L. Sotheran, Pauline Thomas, Stanley R. Yancovitz, Donna Mildvan, et al. "HIV-1 Infection among Intravenous Drug Users in Manhattan, New York City, from 1977 through 1987." *Journal of the American Medical Association* 261, no. 7 (1989): 1008–12.

Dickenson, Donald E. "Your Immune System and Nutrition." *Advocate*, January 20, 1983, 33–41.

"Did You Hear . . . ?" *New York Native*, December 21, 1987, 4.

"A Discussion on the Etiology and Epidemiology of Typhoid (Enteric) Fever: Discussion." *Proceedings of the Royal Society of Medicine* 1 (1907–8): 227–28.

Disman, Christopher. "The San Francisco Bathhouse Battles of 1984: Civil Liberties, AIDS Risk, and Shifts in Health Policy." *Journal of Homosexuality* 44, no. 3–4 (2003): 71–129.

"Dissemination of Enteric Fever Due to a 'Typhoid Carrier.'" *Lancet* 171, no. 4404 (1908): 246–47.

"Doc Confirms 'Patient Zero' Began Plague." *New York Post,* October 12, 1987.

d'Ombrain, Nicholas. "Public Inquiries in Canada." *Canadian Public Administration* 40, no. 1 (1997): 86–107.

Donovan, Jenny L., and David R. Blake. "Patient Non-Compliance: Deviance or Reasoned Decision-Making?" *Social Science and Medicine* 34, no. 5 (1992): 507–13.

Drew, W. Lawrence, Lawrence Mintz, Richard C. Miner, Michael Sands, and Barbara Ketterer. "Prevalence of Cytomegalovirus Infection in Homosexual Men." *Journal of Infectious Diseases* 143, no. 2 (1981): 188–92.

Dritz, Selma K. "Charting the Epidemiological Course of AIDS, 1981–1984." Oral history conducted in 1992 by Sally Smith Hughes. In *The AIDS Epidemic in San Francisco: The Medical Response, 1981–1984, Volume I,* Regional Oral History Office, Bancroft Library, University of California, Berkeley, 1995. Online Archive of California, 2009. http://content.cdlib.org/ark:/13030/kt2m3n98v1/.

Duberman, Martin B. *Stonewall.* New York: Plume, 1994.

Duffin, Jacalyn. "AIDS, Memory and the History of Medicine: Musings on the Canadian Response." *Genitourinary Medicine* 70, no. 1 (1994): 64–69.

"DUGAS (Gaétan)." *Le Soleil,* March 31, 1984, sec. Décès et avis divers, H-14.

Duggan, Lisa, and Nan D. Hunter. *Sex Wars: Sexual Dissent and Political Culture.* London: Routledge, 1995.

Dullea, Georgia. "A Father and a Son, Growing Up Again: At Home with Robert and Ian MacNeil." *New York Times*, May 5, 1994.

Dunbar, R. I. M., Ben Teasdale, Jackie Thompson, Felix Budelmann, Sophie Duncan, Evert van Emde Boas, and Laurie Maguire. "Emotional Arousal When Watching Drama Increases Pain Threshold and Social Bonding." *Royal Society Open Science* 3 (September 21, 2016). doi: 10.1098/rsos.160288.

Durrell, Don, Don Larventz, and Barry Spillman, *A Gablevision Special on A.I.D.S.* Television program first broadcast April 2, 1983. Vancouver: Video Out Distribution, 2013. DVD.

Eckert, Edward A. "Spatial and Temporal Distribution of Plague in a Region of Switzerland in the Years 1628 and 1629." *Bulletin of the History of Medicine* 56, no. 2 (1982): 175–94.

Eicher, Diane. "New AIDS Book Chronicles the Epidemic." *Denver Post*, November 13, 1987, 1E, 4E.

Elliman, Donald M. Jr. "Publisher's Letter." *People*, December 28, 1987. http://people.com/archive/publishers-letter-vol-28-no-26/feed/.

Emke, Ivan. "Around the Bush Yet Again: Reflection on Reckless Vectors, Past and Present." *Sexuality Research and Social Policy* 2, no. 2 (2005): 95–98.

———. "Speaking of AIDS in Canada: The Texts and Contexts of Official, Counter-Cultural and Mass Media Discourses Surrounding AIDS." DPhil thesis, Carleton University, 1991.

Engel, Margaret. "AIDS and Prejudice: One Reporter's Account of the Nation's Response." *Washington Post*, December 1, 1987, sec. Health, Z10.

Epstein, Steven. *Impure Science: AIDS, Activism, and the Politics of Knowledge*. Berkeley: University of California Press, 1996.

Erasmus, Desiderius. *Collected Works of Erasmus: Colloquies*. Translated and annotated by Craig R. Thompson. Toronto: University of Toronto Press, 1997.

Etheridge, Elizabeth W. *Sentinel for Health: A History of the Centers for Disease Control*. Berkeley: University of California Press, 1992.

Evans, S. W. *VD Case-Finding Manual: For Use in Training Programs*. Trial ed. Raleigh, NC: VD Education Institute, 1945.

"The Face of AIDS: One Year in the Epidemic." *Newsweek*, August 10, 1987.

Faderman, Lilian, and Stuart Timmons. *Gay L.A.: A History of Sexual Outlaws, Power Politics, and Lipstick Lesbians*. New York: Basic Books, 2006.

Fain, Nathan. "Is Our 'Lifestyle' Hazardous to Our Health? Part II," *Advocate*, April 1, 1982, 17–21.

Fairchild, Amy L. "The Democratization of Privacy: Public-Health Surveillance and Changing Perceptions of Privacy in Twentieth-Century America." In *History and Health Policy in the United States: Putting the Past Back In*, edited by Rosemary A. Stevens, Charles E. Rosenberg, and Lawton R. Burns, 111–29. London: Rutgers University Press, 2006.

Farmer, Paul. *AIDS and Accusation: Haiti and the Geography of Blame*. Rev. ed. Berkeley: University of California Press, 2006.

Fayerman, Pamela. "AIDS Doctor Faces Permanent Ban: Michael Maynard Is Accused of Sexual Misconduct." *Vancouver Sun*, March 6, 2003, A1.

Fee, Elizabeth. "Sin versus Science: Venereal Disease in Twentieth-Century Baltimore." In Fee and Fox, *AIDS: The Burdens of History*, 121–46.

Fee, Elizabeth, and Daniel M. Fox, eds. *AIDS: The Burdens of History*. Berkeley: University of California Press, 1988.

———. *AIDS: The Making of a Chronic Disease*. Berkeley: University of California Press, 1992.

Feldstein, Mark. "Not after Reporters . . . Just Their Sources." *News Media and the Law* 30, no. 2 (Summer 2006). http://www.rcfp.org/browse-media-law -resources/news-media-law/news-media-and-law-summer-2006/not-after -reporters-just-th.

Felknor, Bill. "Laboratory Scientist Draws 'Atoms-In-Depth' Using Computer-Oriented Graphic Technique." *News: Oak Ridge National Laboratory*, April 2, 1965, 1. http://www.umass.edu/molvis/francoeur/ortep/ortepnews .html.

Fettner, Ann Giudici, and William A. Check. *The Truth about AIDS*. Rev. ed. New York: Henry Holt, 1985.

Fidler, David P. "From International Sanitary Conventions to Global Health Security: The New International Health Regulations." *Chinese Journal of International Law* 4, no. 2 (2005): 325–92.

Fine, Gary Alan. "Welcome to the World of AIDS: Fantasies of Female Revenge." *Western Folklore* 46, no. 3 (1987): 192–97.

"'First AIDS Patient' Story Dismissed," *Gazette* [Montreal], October 17, 1987.

Fletcher, Robert. *A Tragedy of the Great Plague of Milan in 1630*. Baltimore: Lord Baltimore Press, 1898. Ebook and Texts Archive, https://ia800207.us .archive.org/9/items/atragedygreatpl00fletgoog/atragedygreatpl00fletgoog .pdf.

Foege, William H. "Centers for Disease Control." *Journal of Public Health Policy* 2, no. 1 (1981): 8–18.

Foucault, Michel. *The Birth of the Clinic: An Archaeology of Medical Perception*. Translated by A. M. Sheridan Smith. London: Pantheon Books, 1973.

———. *Madness and Civilization*. Translated by Richard Howard. New York: Pantheon Books, 1965.

———. *The Will to Knowledge*. Vol. 1 of *The History of Sexuality*. Translated by Robert Hurley. 1978. Reprint, London: Penguin, 1998.

Fourlanty, Éric. "Zero Patience." *Voir*, March 10, 1994.

Friedman-Kien, Alvin E., Linda J. Laubenstein, Pablo Rubinstein, Elena Buimovici-Klein, Michael Marmor, Rosalyn Stahl, Ilya Spigland, et al. "Disseminated Kaposi's Sarcoma in Homosexual Men." *Annals of Internal Medicine* 96, no. 6, part 1 (1982): 693–700.

Fuerst, Mark. "'Shell-Shocked' Gays Told 'Wear Condoms': Homosexual Practices Linked to Kaposi's Risk." *Medical Post*, April 19, 1983.

The Fungus Queen. "Fungus." Letter to the editor. *Bay Area Reporter* [San Francisco], November 18, 1982, 8.

"GATE Sponsors Informational Program on AIDS." *Fine Print* [Edmonton], May 1983, 21.

Gavner, Bernard. "US Wages War on Rise in VD: Medical Sleuths Have Job of Tracking Down Disease." *Niagara Falls Gazette*, April 23, 1961, 9A.

Gay Men's Health Crisis. "Another Epidemic: Acquired Immune Deficiency." *Bay Area Reporter* [San Francisco], August 5, 1982.

———. "Late Evidence on Contagious Causes." *G.M.H.C. Newsletter*, July 1982, 2.

Gay Men with AIDS. "A Warning to Gay Men with AIDS." *New York Native*, November 22, 1982, 16.

Geary, Jim. "Who Should Look at Whom." *Bay Area Reporter* [San Francisco], September 30, 1982, 7.

Gelman, Anna C., Jules E. Vandow, and Nathan Sobel. "Current Status of Venereal Disease in New York City: A Survey of 6,649 Physicians in Solo Practice." *American Journal of Public Health* 53, no. 12 (1963): 1903–18.

General Medical Council. *Confidentiality.* October 12, 2009. http://www.gmc-uk.org/static/documents/content/Confidentiality_-_English_1015.pdf.

Gever, Martha. "Pictures of Sickness: Stuart Marshall's *Bright Eyes*." In Crimp, *AIDS: Cultural Analysis, Cultural Activism*, 108–26.

Gilbertson, Fred. "Forum Fans Fears." *Vancouver Gay Community Centre News*, April 1983, 41–43.

Giles-Vernick, Tamara, Ch. Didier Gondola, Guillaume Lachenal, and William H. Schneider. "Social History, Biology, and the Emergence of HIV in Colonial Africa." *Journal of African History* 54 (2013): 11–30.

Gilman, Sander L., "AIDS and Syphilis: The Iconography of Disease." In Crimp, *AIDS: Cultural Analysis, Cultural Activism*, 87–107.

Gilman, Sander L., and Dorothy Nelkin. "Placing Blame for Devastating Disease." *Social Research* 55, no. 3 (1988): 361–78.

Ginzburg, Carlo. *The Cheese and the Worms: The Cosmos of a Sixteenth-Century Miller.* Translated by John Tedeschi and Anne Tedeschi. Baltimore: Johns Hopkins University Press, 1980.

———. *Ecstasies: Deciphering the Witches' Sabbath.* Translated by Raymond Rosenthal. New York: Pantheon Books, 1991.

Gladwell, Malcolm. *The Tipping Point: How Little Things Can Make a Big Difference.* New York: Little, Brown, 2000.

Goddu, Teresa A. "Vampire Gothic." *American Literary History* 11, no. 1 (1999): 125–41.

Goedert, James J., William C. Wallen, Dean L. Mann, Douglas M. Strong, Carolyn Y. Neuland, Mark H. Greene, Christine Murray, et al. "Amyl Nitrite May Alter T Lymphocytes in Homosexual Men." *Lancet* 319, no. 8269 (1982): 412–16.

Goffman, Erving. *Asylums: Essays on the Social Situation of Mental Patients and Other Inmates.* Garden City, NY: Anchor Books, 1961.

Goldstein, Diane E. *Once Upon a Virus: AIDS Legends and Vernacular Risk Perception.* Logan: Utah State University Press, 2004.

Goldstein, Richard. "Heartsick: Fear and Loving in the Gay Community." *Village Voice*, June 28, 1983, 1, 9–12.

Golinski, Jan. *Making Natural Knowledge: Constructivism and the History of Science.* London: University of Chicago Press, 2005.

Goodman, Herman. "An Epidemic of Genital Chancres from Perversion." *American Journal of Syphilis, Gonorrhea, and Venereal Diseases* 28 (1944): 310–14.

Gorman, Christine. "Strange Trip Back to the Future: The Case of Robert R. Spurs New Questions about AIDS." *Time*, November 9, 1987, 75.

Gostin, Lawrence O. *The AIDS Pandemic: Complacency, Injustice, and Unfilled Expectations.* London: University of North Carolina Press, 2004.

Gottlieb, Michael S., H[oward] M. Schanker, P[eng] T. Fan, A[ndrew] Saxon, J[oel] D. Weisman, and I[rving] Pozalski [*sic*]. "*Pneumocystis* Pneumonia—Los Angeles." *MMWR* 30 (1981): 250–52. https://www.cdc.gov/mmwr/preview/mmwrhtml/june_5.htm.

Gottlieb, Michael S., Jerome E. Groopman, Wilfred M. Weinstein, John L. Fahey, and Roger Detels. "UCLA Conference: The Acquired Immunodeficiency Syndrome." *Annals of Internal Medicine* 99 (1983): 208–20.

Gould, Deborah B. *Moving Politics: Emotion and ACT UP's Fight against AIDS.* Chicago: University of Chicago Press, 2009.

Graveline, Carole, Jean Robert, and Réjean Thomas. *Les préjugés plus forts que la mort: le sida au Québec.* Montreal: VLB Editeur, 1998.

Greenberg, David F. *The Construction of Homosexuality.* Chicago: University of Chicago Press, 1988.

Greene, Jeremy A. "Therapeutic Infidelities: 'Noncompliance' Enters the Medical Literature, 1955–1975." *Social History of Medicine* 17, no. 3 (2004): 327–43.

Gregg, Sandra R. "City's TB Clinic Survives by Borrowing Everything." *Washington Post*, May 25, 1981, B1.

Greyson, John. "Liberace's Music Helped Cure Me." In *Urinal and Other Stories*, by John Greyson, 252–71. Toronto: Art Metropole and the Power Plant, 1993.

Griffin, Kevin C. "A Community Mourns BC Activist's Death." *Body Politic*, July/August 1983, 10.

Grimson, Roger C., and William W. Darrow. "Association between Acquired Immune Deficiency Syndrome and Sexual Contact: An Analysis of the Incidence Pattern." In *Infectious Complications of Neoplastic Disease: Controversies in Management*, edited by Arthur E. Brown and Donald Armstrong, 221–27. New York: Yorke Medical Books, 1985.

Grmek, Mirko D. *History of AIDS: Emergence and Origin of a Modern Pandemic*. Translated by Russell C. Maulitz and Jacalyn Duffin. Princeton, NJ: Princeton University Press, 1990.

Grover, Jan Zita. "AIDS: Keywords." In Crimp, *AIDS: Cultural Analysis, Cultural Criticism*, 17–30.

Hamer, W. H. "A Discussion on the Etiology and Epidemiology of Typhoid (Enteric) Fever: The Relation of the Bacillus typhosus to Typhoid Fever." *Proceedings of the Royal Society of Medicine* 1 (1907–8): 204–18.

Hanson, Ellis. "Undead." In *Inside/Out: Lesbian Theories, Gay Theories*, edited by Diana Fuss, 324–40. London: Routledge, 1991.

Harden, Victoria. *AIDS at 30: A History*. Dulles, VA: Potomac Books, 2012.

Hardy, Anne. "Methods of Outbreak Investigation in the 'Era of Bacteriology' 1880–1920." *Sozial-und Präventivmedizin/Social and Preventive Medicine* 46, no. 6 (2001): 355–60.

Haseltine, Nate. "Complacency Slowed Anti-Syphilis Drive in US, Health Chief Admits." *Washington Post*, September 5, 1962, A3.

———. "Meeting the Health Threat of Mexican Migrants." *Washington Post*, February 25, 1959, B7.

Hastings, Deborah. "Shilts Says Film Version of His Book Still Alive." *Indiana Gazette*, October 30, 1991, 31.

Hayday, Matthew. "Confusing and Conflicting Agendas: Federalism, Official Languages and the Development of the Bilingualism in Education Program in Ontario, 1970–1983." *Journal of Canadian Studies* 36, no. 1 (2001): 50–79.

Heagerty, John Joseph. *Four Centuries of Medical History in Canada and a Sketch of the Medical History of Newfoundland*. Toronto: Macmillan Canada, 1928.

Heaphy, Brian. "Silence and Strategy: Researching AIDS/HIV Narratives in the Flow of Power." In *Meddling with Mythology: AIDS and the Social Construction of Knowledge*, edited by Rosaline S. Barbour and Guro Huby, 20–36. London: Routledge, 1998.

Heller, Jean. "Syphilis Victims in US Study Went Untreated for 40 Years." *New York Times*, July 26, 1972, 1, 8.

Hellman, Ronald E. "Facing Up to Compulsive Lifestyles." In *Gay Life: Leisure, Love, and Living for the Contemporary Gay Male*, edited by Eric E. Rofes, 30–39. Garden City, NY: Doubleday, 1986.

Helquist, Michael. "What to Expect at the KS Clinic," *Coming Up!* March 1983.

Helquist, Michael, and Rick Osmon. "Sex and the Baths: A Not-So-Secret Report." *Journal of Homosexuality* 44, no. 3/4 (2003): 153–75.

Henderson, Randi. "Speaking Out on AIDS." *Baltimore Sun*, March 29, 1988, 1C, 3C.

Henig, Robin Marantz. "AIDS: A New Disease's Deadly Odyssey." *New York Times*, February 6, 1983, SM28–30, SM32, SM36, SM38, SM42, SM44.

Herrup, Cynthia B. *A House in Great Disorder: Sex, Law, and the 2nd Earl of Castlehaven.* Oxford: Oxford University Press, 1999.

Hessol, Nancy A., Beryl A. Koblin, Godfried J. P. van Griensven, Peter Bacchetti, Jennifer Y. Liu, Cladd E. Stevens, Roel A. Coutinho, et al. "Progression of Human Immunodeficiency Virus Type 1 (HIV-1) Infection among Homosexual Men in Hepatitis B Vaccine Trial Cohorts in Amsterdam, New York City, and San Francisco, 1978–1991." *American Journal of Epidemiology* 139, no. 11 (1994): 1077–87.

Hewlett, Mary. "The French Connection: Syphilis and Sodomy in Late-Renaissance Lucca." In Siena, *Sins of the Flesh*, 239–60.

Higgins, Gerald L. "The History of Confidentiality in Medicine: The Physician-Patient Relationship." *Canadian Family Physician* 35 (April 1989): 921–26, 14.

Holleran, Andrew. *Dancer from the Dance.* 1978. Reprint, New York: Perennial, 2001.

———. "Journal of the Plague Year." *Christopher Street*, November 1982, 15–21.

Holt, Patricia. "Behind the Tragedy of AIDS." *San Francisco Chronicle*, October 18, 1987, sec. Review, 1, 8, 10.

"Homosexual Linked to 40 AIDS Cases May Have Carried Infection." *Los Angeles Times*, March 27, 1984, 10.

Hooper, Edward. "The Allegation That *The River* Has Damaged Modern Attempts to Eradicate Polio." *AIDS Origins* (blog). October 15, 2004. http://www.aidsorigins.com/allegation-river-has-damaged-modern-attempts-eradicate-polio#sthash.jVToYIPR.dpuf.

———. "Michael Worobey's Wobbly Research into the Early History of HIV." *AIDS Origins* (blog). March 19, 2008. http://www.aidsorigins.com/michael-worobey-wobbly-research-early-history-hiv.

———. "The Origins of the AIDS Pandemic: A Quick Guide to the Principal Theories and the Alleged Refutations." *AIDS Origins* (blog). April 25, 2012. http://www.aidsorigins.com/origins-aids-pandemic.

———. *The River: A Journey Back to the Source of HIV and AIDS.* London: Allen Lane, 1999.

Hooper, Edward, and William D. Hamilton. "1959 Manchester Case of Syndrome Resembling AIDS." *Lancet* 348 (1996): 1363–65.

Houston, Andrea. "Ford to Pass on Pride, but Barbara Hall Shows Longstanding Solidarity." *Daily Xtra,* June 21, 2011, http://www.dailyxtra.com/toronto/news-and-ideas/news/ford-pass-pride-barbara-hall-shows-longstanding-solidarity-5088.

Howard, John. *Men Like That: A Southern Queer History.* Chicago: University of Chicago Press, 1999.

Hughes, Sally Smith. "The Kaposi's Sarcoma Clinic at the University of California, San Francisco: An Early Response to the AIDS Epidemic." *Bulletin of the History of Medicine* 71, no. 4 (1997): 651–88.

Humphreys, Margaret. "No Safe Place: Disease and Panic in American History." *American Literary History* 14, no. 4 (2002): 845–65.

———. *Yellow Fever and the South.* New Brunswick, NJ: Rutgers University Press, 1992.

Hussain, Misha. "Hunger and Frustration Grow at Ebola Ground Zero in Guinea." Reuters, March 3, 2015. http://uk.reuters.com/article/us-health-ebola-guinea-village-idUKKBN0LZ1R220150303.

Hydén, Lars-Christer. "Illness and Narrative." *Sociology of Health and Illness* 19, no. 1 (1997): 48–69.

"Ideas." Part 1 of an eight-part radio documentary about the science and politics of AIDS. Hosted by Lister Sinclair and produced by Max Allen. *Ideas,* Canadian Broadcasting Corporation Radio series, first broadcast on October 13, 1987. Audiocassette. Transcript available through Vancouver Public Library, https://vpl.bibliocommons.com/item/show/480700038_the_aids_campaign?active_tab=bib_info.

Iliffe, John. *The African AIDS Epidemic: A History.* Oxford: James Currey, 2006.

Illich, Ivan. *Medical Nemesis: The Expropriation of Health.* London: Calder and Boyars, 1975.

"International Notes—Quarantine Measures: Smallpox—Stockholm, Sweden, 1963." *MMWR* 45, no. 25 (1996): 538–45.

Jaffe, Harold W. "The Early Days of the HIV-AIDS Epidemic in the USA." *Nature Immunology* 9, no. 11 (2008): 1201–3.

Jay, Karla, and Allen Young. *The Gay Report: Lesbians and Gay Men Speak Out about Sexual Experiences and Lifestyles.* New York: Summit Books, 1979.

Jewkes, Rachel. "Child Sexual Abuse and HIV Infection." In *Sexual Abuse of Young Children in Southern Africa,* edited by Linda Richter, Andrew Dawes, and Craig Higson-Smith, 130–42. Cape Town: HSRC Press, 2004.

Johnson, Diane, and John F. Murray. "AIDS without End." *New York Review of Books* 35, no. 13 (1988): 57–63.

Johnston, David. "Africans Asking: Did Canada Give AIDS to World?" *Montreal Gazette,* June 3, 1989.

Joint United Nations Programme on HIV/AIDS. *AIDS by the Numbers 2015.*

Geneva: UNAIDS, 2015. http://www.unaids.org/sites/default/files/media
_asset/AIDS_by_the_numbers_2015_en.pdf.

———. *Outlook 30*. Geneva: UNAIDS, 2011.http://www.unaids.org/sites/default/
files/media_asset/20110607_JC2069_30Outlook_en_0.pdf .

Jones, D. *A Sermon Upon the Dreadful Fire of London, Preach'd in the Parish-
church of St. Dunstan in the West in London, on Thursday, September 2. 1703*
London, 1703. Facsimilie, Eighteenth Century Collections Online digital library, http://find.galegroup.com/ecco/infomark.do?&source=gale&prodId=
ECCO&userGroupName=cambuni&tabID=T001&docId=CW3321184722
&type=multipage&contentSet=ECCOArticles&version=1.0&docLevel=
FASCIMILE.

Jones, James H. *Bad Blood: The Tuskegee Syphilis Experiment*. Rev. and expanded ed. New York: Free Press, 1993. First published 1981.

Jones, James W. "Discourses on and of AIDS in West Germany, 1986–90." *Journal of the History of Sexuality* 2, no. 3 (1992): 439–68.

Jordanova, Ludmilla. *Defining Features: Scientific and Medical Portraits 1660–
2000*. London: Reaktion Books with National Portrait Gallery, London,
2000.

———. "The Social Construction of Medical Knowledge." *Social History of Medicine* 8, no. 3 (1995): 361–81.

Joyce, Rob. *"Proud* Lives." *Q Magazine* [Vancouver], May 1988, 13–15, 17.

Kahn, Arthur D. *AIDS, The Winter War*. Philadelphia: Temple University Press,
1993.

Kaiser, Charles. *The Gay Metropolis*. London: Weidenfeld and Nicholson, 1998.

Kalmuk, Michael. "An Apology Owed to Brown Family." *Vancouver Sun*,
June 22, 1989, A18, ProQuest (243552753).

Kanabus, Annabel, and Sarah Allen, and updated by Bonita de Boer. "The
Origin of AIDS and HIV and the First Cases of AIDS." AVERT, updated
May 12, 2005, http://web.archive.org/web/20050527223015/http://www.avert
.org/origins.htm.

Kanee, B., and C. L. Hunt. "Homosexuality as a Source of Venereal Disease."
Canadian Medical Association Journal 65, no. 2 (1951): 138–40.

Katz, Jonathan Ned. *Gay American History: Lesbians and Gay Men in the USA*.
New York: Thomas Y. Crowell, 1976.

Kelley, Ken. "The Interview: Randy Shilts." *San Francisco Focus* 36, no. 6
(1989): 64–66, 94–108, 110–13.

Kellman, Steven G. "From Oran to San Francisco: Shilts Appropriates Camus."
College Literature 24, no. 1 (1997): 202–12.

Kennedy, Elizabeth Lapovsky, and Madeline D. Davis. *Boots of Leather, Slippers of Gold: The History of a Lesbian Community*. New York: Routledge,
1993.

Kiley, Sam. "Third Nun Dies as Zaire Tracks Down Killer Virus." *Times* [London], May 13, 1995.

Kingston, Tim. "Controversy Follows Shilts And 'Zero' to London." *Coming Up!* April 1988, 11.

Kinsella, James. *Covering the Plague: AIDS and the American Media*. London: Rutgers University Press, 1989.

Kinsman, Gary. "Managing AIDS Organizing: 'Consultation,' 'Partnership' and 'Responsibility' as Strategies of Regulation." In *Organizing Dissent: Contemporary Social Movements in Theory and Practice*, 2nd ed., edited by William K. Carroll, 213–39. Toronto: Garamond Press, 1997.

———. *The Regulation of Desire: Homo and Hetero Sexualities*. 2nd ed. Montreal: Black Rose Books, 1996.

———. "Vectors of Hope and Possibility: Commentary on Reckless Vectors." *Sexuality Research and Social Policy* 2, no. 2 (2005): 99–105.

———. "Wolfenden in Canada: Within and beyond Official Discourse in Law Reform Struggles." In *Human Rights, Sexual Orientation and Gender Identity in the Commonwealth: Struggles for Decriminalisation and Change*, edited by Corinne Lennox and Matthew Waites, 183–205. London: School of Advanced Study, University of London, 2013.

Kirkus Reviews. Unsigned review of *And the Band Played On: Politics, People, and the AIDS Epidemic*, by Randy Shilts. September 1, 1987, 1303–4.

Kirp, David L. "Politics Is Latest AIDS Sideshow." *Lodi* [CA] *News-Sentinel*, July 9, 1987, 4. https://news.google.com/newspapers?id=BLM0AAAAIBAJ &sjid=YiEGAAAAIBAJ&dq=aids%20kirp&pg=3276%2C926014.

Klooster, Wim. "Slave Revolts, Royal Justice, and a Ubiquitous Rumor in the Age of Revolutions." *William and Mary Quarterly*, 3rd ser., 71, no. 3 (2014): 401–24.

Klovdahl, Alden S. "A Note on Images of Networks." *Social Networks* 3 (1981): 197–214.

———. "Social Networks and the Spread of Infectious Diseases: The AIDS Example." *Social Science and Medicine* 21, no. 11 (1985): 1203–16.

Knabe, Susan, and Wendy Gay Pearson. *Zero Patience: A Queer Film Classic*. Vancouver: Arsenal Pulp Press, 2011.

Koblin, Beryl A., Birgit H. B. van Benthem, Susan P. Buchbinder, Leigh Ren, Eric Vittinghoff, Cladd E. Stevens, Roel A. Coutinho, and Godfried J. P. van Griensven. "Long-Term Survival after Infection with Human Immunodeficiency Virus Type 1 (HIV-1) among Homosexual Men in Hepatitis B Vaccine Trial Cohorts in Amsterdam, New York City, and San Francisco, 1978–1995." *American Journal of Epidemiology* 150, no. 10 (1999): 1026–30.

Koprowski, Hilary. "Hypotheses and Facts." *Philosophical Transactions of the Royal Society of London B: Biological Sciences* 356, no. 1410 (2001): 832.

Kramer, Larry. *Reports from the Holocaust: The Making of an AIDS Activist.* New York: St. Martin's Press, 1989.

Kraut, Alan M. *Silent Travelers: Germs, Genes, and The "Immigrant Menace."* New York: Johns Hopkins University Press, 1995.

Krever, Horace. *Commission of Inquiry on the Blood System in Canada, Final Report.* 3 vols. Ottawa: The Commission, 1997.

Krueger, Ron. "He Eats, Thinks and Drinks Ideas: Randy Shilts and Young Americans for Freedom." *Beacon-News* [Aurora, IL], January 23, 1968.

Kumar, Abhishek, Vern Paxson, and Nicholas Weaver. "Exploiting Underlying Structure for Detailed Reconstruction of an Internet-Scale Event." Paper presented at the Fifth ACM SIGCOMM Conference on Internet Measurement, Berkeley, CA, October 19–21, 2005. https://www.usenix.org/legacy/event/imc05/tech/full_papers/kumar/kumar.pdf.

Kusukawa, Sachiko. "Illustrating Nature." In *Books and the Sciences in History,* edited by Marina Frasca-Spada and Nicholas Jardine, 90–113. Cambridge: Cambridge University Press, 2000.

Lacayo, Richard. "Assault with a Deadly Virus." *Time,* July 20, 1987, 57.

Lacey, Marc. "From Édgar, 5, Coughs Heard Round the World." *New York Times,* April 29, 2009.

Lalonde, Michelle, and Andre Picard. "AIDS Activists Disrupt Opening of Conference." *Globe and Mail* [Toronto], June 5, 1989.

Lanzaratta, Philip A. "Why Me?" *Christopher Street,* April 1982, cover, 15–16.

———. "Surviving AIDS." *Christopher Street,* October 1984, 30–35.

Last, John M., ed. *A Dictionary of Epidemiology.* New York: Oxford University Press, 1983.

Latour, Bruno, and Steve Woolgar. *Laboratory Life: The Social Construction of Scientific Facts.* London: Sage, 1979.

Lautens, Trevor. "As I Like It." *Vancouver Sun,* June 7, 1989, A11, ProQuest (243565235).

Lavoie, René. "Deux solitudes: les organismes sida et la communauté gaie." In *Sortir de l'ombre: histoires des communautés lesbienne et gaie de Montréal,* edited by Irène Demczuk and Frank W. Remiggi, 337–62. Montreal: VLB Éditeur, 1998.

Lawrence, Susan C. *Privacy and the Past: Research, Law, Archives, Ethics.* New Brunswick, NJ: Rutgers University Press, 2016.

Lazier, Jerry A. "Aunt Mary Shilts." *Bay Area Reporter* [San Francisco], January 14, 1988, 8.

———. "Gay Aunt Mary." *Coming Up!* February 1988, 3.

Leavitt, Judith Walzer. *Typhoid Mary: Captive to the Public's Health.* Boston: Beacon Press, 1996.

Ledwell, Tony. Associated Press newswire, March 3, 1977, Nexis UK.

Lee, Lisa M., and Christina Zarowsky. "Foundational Values for Public Health." *Public Health Reviews* 36, no. 2 (2015): 1–9.

LeFebour, Patricia A., and Douglas Elliott. "Inquiry into the Blood System in Canada: The Krever Commission." *Canadian HIV/AIDS Policy and Law Newsletter* 1, no. 3 (1995). http://www.aidslaw.ca/site/download/9189/.

Leishman, Katie. "The Writing Cure." *New York Times*, March 5, 1994, 23.

Leo, John. "The Real Epidemic: Fear and Despair." *Time*, July 4, 1983, 56–58.

Lerner, Barron H. "Ill Patient, Public Activist: Rose Kushner's Attack on Breast Cancer Chemotherapy." *Bulletin of the History of Medicine* 81, no. 1 (2007): 224–40.

Levine, Carol. "Ethics and Epidemiology in the Age of AIDS." In *Ethics and Epidemiology*, edited by Steven S. Coughlin and Tom L. Beauchamp, 239–54. Oxford: Oxford University Press, 1996.

Levy, Jay A. "HIV Pathogenesis: 25 Years of Progress and Persistent Challenges." *AIDS* 23, no. 2 (2009): 147–60.

Lewis, Bill. "Case May Set Precedent, Decision Expected Feb 14." *Body Politic*, February 1979, 7–9.

Leznoff, Maurice, and William A. Westley. "The Homosexual Community." *Social Problems* 3, no. 4 (1956): 257–63.

Liclair, Christian. "Silence=Death-Project." *The Nomos of Images* (blog), ISSN: 2366-9926, December 30, 2015. http://nomoi.hypotheses.org/198.

Lie, Anne Kveim. "Origin Stories and the Norwegian Radesyge." *Social History of Medicine* 20, no. 3 (2007): 563–79.

Lorch, Paul. "The Cast [*sic*] against Fear." *Bay Area Reporter* [San Francisco], November 4, 1982, 6.

———. "KS Diagnosis, Takes Life." *Bay Area Reporter* [San Francisco], December 23, 1982, 1, 15.

Luke, Douglas A., and Jenine K. Harris. "Network Analysis in Public Health: History, Methods, and Applications." *Annual Review of Public Health* 28, no. 1 (2007): 69–93.

Luker, Ralph E. "Shilts, Randy Martin." In *American National Biography Online*. Oxford University Press, 2000–2010. Article published 2000. http://www.anb.org/articles/16/16–03326.html.

Luther, Martin. *Luther: Letters of Spiritual Counsel.* Edited and translated by Theodore G. Tappert. London: SCM Press, 1955.

Lynch, Michael. "Living with Kaposi's." *Body Politic*, November 1982, 31–37.

———. "The Power of Names." *Xtra!* February 26, 1988.

Lynch, Michael, and Steve Woolgar, eds. *Representation in Scientific Practice.* Cambridge, MA: MIT Press, 1990.

Maberry, Jonathan. *Patient Zero.* New York: St. Martin's Griffin, 2009.

Mackinnon, Martha, Keel Cottrelle, and Horace Krever. "Legal and Social Aspects of AIDS in Canada." In *AIDS: A Perspective for Canadians: Back-*

ground Papers, edited by Royal Society of Canada, 347–407. Ottawa: Royal Society of Canada, 1988.

"The Man Who Gave Us AIDS: Triggered 'Gay Cancer' Epidemic." *New York Post*, October 6, 1987.

Markel, Howard. "Journals of the Plague Years: Documenting the History of the AIDS Epidemic in the United States." *American Journal of Public Health* 91, no. 7 (2001): 1025–28.

——. *Quarantine! East European Jewish Immigrants and the New York City Epidemics of 1892*. London: Johns Hopkins University Press, 1997.

Markel, Howard, and Alexandra Minna Stern. "The Foreignness of Germs: The Persistent Association of Immigrants and Disease in American Society." *Milbank Quarterly* 80, no. 4 (2002): 757–88.

Marko, Jim. "'Advocate' Employee Claims EST Training Refusal Led to Firing." *Arizona Gay News* [Tucson], April 21, 1978.

Marks, Neil Alan. "New York Gaycult, the Jewish Question . . . and Me." *Christopher Street*, November 1981, 8–21.

Martin, Brian. "The Politics of a Scientific Meeting: The Origin-of-AIDS Debate at the Royal Society." *Politics and the Life Sciences* 20, no. 2 (2001): 119–30.

Mass, Lawrence. "Cancer as Metaphor." *New York Native*, August 24, 1981, 13.

Mathieson, Cynthia M., and Henderikus J. Stam. "Renegotiating Identity: Cancer Narratives." *Sociology of Health and Illness* 17, no. 3 (1995): 283–306.

Maupassant, Guy de. *The Complete Short Stories of Guy de Maupassant*. New York: P. F. Collier and Son, 1903.

——. *Correspondance / Guy de Maupassant*. Edited by Jacques Suffel. 3 vols. Geneva : Edito-service, 1973.

Mbali, Mandisa. *South African AIDS Activism and Global Health Politics*. London: Palgrave Macmillan, 2013.

McAllister, Marie E. "Stories of the Origin of Syphilis in Eighteenth-Century England: Science, Myth, and Prejudice." *Eighteenth-Century Life* 24, no. 1 (2000): 22–44.

McArthur, James B. "As the Tide Turns: The Changing HIV/AIDS Epidemic and the Criminalization of HIV Exposure." *Cornell Law Review* 94, no. 3 (2009): 707–41.

McCaskell, Tim. "A Brief History of AIDS Activism in Canada." *Socialist Worker*, November 24, 2012, http://www.socialist.ca/node/1453.

McGough, Laura J. *Gender, Sexuality, and Syphilis in Early Modern Venice: The Disease That Came to Stay*. Basingstoke, UK: Palgrave Macmillan, 2011.

——. "Quarantining Beauty: The French Disease in Early Modern Venice." In Siena, *Sins of the Flesh*, 211–37.

McGovern, Michael. "The Man Who Flew Too Much: AIDS Traced to Sexy Steward." *Daily News* [New York], October 7, 1987, 18.

McGrath, Cathleen, Jim Blythe, and David Krackhardt. "The Effect of Spatial Arrangement on Judgments and Errors in Interpreting Graphs." *Social Networks* 19 (1997): 223–42.

McKay, Richard Andrew. "Before HIV: Venereal Disease among Homosexually Active Men in England and North America." In *The Routledge History of Disease*, edited by Mark Jackson, 441–59. London: Routledge, 2017. http://www.tandfebooks.com/userimages/ContentEditor/1489134497468/9780415720014_oachapter24.pdf.

———. "The Emergence of the 'Patient Zero' Concept in the North American AIDS Epidemic." MSc diss., University of Oxford, 2005.

———. "'Patient Zero': The Absence of a Patient's View of the Early North American AIDS Epidemic." *Bulletin of the History of Medicine* 88, no. 1 (Spring 2014): 161–94. Published by The Johns Hopkins University Press. DOI:10.1353/bhm.2014.0005.

———. "'Patient Zero' Research." Letter to the editor. *San Francisco Bay Times*, July 5, 2007.

———. "Sex and Skin Cancer: Kaposi's Sarcoma Becomes the 'Stigmata of AIDS,' 1979–83." In *A Medical History of Skin: Scratching the Surface*, edited by Jonathan Reinarz and Kevin Siena, 113–27. London: Pickering and Chatto, 2013.

McKusick, Leon, William Horstman, and Thomas J. Coates. "AIDS and Sexual Behavior Reported by Gay Men in San Francisco." *American Journal of Public Health* 75, no. 5 (1985): 493–96.

McLean, Matthew. *The Cosmographia of Sebastian Münster: Describing the World in the Reformation*. Aldershot, UK: Ashgate, 2007.

"MDs Doubt Claim Canadian Carried AIDS to Continent." *Toronto Star*, October 7, 1987, A2, LexisNexis News.

"Medical Caution and Political Judgment." *Body Politic* [Toronto], May 1983, 8.

Metcalfe, Robin. "Light in the Loafers: The Gaynor Photographs of Gaëtan [*sic*] Dugas and the Invention of Patient Zero." In *Image and Inscription: An Anthology of Contemporary Canadian Photography*, edited by Robert Bean, 65–75. Toronto: YYZ Books and Gallery 44 Centre for Contemporary Photography, 2005.

Meyerowitz, Joanne. "*AHR Forum:* Transnational Sex and U.S. History." *American Historical Review* 114, no. 5 (2009): 1273–86.

———. *How Sex Changed: A History of Transsexuality in the United States*. London: Harvard University Press, 2002.

Meyerson, Beth E., Frederick A. Martich, and Gerald P. Naehr. *Ready to Go: The History and Contributions of US Public Health Advisors*. Research Triangle Park, NC: American Social Health Association, 2008.

Miller, James. "AIDS in the Novel: Getting It Straight." In *Fluid Exchanges:*

Artists and Critics in the AIDS Crisis, edited by James Miller, 257–71. Toronto: University of Toronto Press, 1992.

Minton, Henry L. *Departing from Deviance: A History of Homosexual Rights and Emancipatory Science in America*. London: University of Chicago Press, 2002.

Montgomery, Charlotte. "Begin Appoints Advisers to Study AIDS." *Globe and Mail* [Toronto], August 16, 1983, 8.

Montréal Ce Soir [nightly television news program]. Presented by Marie-Claude Lavallée, Philippe Bélisle, Réal d'Amours, and Charles Tisseyre. Radio-Canada, broadcast October 7, 1987. DVD, 08:50.

Moore, Karen. "Patient Zero Excerpt Showed Bad Judgment." *Toronto Star*, December 29, 1987, A16, ProQuest (435693482).

Moore, R. I. *The Formation of a Persecuting Society: Authority and Deviance in Western Europe, 950–1250*. 2nd ed. Oxford: Basil Blackwell, 2007. First published in 1987.

Morens, David M., Gregory K. Folkers, and Anthony S. Fauci. "The Challenge of Emerging and Re-Emerging Infectious Diseases." *Nature* 430 (July 8, 2004): 242–49.

Morris, Rosalind C. *Can the Subaltern Speak? Reflections on the History of an Idea*. New York: Columbia University Press, 2010.

Moss, Andrew R. "AIDS Epidemiology: Investigating and Getting the Word Out." Oral history interview conducted in 1992 by Sally Smith Hughes. In *The AIDS Epidemic in San Francisco: The Medical Response, 1981–1984*, *Volume II*. Regional Oral History Office, Bancroft Library, University of California–Berkeley, 1996. Online Archive of California, 2009. http://ark.cdlib.org/ark:/13030/kt7b69n8jn.

———. "AIDS without End." Letter to the editor. *New York Review of Books* 35, no. 19 (December 8, 1988): 60.

"The Most Memorable Books of the Last 25 Years." *USA Today*. April 9, 2007. http://www.usatoday.com/life/top25-books.htm.

Mullins, Luke. "Rep. John Mica on Fannie/Freddie Special Prosecutor." *The Home Front* (blog), *US News and World Report*, October 29, 2008. http://money.usnews.com/money/blogs/the-home-front/2008/10/29/rep-john-mica-on-fanniefreddie-special-prosecutor.html.

Münster, Sebastian. *Cosmographia, beschreibung aller lender. . . .* Basel: Henrichum Petri, 1544.

———. *Cosmographia, das ist: Beschreibung der gantzen Welt. . . .* Basel: Henricpetrinischen, 1628.

———. *Cosmographiae universalis libri VI in quibus. . . .* Basle: H. Petrus, 1552.

———. *Cosmographei: oder beschreibung aller länder. . . .* Basel, 1550.

———. *Cosmographey: das ist Beschreibung aller Länder. . . .* Basel: Sebastianum Henricpetri, 1614.

Murphy, Timothy F. *Ethics in an Epidemic: AIDS, Morality, and Culture.* Berkeley: University of California Press, 1994.

Myers, David. "Doctors Warn Gays." *Vancouver Gay Community Centre News,* April 1983, 43–44.

Nahmias, A. J., J. Weiss, X. Yao, F. Lee, R. Kodsi, M. Schanfield, T. Matthews, et al. "Evidence for Human Infection with an HTLV-III/LAV-like Virus in Central Africa, 1959." *Lancet* 1 (1987): 1279–80.

Name Withheld on Request. "KS Puzzles." *Bay Area Reporter* [San Francisco], July 1, 1982.

Naphy, William G. *Plagues, Poisons, and Potions: Plague-Spreading Conspiracies in the Western Alps, c. 1530–1640.* Manchester, UK: Manchester University Press, 2002.

———. "Plague-Spreading and a Magisterially Controlled Fear." In *Studies in Early Modern European History,* edited by William G. Naphy and Penny Roberts, 28–43. Manchester, UK: Manchester University Press, 1997.

———. *Sex Crimes: From Renaissance to Enlightenment.* Stroud: Tempus, 2002.

Nattrass, Nicoli. *The AIDS Conspiracy: Science Fights Back.* New York: Columbia University Press, 2012.

Nelkin, Dorothy. "Promotional Metaphors and Their Popular Appeal." *Public Understanding of Science* 3, no. 1 (1994): 25–31.

Newsome, W. Jake. "Migrating Memories: Transatlantic Commemoration of the Nazis' Homosexual Victims in West Germany and the United States." Paper presented at the annual meeting of the American Historical Association, Atlanta, January 10, 2016.

Newton, Esther. *Cherry Grove, Fire Island: Sixty Years in America's First Gay and Lesbian Town.* Boston: Beacon, 1993.

Nichols, Stuart. "For Patients, For Ourselves." *New York Native,* October 11, 1982, 15.

Noel, Grégoire E. "Another Case of AIDS in the Pre-AIDS Era." *Reviews of Infectious Diseases* 10, no. 3 (1988): 668–69.

Nohl, Johannes. *The Black Death: A Chronicle of the Plague.* Translated by C. H. Clarke. London: George Allen and Unwin, 1926.

Nordwind, Richard. "Doctor Helped Track Down Sexual Link Between Cluster of 40 AIDS Victims." *Los Angeles Herald Examiner,* March 28, 1984, A6.

"Northwest Personality: Randy Shilts." *Northwest Gay Review,* December–January (1974): 6–7.

"Notes on Fashion." *New York Times,* June 16, 1981, B14.

Nungesser, Lon G. *Epidemic of Courage: Facing AIDS in America.* New York: St. Martin's Press, 1986.

———. Letter to the editor. *Coming Up!* May 1988, 2–3.

Nutton, Vivian. "The Seeds of Disease: An Explanation of Contagion and Infection from the Greeks to the Renaissance." *Medical History* 27, no. 1 (1983): 1–34.

O'Brien, Raymond C. "AIDS: Perspective on the American Family." *Villanova Law Review* 34, no. 2 (1989): 209–79.

———. "A Legislative Initiative: The Ryan White Comprehensive AIDS Resource Emergency Act of 1990." *Journal of Contemporary Health Law and Policy* 7 (1991): 183–206.

Olson, Wyatt. "The Protection Racket: And the Band Plays On." *Broward–Palm Beach New Times*, February 2, 2006, 1–5. http://www.newtimesbpb .com/Issues/ 2006–02–02/news/feature_1.html.

O'Neill, Patrick. "Gay Reporter's AIDS Exposé Vents Anger over Epidemic." *Oregonian* [Portland], November 18, 1987, B1, B4.

Oppenheimer, Gerald M. "Causes, Cases, and Cohorts: The Role of Epidemiology in the Historical Construction of AIDS." In *AIDS: The Making of a Chronic Disease,* edited by Elizabeth Fee and Daniel M. Fox, 49–76. Berkeley: University of California Press, 1992.

———. "In the Eye of the Storm: The Epidemiological Construction of AIDS." In Fee and Fox, *AIDS: The Burdens of History*, 267–300.

Ortleb, Charles L. "Randy Shilts's Agenda." *New York Native*, October 19, 1987, 5.

———. "Scientist Zero." *Christopher Street*, March 1989.

Osborne, Robert. "Rambling Reporter." *Hollywood Reporter*, September 25, 1987.

"An Outbreak of Enteric Fever and Human 'Carriers.'" *Lancet* 171, no. 4409 (1908): 685.

Padron, Jeanne. "Man of the Year?" Letter to the editor. *Time*, December 14, 1987.

Parascandola, John. *Sex, Sin, and Science: A History of Syphilis*. Westport, CT: Praeger, 2008.

"Park Renaming to Honour Former City of Toronto Mayor, Barbara Hall." City of Toronto. July 14, 2014. http://wx.toronto.ca/inter/it/newsrel.nsf/bydate/ 52ED80777CB64FAB85257D150057C547.

Park, William H. "Typhoid Bacilli Carriers." *Journal of the American Medical Association* 51, no. 12 (1908): 981–82.

Patel, Pragna, Craig B. Borkowf, John T. Brooks, Arielle Lasry, Amy Lansky, and Jonathan Mermin. "Estimating Per-Act HIV Transmission Risk: A Systematic Review." *AIDS* 28 (2014): 1509–19.

Paterson, Timothy Murray. "Tainted Blood, Tainted Knowledge: Contesting Scientific Evidence at the Krever Inquiry." PhD thesis, University of British Columbia, 1999. doi: 10.14288/1.0089863.

"Patient Zero." In *Mosby's Medical Dictionary*, 9th ed., edited by Marie T. O'Toole. St. Louis: Mosby Elsevier, 2013.

"Patient Zero." *People*, December 28, 1987, 47.

Patton, Cindy. *Globalizing AIDS*. Minneapolis: University of Minnesota Press, 2002.

———. *Inventing AIDS*. New York: Routledge, 1990.

———. *Sex and Germs: The Politics of AIDS*. Boston: South End Press, 1985.

Pauwels, Luc. "A Theoretical Framework for Assessing Visual Representational Practices in Knowledge Building and Science Communications." In Pauwels, *Visual Cultures of Science*, 1–25.

———, ed. *Visual Cultures of Science: Rethinking Representational Practices in Knowledge Building and Science Communication*. Lebanon, NH: Dartmouth College Press / University Press of New England, 2006.

Pearce, Richard B. "'AIDS' Topic of Local Conference: Causes, Spread, and Possible Cures Discussed." *Bay Area Reporter* [San Francisco], November 4, 1982.

———. "Gay Compromise Syndrome: The Battle Widens." *Bay Area Reporter* [San Francisco], July 8, 1982, 15.

———. "Parasites and Immune Suppression: An AIDS Connection?" *BAR*, December 30, 1982.

Pearhouse, Richard. "Legislation Contagion: The Spread of Problematic New HIV Laws in Africa." Paper presented at the Seventeenth International AIDS Conference, Mexico City, August 6, 2008.

Pedler, Gary. "The Cauldron Part II: Interview with the Owners." *Bay Area Reporter* [San Francisco], April 22, 1982, 14–16.

Pelling, Margaret. *Cholera, Fever and English Medicine, 1825–1865*. Oxford: Oxford University Press, 1978.

———. "The Meaning of Contagion: Reproduction, Medicine and Metaphor." In *Contagion: Historical and Cultural Studies*, edited by Alison Bashford and Claire Hooker, 15–38. London: Routledge, 2001.

Pepin, Jacques. *The Origins of AIDS*. Cambridge: Cambridge University Press, 2011.

Perigard, Mark A. "They Fiddled While Rome Burned—A San Francisco AIDS Reporter's Wide-Ranging Critique." *Bay Windows* [Boston], November 12–18, 1987, 1, 6.

Perlman, David. "A War against 'Gay Plague.'" *San Francisco Chronicle*, November 17, 1982, 1, 5–6.

Persky, Stan. "AIDS and the State." *This Magazine* 22, no. 1, March/April (1990): 10–14.

Philadelphia. Directed by Jonathan Demme. TriStar Pictures, 1993. Burbank, CA: Columbia TriStar Home Video, 1997. DVD.

Picard, André. *The Gift of Death: Confronting Canada's Tainted-Blood Tragedy*. Rev. ed. Toronto: HarperPerennial, 1998. First published 1995.

———. "Hearings to Mix Blood, Politics and Drama." *Globe and Mail* [Toronto], February 14, 1994, A5.

Picard, André, and Anne McIlroy. "Tainted Blood Tragedy: Never Again." *Globe and Mail* [Toronto], November 27, 1997, A1, A14.

Pietsch, Theodore W. *Trees of Life: A Visual History of Evolution.* Baltimore: Johns Hopkins University Press, 2012.

Piot, Peter, Henri Taelman, Kapita Bila Minlangu, N. Mbendi, K. Ndangi, Kayembe Kalambayi, Chris Bridts, et al. "Acquired Immunodeficiency Syndrome in a Heterosexual Population in Zaire." *Lancet* 324, no. 8394 (1984): 65–69.

———. *No Time to Lose: A Life in Pursuit of Deadly Viruses.* New York: W. W. Norton, 2012.

Plotkin, Stanley A. "Chimpanzees and Journalists." *Vaccine* 22 (2004): 1829–30.

Porter, Roy. "The Patient's View: Doing Medical History from Below." *Theory and Society* 14, no. 2 (1985): 175–98.

Povinelli, Elizabeth A., and George Chauncey. "Thinking Sexuality Transnationally." *GLQ: A Journal of Lesbian and Gay Studies* 5, no. 4 (1999): 439–50.

"Presentations at the NCAB Meeting, December 1, 1982." Meeting transcript. December 1, 1982. http://history.nih.gov/NIHInOwnWords/assets/media/pdf/unpublished/unpublished_38.pdf.

Presidential Commission on the Human Immunodeficiency Virus Epidemic. *Report of the Presidential Commission on the Human Immunodeficiency Virus Epidemic.* Washington, DC: US Government Printing Office, 1988.

"Prevention of Acquired Immune Deficiency Syndrome (AIDS): Report of Inter-Agency Recommendations." *MMWR* 32, no. 8 (1983): 101–3.

Pullan, Brian. "Plague and Perceptions of the Poor in Early Modern Italy." In *Epidemics and Ideas: Essays on the Historical Perception of Pestilence*, edited by Terence Ranger and Paul Slack, 101–24. Cambridge: Cambridge University Press, 1992.

Qualtiere, Louis F., and William W. E. Slights. "Contagion and Blame in Early Modern England: The Case of the French Pox." *Literature and Medicine* 22, no. 1 (2003): 1–24.

Quétel, Claude. *History of Syphilis.* Translated by Judith Braddock and Brian Pike. Cambridge: Polity Press, 1992.

"Quotes of the Week." *US News and World Report*, October 19, 1987, 7.

Raeburn, Paul. "40 AIDS Cases in 10 Cities Linked to One Carrier." Associated Press newswire, March 27, 1984, LexisNexis News.

Rawlinson, H. Graham, and J. L. Granatstein. *The Canadian 100: The 100 Most Influential Canadians of the 20th Century.* Toronto: Little, Brown Canada, 1997.

Rayside, David M., and Evert A. Lindquist. "Canada: Community Activism,

Federalism, and the New Politics of Disease." In *AIDS in the Industrialized Democracies: Passions, Politics, and Policies,* edited by Ronald Bayer and David L. Kirp, 49–98. New Brunswick, NJ: Rutgers University Press, 1992.

"Reckless Vectors: The Infecting 'Other' In HIV/AIDS Law." *Sexuality Research and Social Policy* 2, no. 2 (2005): 1–105.

The Red Queen [Arthur Evans]. "S'not What You Think." *Bay Area Reporter* [San Francisco], April 29, 1982, 8.

Reporters Committee for Freedom of the Press. *The First Amendment Handbook.* 7th ed. Arlington, VA: Reporters Committee for Freedom of the Press, 2011. http://www.rcfp.org/rcfp/orders/docs/FAHB.pdf.

Reverby, Susan M. *Examining Tuskegee: The Infamous Syphilis Study and Its Legacy.* Chapel Hill: University of North Carolina Press, 2009.

Reynolds, L. D. "The Medieval Tradition of Seneca's *Dialogues.*" *Classical Quarterly* 18, no. 2 (1968): 355–72.

Risse, Guenter B. "Epidemics and History: Ecological Perspectives and Social Responses." In Fee and Fox, *AIDS: The Burdens of History,* 33–66.

Roberts, Cokie, and Steven V. Roberts. "The Venereal Disease Pandemic." *New York Times,* November 7, 1971, SM62–81.

Robertson, Mark L. "An Annotated Chronology of the History of AIDS in Toronto: The First Five Years, 1981–1986." *Canadian Bulletin of Medical History* 22, no. 2 (2005): 313–51.

Robins, Mar. "Saving Gayblevision, Vancouver's first gay TV show." *Daily Xtra* [Vancouver], December 3, 2014. http://www.dailyxtra.com/vancouver/news-and-ideas/news/saving-gayblevision-vancouver's-first-gay-tv-show-96656.

Rocke, Michael. *Forbidden Friendships: Homosexuality and Male Culture in Renaissance Florence.* New York: Oxford University Press, 1996.

Rodriguez, Johnette. "AIDS: Reporter Randy Shilts Chronicles the Deadly Epidemic." *NewPaper* [Providence, RI], February 3–10, 1988, sec. NewSection, 1, 4.

Rosenberg, Charles E. *The Cholera Years: The United States in 1832, 1849, and 1866, with a New Afterword.* London: University of Chicago Press, 1987. First published 1962.

———. "Disease and Social Order in America: Perceptions and Expectations." In Fee and Fox, *AIDS: The Burdens of History,* 12–32.

———. *Explaining Epidemics and Other Studies in the History of Medicine.* Cambridge: Cambridge University Press, 1992.

Rosen, George. *A History of Public Health.* Expanded ed. Baltimore: Johns Hopkins University Press, 1993. First published 1958.

Ross, Roger. "Media Finds Easy Target in Dead Man: Friends Angry That Gaetan Dugas Is Labelled Patient Zero." *Q Magazine* [Vancouver], December 15, 1987, 5.

Rothenberg, David. "Unfit to Print." *New York Native,* May 10, 1982, 11.

Rovner, Sandy. "Healthtalk: For Everywoman." *Washington Post,* September 12, 1980, F5.

Roy, André L. "Un montréalais contamine les USA!' *Sortie* [Montreal], November 1987, 6.

Rubin, Gayle S. "Elegy for the Valley of Kings: AIDS and the Leather Community in San Francisco, 1981–1996." In *In Changing Times: Gay Men and Lesbians Encounter HIV/AIDS,* edited by Martin P. Levine, Peter M. Nardi, and John H. Gagnon, 101–44. Chicago: University of Chicago Press, 1997.

———. "Thinking Sex: Notes for a Radical Theory of the Politics of Sexuality." In *Culture, Society and Sexuality: A Reader,* edited by Peter Aggleton and Richard Parker, 143–78. London: UCL Press, 1999.

Ruggiero, Guido. *The Boundaries of Eros: Sex Crime and Sexuality in Renaissance Venice.* Oxford: Oxford University Press, 1985.

Rundall, Thomas G., and Kathryn A. Phillips. "Informing and Educating the Electorate about AIDS." *Medical Care Review* 47, no. 1 (1990): 3–13.

Russell, Bill. "Epitaph for the Sexual Revolution." *Christopher Street,* December 1982, 52–53.

Ryan White CARE Act of 1990. Pub. L. No. 101–381, 104 Stat. 576 (1990). https://history.nih.gov/research/downloads/PL101-381.pdf.

Rydström, Jens. *Sinners and Citizens: Bestiality and Homosexuality in Sweden, 1880–1950.* London: University of Chicago Press, 2003.

Sabatier, Renée. *Blaming Others: Prejudice, Race and Worldwide AIDS.* London: Panos Institute, 1988.

Sachs, Ralph R. "Effect of Urbanization on the Spread of Syphilis." In *Proceedings of World Forum on Syphilis and Other Treponematoses,* by US Department of Health, Education, and Welfare, 153–56. Washington, DC: US Government Printing Office, 1964.

Saleh, Lena D., and Operario, Don. "Moving Beyond 'the Down Low': A Critical Analysis of Terminology Guiding HIV Prevention Efforts for African American Men Who Have Secretive Sex with Men." *Social Science and Medicine* 68 (2009): 390–95.

San Francisco AIDS Foundation. "The Stages of HIV Disease." The Body: The Complete Online HIV/AIDS Resource. August 22, 2008. http://www.thebody.com/content/whatis/art2506.html.

Schechter, Martin T., William J. Boyko, Eric Jeffries, Brian Willoughby, Rod Nitz, and Peter Constance. "The Vancouver Lymphadenopathy-AIDS Study: 1. Persistent Generalized Lymphadenopathy." *Canadian Medical Association Journal* 132 (1985): 1273–79.

S[c]hoonmaker, L. Craig. "Local 'Phobe." Letter to the editor. *New York Native,* October 24, 1983, 5.

Seidman, Steven. "Transfiguring Sexual Identity: AIDS and the Contemporary Construction of Homosexuality." *Social Text* 19–20 (Autumn 1988): 187–205.

Semple, Ellen Churchill. "Domestic and Municipal Waterworks in Ancient Mediterranean Lands." *Geographic Review* 21, no. 3 (1931): 466–74.

Seneca. *Seneca: Moral Essays.* 3 vols. Translated by John W. Basore. London: William Heinemann, 1928.

Shepard, Benjamin Heim. *White Nights and Ascending Shadows: An Oral History of the San Francisco AIDS Epidemic.* London: Cassell, 1997.

Sherman, Grayson [G. D. S.]. "Oh Come All Ye Faithful." *Fine Print* [Edmonton], February 1983, 17.

Shevory, Thomas. *Notorious H.I.V.: The Media Spectacle of Nushawn Williams.* Minneapolis: University of Minnesota Press, 2004.

"Shilts: 'Incredible Programs We Could Do.'" *Oregon Daily Emerald* [Eugene], March 30, 1973, 6.

Shilts, Randy. ——*And the Band Played On: Politics, People, and the AIDS Epidemic.* New York: St. Martin's Press, 1987.

——. "The Decade's Best-Kept Medical Secret: Hepatitis Doesn't Come from Needles." *Advocate,* January 12, 1977, 23–26.

——. "House Panel's Ideas on AIDS Research Financing," *San Francisco Chronicle,* December 6, 1983.

——. "How AIDS Is Changing Gay Lifestyles," *San Francisco Chronicle,* May 2, 1983, 1, 5, 7.

——. "Longer Incubation Period Reported: New Fears about Spread of AIDS." *San Francisco Chronicle,* April 18, 1985, 4.

——. *The Mayor of Castro Street: The Life and Times of Harvey Milk.* New York: St. Martin's Press, 1982.

——. "Memos Show Administration Falsified AIDS Funding Needs." *New York Native,* December 19, 1983, 18, 19, 64.

——. "Patient Zero." *Chicago Tribune,* November 1, 1987, sec. Tempo, 1, 4, 5.

——. "Patient Zero: The Man Who Brought the AIDS Epidemic to California." *California Magazine,* October 1987, cover, 96–99, 149–51, 160.

——. "Some AIDS Patients Still Going to the Baths." *San Francisco Chronicle,* November 15, 1983, 4.

——. "The Strange, Deadly Diseases That Target Gay Men." *San Francisco Chronicle,* May 13, 1982, 6–7.

——. "Study of S.F. Neighborhoods: Startling Finding on 'Gay Disease,'" *San Francisco Chronicle,* March 23, 1983, 2.

Siena, Kevin, ed. *Sins of the Flesh: Responding to Sexual Disease in Early Modern Europe.* Toronto: Centre for Reformation and Renaissance Studies, 2005.

——. "The Strange Medical Silence on Same-Sex Transmission of the Pox, c. 1660–1760." In Borris and Rousseau, *Sciences of Homosexuality in Early Modern Europe,* 115–33.

Silversides, Ann. *AIDS Activist: Michael Lynch and the Politics of Community.* Toronto: Between the Lines, 2003.

Singer, Eleanor, Theresa F. Rogers, and Mary Corcoran. "The Polls—A Report: AIDS." *Public Opinion Quarterly* 51, no. 4 (1987): 580–95.

Sipchen, Bob. "The AIDS Chronicles: Randy Shilts Writes the Biography of an Epidemic and Finds More Bunglers Than Heroes." *Los Angeles Times,* October 9, 1987, V1, V8-V9.

Sister Boom Boom. "Sis Boom Bah." *Bay Area Reporter* [San Francisco], May 20, 1982, 6.

Skowronski, Danuta M., Martin Petric, Patricia Daly, Robert A. Parker, Elizabeth Bryce, Patrick W. Doyle, Michael A. Noble, et al. "Coordinated Response to SARS, Vancouver, Canada." *Emerging Infectious Diseases* 12, no. 1 (2006): 155–58.

Slack, Paul. *The Impact of Plague in Tudor and Stuart England.* London: Routledge and Kegan Paul, 1985.

Smith, Liz. "Movie Deal for Shilts' 'Mayor of Castro Street.'" *San Francisco Chronicle,* October 13, 1987, E1.

Sontag, Susan. *Illness as Metaphor.* New York: Farrar, Straus and Giroux, 1978.

———. *Illness as Metaphor and AIDS and Its Metaphors.* New York: Picador USA, 1990.

Soper, George A. "The Work of a Chronic Typhoid Germ Distributor." *Journal of the American Medical Association* 48 (1907): 2019–22.

Spence, James R. "The Law of Crime against Nature." *North Carolina Law Review* 32, no. 3 (1954): 312–24.

Spencer, Frank. "AIDS: A Failure to Respond." *Hartford Courant,* October 30, 1987, C1, C7.

Stackpool-Moore, Lucy. *Verdict on a Virus: Public Health, Human Rights and Criminal Law.* London: International Planned Parenthood Federation, 2008. http://www.ippf.org/resource/Verdict-Virus-Public-health-human-rights-and -criminal-law.

Stanton, Keith. "Hugs Instead of Kisses." Letter to the editor. *Bay Area Reporter* [San Francisco], October 14, 1982, 6.

Steacy, Anne, and Lisa Van Dusen. "'Patient Zero' and the AIDS Virus." *Maclean's,* October 19, 1987, 53.

Stebbing, Justin, and Graeme Moyle. "The Clades of HIV: Their Origins and Clinical Significance." *AIDS Reviews* 5, no. 4 (2003): 205–13.

Steele, Derek G. "The Evolution of the Canadian AIDS Society: A Social Movement Organization as Network, Coalition and Umbrella Organization." DPhil thesis, McGill University, 2000.

Steele, Scott. "AIDS, the Musical: Zero Patience." *Maclean's,* March 7, 1994, 60.

Steinbrook, Robert. "The *Times* Poll: 42% Would Limit Civil Rights in AIDS Battle." *Los Angeles Times,* July 31, 1987, B1, B21.

Stein, Marc. *City of Sisterly and Brotherly Loves: Lesbian and Gay Philadelphia, 1945–72.* Philadelphia: Temple University Press, 2004.
———. "Theoretical Politics, Local Communities: The Making of US LGBT Historiography." *GLQ: A Journal of Lesbian and Gay Studies* 11, no. 4 (2005): 605–25.
Stern, Nora. "'The Band Played On'—Story of First AIDS Victim Was Overly-Sensational." *Seattle Times,* November 12, 1987, A19, NewsBank (469938).
Stewart, H. C., R. S. Gass, and Ruth R. Puffer. "Tuberculosis Studies in Tennessee: A Clinic Study with Reference to Epidemiology within the Family." *American Journal of Public Health and the Nation's Health* 26, no. 7 (1936): 689–96.
Stewart, Karl. "A Full Knight." *Bay Area Reporter* [San Francisco], December 23, 1982, 29.
Stewart, Noah. "A Friend's Death." *Angles,* May 1984, 17.
Stinton, Michael, and Anne Eaton. "The Monster Who Gave Us AIDS." *Star* [Tarrytown, NY], October 27, 1987, 6–7.
Strassler, Robert B., ed. *The Landmark Thucydides: A Comprehensive Guide to the Peloponnesian War.* New York: Touchstone, 1996.
Streitfeld, David. "Book Report." *Washington Post,* January 24, 1988, B015.
Streitmatter, Rodger. *Unspeakable: The Rise of the Gay and Lesbian Press in America.* Boston: Faber and Faber, 1995.
Sturken, Marita. *Tangled Memories: The Vietnam War, the AIDS Epidemic, and the Politics of Remembering.* Berkeley: University of California Press, 1997.
Sullivan, Kathleen M., and Martha A. Field. "AIDS and the Coercive Power of the State." *Harvard Civil Rights–Civil Liberties Law Review* 23, no. 1 (1988): 139–97.
———. "AIDS and the Criminal Law." *Law, Medicine and Health Care* 15, no. 1–2 (1987): 46–60.
Susser, Mervyn. "Epidemiology in the United States after World War II: The Evolution of Technique." *Epidemiologic Reviews* 7, no. 1 (1985): 147–77.
Susser, Mervyn, and Ezra Susser. "Choosing a Future for Epidemiology: I. Eras and Paradigms." *American Journal of Public Health* 86, no. 5 (1996): 668–73.
Swenson, Robert M. "Plagues, History, and AIDS," *American Scholar* 57, no. 2 (Spring 1988): 183–200.
Szabo, Jason. "Re-Birthing Pains: Protease Inhibitors, The 'Lazarus Syndrome,' and the Transformation of the Acquired Immunodeficiency Syndrome." Paper presented at the 82nd annual meeting of the American Association for the History of Medicine, Cleveland, OH, April 26, 2009.
Szasz, Thomas. *The Myth of Mental Illness: Foundations of a Theory of Personal Conduct.* New York: Dell, 1961.
Taravella, Steve. "'A Story of Prejudice': Author Chronicles Politics behind AIDS Policies." *Modern Healthcare,* January 1, 1988, 76.

Tasker, Fred, and Jacqueline Charles. "Disease Research: Scientists Trace AIDS through Haiti; Findings Draw Anger." *Miami Herald*, October 31, 2007, 1A.

Task Force on Kaposi's Sarcoma and Opportunistic Infections, CDC, "A Cluster of Kaposi's Sarcoma and *Pneumocystis carinii* Pneumonia among Homosexual Male Residents of Los Angeles and Range Counties, California." *MMWR* 31, no. 23 (1982): 305–7.

Terry, Jennifer. *An American Obsession: Science, Medicine and Homosexuality in Modern Society.* London: University of Chicago Press, 1999.

——. "The Seductive Power of Science in the Making of Deviant Subjectivity." In *Science and Homosexualities*, edited by Vernon A. Rosario, 271–96. New York: Routledge, 1997.

Tesher, Ellie. "Blood Drama Unmasks Bland 'Stars.'" *Toronto Star*, October 13, 1995, A2, ProQuest (1357140608).

——. "Blood Inquiry a Sorry Litany of Errors." *Toronto Star*, September 8, 1995, A2, ProQuest (1355573880).

Thomas, David J. "An Interview with Randy Shilts." *Christopher Street*, February 1982, 28–35.

Thompson, Paul, and Rob Perks. *An Introduction to the Use of Oral History in the History of Medicine.* London: National Life Story Collection, 1993.

Tiemeyer, Phil. *Plane Queer: Labor, Sexuality, and AIDS in the History of Male Flight Attendants.* Berkeley: University of California Press, 2013.

Tomes, Nancy. "Oral History in the History of Medicine." *Journal of American History* 78, no. 2 (1991): 607–17.

——. "The Making of a Germ Panic, Then and Now." *American Journal of Public Health* 90, no. 2 (2000): 191–98.

Toumey, Christopher P. "Conjuring Medical Science: The 1986 Referendum on AIDS/HIV Policy in California." *Medical Anthropology Quarterly* 11, no. 4 (1997): 477–97.

Trebilcock, Michael J., and Lisa Austin. "The Limits of the Full Court Press: Of Blood and Mergers." *University of Toronto Law Journal* 48, no. 1 (Winter 1998): 1–59.

Treichler, Paula A. "AIDS, Gender, and Biomedical Discourse: Current Contests for Meaning." In Fee and Fox, *AIDS: The Burdens of History*, 190–266.

——. "AIDS, Homophobia, and Biomedical Discourse: An Epidemic of Signification." In *AIDS: Cultural Analysis, Cultural Activism,* edited by Douglas Crimp, 31–70. Cambridge, MA: MIT Press, 1988.

——. *How to Have Theory in an Epidemic: Cultural Chronicles of AIDS.* London: Duke University Press, 1999.

"The Trial of Mervin Lord Audley, Earl of Castlehaven, for a Rape and Sodomy, on the 25th of April 1631." In *A Complete Collection of State-Trials, and Proceedings for High-Treason, and Other Crimes and Misdemeanours.* 4th ed. 11 vols. London, 1776. Facsimile, Eighteenth Century Collections Online

digital library, http://find.galegroup.com/ecco/infomark.do?&contentSet=
ECCOArticles&type=multipage&tabID=T001&prodId=ECCO&docId
=CW3325058195&source=gale&userGroupName=oxford&version=1.0&
docLevel=FASCIMILE.

Trouillot, Michel-Rolph. "Silencing the Past: Layers of Meaning in the Haitian
Revolution." In *Between History and Histories: The Making of Silences and
Commemorations*, edited by Gerald M. Sider and Gavin A. Smith, 31–61. To-
ronto: University of Toronto Press, 1997.

Trout, Hank. "S & M Distinctions." *Bay Area Reporter* [San Francisco], July 1,
1982, 8.

Tsang T., T. Lai-Yin, L. Pak-Yin, M. Lee, J.-S. Wu, Y.-C. Wu, I.-H. Chiang, et al.
"Update: Outbreak of Severe Acute Respiratory Syndrome—Worldwide,
2003." *MMWR* 52 (2003): 241–48. https://www.cdc.gov/mmwr/preview/
mmwrhtml/mm5212a1.htm.

Udesky, Laurie. "Randy Shilts." *Progressive* 55, no. 5 (1991): 30–34.

UNAIDS. *AIDS by the Numbers 2015*. Geneva: UNAIDS, 2015,.http://www
.unaids.org/sites/default/files/media_asset/AIDS_by_the_numbers_2015_en
.pdf.

United in Anger: A History of ACT UP. Directed by Jim Hubbard and produced
by Jim Hubbard and Sarah Schulman, 2012. New York: United in Anger,
2014. DVD.

"Un Québécois responsable de la propagation du SIDA en Amérique? IMPOS-
SIBLE DE L'AFFIRMER—Des spécialistes." *Le Journal de Montréal*, October 8,
1987, 2.

US Department of Health and Human Services. "Modifications to the HIPAA
Privacy, Security, Enforcement, and Breach Notification Rules under the
Health Information Technology for Economic and Clinical Health Act and
the Genetic Information Nondiscrimination Act; Other Modifications to the
HIPAA Rules; Final Rule." *Federal Register* 78, no. 17 (2013): 5613–14.

US Department of Health, Education, and Welfare. *Venereal Disease Branch
Field Manual*. Atlanta: Communicable Disease Center, 1962.

Van Gelder, Lindsy. "Death in the Family." *Rolling Stone*, February 3, 1983, 18.

Verbatim Transcripts of Commission of Inquiry on the Blood System in Canada.
247 vols. Gloucester, ON: International Rose Reporting, 1997. CD-ROM.

Verghese, Abraham. *My Own Country: A Doctor's Story*. New York: Vintage
Books, 1994.

"Virus Linked to Cancer Outbreak in Gay Community." *Bay Area Reporter*
[San Francisco], August 26, 1982.

Voltaire. *Candide, Zadig, and Selected Stories*. Translated by Donald M. Frame.
New York: New American Library, 1963.

Wain-Hobson, Simon, Céline Renoux-Elbé, Jean-Pierre Vartanian, and Andreas Meyerhans. *Contagious: Cultures, Carriers, and the Outbreak Narrative*. London: Duke University Press, 2008.

——. "Network Analysis of Human and Simian Immunodeficiency Virus Sequence Sets Reveals Massive Recombination Resulting in Shorter Pathways." *Journal of General Virology* 84, no. 4 (2003): 885–95.

Wald, Priscilla. *Contagious: Cultures, Carriers, and the Outbreak Narrative*. London: Duke University Press, 2008.

Warner, Tom. *Never Going Back: A History of Queer Activism in Canada*. Toronto: University of Toronto Press, 2002.

Washer, Peter. "Representations of SARS in the British Newspapers." *Social Science and Medicine* 59 (2004): 2561–71.

Watney, Simon. *Policing Desire: Pornography, AIDS and the Media*. 3rd ed. Minneapolis: University of Minnesota Press, 1997. First published 1987.

Weait, Matthew. "Taking the Blame: Criminal Law, Social Responsibility and the Sexual Transmission of HIV." *Journal of Social and Family Law* 23, no. 4 (2001): 441–57.

Weeks, Jeffrey. *Making Sexual History*. Cambridge: Polity Press, 2000.

Weir, John. "Reading Randy." *Out*, August–September 1993, 45–49.

Weir, Lorna, and Eric Mykhalovskiy. "The Geopolitics of Global Public Health Surveillance in the Twenty-First Century." In *Medicine at the Border: Disease, Globalization and Security, 1850 to the Present*, edited by Alison Bashford, 240–63. Basingstoke, UK: Palgrave Macmillan, 2006.

Weiss, Mike. "Randy Shilts Was Gutsy, Brash and Unforgettable: He Died 10 Years Ago, Fighting for the Rights of Gays in American Society." *San Francisco Chronicle*, February 17, 2004, D1. http://www.sfgate.com/cgi-bin/article .cgi?f=/c/a/2004/02/17/DDGGH50UAU1.DTL.

Whitaker, Rupert. "Thirty Years of AIDS: Triumphs, Failures, and the Unlearned Lessons." Lecture at King's College, London, November 3, 2011. Podcast, MP3 file, 49:10. http://podcast.ulcc.ac.uk/accounts/kings/Humanities _and_Health/3_11_2011_Rupert_Whitaker_Triumphs_failures_and _unlearned_lessons.mp3.

William, Dan. "If AID Is an Infectious Disease . . . A Sexual Syllogism." *New York Native*, August 16, 1982, 33.

Williamson, Judith. "Aids and Perceptions of the Grim Reaper." *Metro* 80 (Spring 1989): 2–6.

Willrich, Michael. *Pox: An American History*. New York: Penguin, 2011.

Wills, Garry. "Randy Shilts: The Rolling Stone Interview." *Rolling Stone*, September 30, 1993, 46–49, 122–23.

Wilson, Craig. "The Chronicler of AIDS: Randy Shilts, Tracking the Epidemic." *USA Today*, October 12, 1987, sec. Life, 1D–2D.

Wilson, Nancy, and Jeri Ann Harvey, "Profile: In Memorium," *Journey*, June/July 1983, 6–7, 31, https://issuu.com/mccchurches/docs/1983-june-july-journey.

Wiltshire, John. "A Patients' History of Medicine." *Clinical Medicine* 7 (2007): 370–73.

Winskell, Kate, and Daniel Enger. "A New Way of Perceiving the Pandemic: The Findings from a Participatory Research Process on Young Africans' Stories about HIV/AIDS." *Culture, Health and Sexuality* 11, no. 4 (2009): 453–67.

Winslow, Charles-Edward Amory. *The Conquest of Epidemic Disease: A Chapter in the History of Ideas.* 1943. Reprint, Madison: University of Wisconsin Press, 1980.

Winter, Jay. "Thinking about Silence." In *Shadows of War: A Social History of Silence in the Twentieth Century*, edited by Efrat Ben-Ze'ev, Ruth Ginio, and Jay Winter, 3–31. Cambridge: Cambridge University Press, 2010.

Withnall, Adam. "Ebola Outbreak's 'Patient Zero' Identified as a Two-Year-Old Boy from Guinea Named Emile Ouamouno." *Independent* [London], October 28, 2014. http://www.independent.co.uk/news/world/africa/ebola -outbreaks-patient-zero-identified-as-a-two-year-old-boy-from-guinea -named-emile-ouamouno-9823513.html.

Woodard, Joe. "Bad Blood and Bad Medicine." *Alberta Report* 21, no. 21 (1994): 26, Academic Search Complete, EBSCOhost (9406077701).

Worobey, Michael, Marlea Gemmel, Dirk E. Teuwen, and Steven M. Wolinsky. "Direct Evidence of Extensive Diversity of HIV-1 in Kinshasa by 1960." *Nature* 455, no. 2 (2008): 661–64.

Worobey, Michael, Thomas D. Watts, Richard A. McKay, Timothy Granade, Dirk E. Teuwen, Beryl A. Koblin, Walid Heneine, et al. "1970s and 'Patient 0' genomes illuminate early HIV/AIDS history in North America." *Nature* 538, no. 7627 (2016): 98–101.

Worth, Heather, Cindy Patton, and Diane Goldstein. "Introduction to Special Issue: Reckless Vectors; The Infecting 'Other' In HIV/AIDS Law." *Sexuality Research and Social Policy* 2 no. 2 (2005): 3–14.

Wright, David, and Renée Saucier. "Madness in the Archives: Anonymity, Ethics, and Mental Health History Research." *Journal of the Canadian Historical Association* 23, no. 2 (2012): 65–90.

Wright, Joe. "'Only Your Calamity': The Beginnings of Activism by and for People with AIDS," *American Journal of Public Health* 103, no. 10 (2013): 1788–98.

X. v. College of Physicians and Surgeons of British Columbia [1990] BCSC, B.C.J. no. 1316 and [1991] B.C.J. no. 2410.

Yarbrough, Jeff. "The Life and Times of Randy Shilts." *Advocate,* June 15, 1993, 32–39.

Young, Philip. "Patient Zero: Man Who Gave the World AIDS." *Northern Echo* [High Wycombe, UK], April 9, 1988.

The Zero Factor. Documentary film in multipart televised documentary series *A*

Time of AIDS. Directed by Anne Moir. Princeton, NJ: Films for the Humanities, 1992. Videocassette (VHS), 60 min.

Zero Patience. Directed by John Greyson. Toronto: Zero Patience Productions, 1993. New York: Strand Releasing Home Video, 2005. DVD.

"Zero Patience [/] A John Greyson Movie Musical." *Xtra!* [Toronto], February 18, 1994, 2.

Zinsser, Hans. *Rats, Lice, and History.* London: George Routledge, 1935.

Zuger, Abigail. "With AIDS, Time to Get beyond Blame." *New York Times,* April 19, 2010, D6.

Index